POLIO

ALSO BY DAVID M. OSHINSKY

Worse Than Slavery:
Parchman Farm and the Ordeal of Jim Crow Justice

A Conspiracy So Immense:
The World of Joe McCarthy

Senator Joseph McCarthy and
the American Labor Movement

The Case of the Nazi Professor
(co-author)

American Passage: A History of the United States
(co-author)

The Oxford Companion to United States History
(co-editor)

POLIO

An American Story

DAVID M. OSHINSKY

OXFORD
UNIVERSITY PRESS

2005

OXFORD
UNIVERSITY PRESS

Oxford University Press, Inc., publishes works that further
Oxford University's objective of excellence in research,
scholarship, and education.

Oxford   New York
Auckland   Cape Town   Dar es Salaam   Hong Kong   Karachi
Kuala Lumpur   Madrid   Melbourne   Mexico City   Nairobi
New Delhi   Shanghai   Taipei   Toronto

With offices in
Argentina   Austria   Brazil   Chile   Czech Republic   France   Greece
Guatemala   Hungary   Italy   Japan   Poland   Portugal   Singapore
South Korea   Switzerland   Thailand   Turkey   Ukraine   Vietnam

Published by Oxford University Press, Inc.
198 Madison Avenue, New York, NY 10016
www.oup.com

Oxford is a registered trademark of Oxford University Press

Library of Congress Cataloging-in-Publication Data
Oshinsky, David M., 1944–
Polio : an American story / David M. Oshinsky.
p. cm.
Includes bibliographical references and index.
ISBN-13: 978-0-19-515294-4
ISBN-10: 0-19-515294-8
1. Poliomyelitis—United States—History—20th century. I. Title.
RC181.U5O83 2005
614.5'49'0973—dc22
2004025249

9 8 7 6 5 4 3 2
Printed in the United States of America
on acid-free paper

For Jane

Her love, her compassion, her sense of family; her extraordinary courage in the face of adversity—all make her the indispensable one.

Contents

POLIO

Introduction

SAN ANGELO in 1949 was pure West Texas, a county seat of 50,000 people between Abilene and the Mexican border at Del Rio, set in a vast landscape of farm fields, oil wells, and cattle ranches trimmed in barbed wire. Like so many other towns of that era, it had sprung to life during World War II, nearly doubling its population with the expansion of a military air base at Goodfellow Field. As thousands of people arrived, and thousands more returned home from the war, San Angelo found itself connected to the larger world in vital, sometimes dangerous, new ways.

The late 1940s were flush years in the United States. A booming economy encouraged Americans to marry, start a family, buy a house, consume. In San Angelo as elsewhere, the pain and sacrifice of the Great Depression and World War II had been replaced by a more optimistic vision of material comfort and economic success. The town continued to prosper and expand. In 1949, the San Angelo *Standard-Times* predicted a golden future, linking prosperity, among other things, to the region's warm climate and "health-giving" reputation.

On May 20, a small blot on this bright picture appeared. The newspaper reported that a local child had come down with poliomyelitis. San Angelo had endured minor outbreaks before. The disease touched down in the late spring, like hailstorms and tornadoes, but had never really spread. There was mild concern, nothing more.

Within days, concern had turned to alarm. Parents began arriving at Shannon Memorial Hospital with "feverish, aching youngsters in their arms." Twenty-five polio cases were confirmed by the medical staff, and the death toll mounted: Esperanza Ramirez, ten months; Billie Doyle Kleghorn, seven; Susan Barr, four; and Donald Shipley, seven. On June 6, the *Standard-Times* reflected the town's growing desperation: "Polio Takes Seventh Life: San Angelo Pastors Appeal for Divine Help in Plague."[1]

Dr. R. E. Elvins, the city health officer, told people what they already knew: polio had "topped epidemic proportions." Employing the usual guidelines for a disease with no known cause or prevention or cure, he recommended that San Angelo's children avoid crowds, wash their hands regularly, get plenty of rest, and stay out of pools and swimming holes. "You can't wave a wand and clear up polio," he said. "It's largely up to individual families."[2]

Elvins had one more suggestion. Since poliovirus was often found in human feces and on the legs of houseflies, he called for a heavy spraying of DDT, singling out the open pit toilets on the "Latin American" and "Negro" side of town. Others were less subtle, blaming the epidemic on the "wetbacks" who migrated north each year to tend San Angelo's livestock and crops.[3]

In early June, with the temperature nudging 100 and the polio count at sixty-one, the city council voted to close all indoor meeting places for a week. "Theater marquees went dark in San Angelo Thursday night," said the *Standard-Times*. "There were no youngsters splashing in the municipal swimming pool during the day. No San Angelo churches will meet Sunday." The lockdown was soon complete. Bars and bowling alleys shut their doors, professional wrestling was canceled at the high school, popular country bands like Snuffy Smith and the Snuff Dippers steered clear of town.

So, too, did everyone else. Tourist traffic disappeared. Rumors spread about catching polio from an uncovered sneeze, from handling money, or from talking on the telephone. "We got to the point no one could comprehend," a local pediatrician noted, "when people would not even shake hands."[4]

For the most part, local residents did what other Americans had been taught to do in a polio epidemic: make filth the enemy and cleanliness the goal. Measures that would have seemed preposterous a few weeks before, such as monitoring the health of migrant workers and banning the sale of livestock within city limits, gained quick public support. "It's bad," said one state health official of San Angelo's predicament. "All I can do is repeat and repeat my warnings—clean up filth and breeding places of flies and insects. And keep on cleaning up."[5]

San Angelo bought two fogging machines to bathe the city in DDT. Twice each day, flatbed trucks would rumble through the streets, spraying the chemical from large hoses while children danced innocently in the mist that trailed behind. As a goodwill gesture, the local Sherwin-Williams store provided DDT at no cost, urging customers to drench the walls and furniture in their homes. ("Bring your own container!" it said.) One hardware store advertised its own brand of insecticide— "Queen City Kill . . . Five times more powerful than DDT." Another promised an even stronger concoction, called "Super-Activated Bug Juice."[6]

Fear of polio became the perfect selling tool. The Hi-Tone Cleaners vowed to disinfect its equipment before each pressing and wash. Local Sani-Flush ads urged a closer scrubbing of the family toilet "when polio's on the rampage." Clorox warned, "It's the dirt you don't see that does the damage." Companies hawked "polio insurance," while chiropractors promised immunity from the disease. "Keep your child's body correctly adjusted," said Dr. Roy Crowder, "and there is no likelihood of polio."[7]

But nothing seemed to work. By mid-June more than half of San Angelo's 160 hospital beds were filled by polio patients, almost all of them children under fifteen. A small staff of doctors and nurses worked exhausting double shifts. Volunteers overcame their fear of contagion to comfort patients, pack their limbs with hot compresses, and watch over those in iron lungs. The ultimate nightmare was a thunderstorm that could knock out the respirators lining the makeshift isolation wards. As one doctor recalled: "An alarm in the hospital was sounded with the appearance of dark clouds in the sky. . . . Pumping the hand lever [of an iron lung] fatigued even the most rugged of men and women after a short time, but others stood by to relieve any tired pumper. No patient died because of the failure of a respirator during a storm."[8]

A half-dozen polio experts arrived, dispatched by the National Foundation for Infantile Paralysis, known to most Americans as the March of Dimes. They took stool and tissue samples from the patients for use, it was said, in a program to assist polio researchers in their quest for a vaccine. They also directed supplies and personnel to San Angelo for those in need of aftercare, including wheelchairs and physical therapists, and provided money for medical bills. The most serious cases were flown to regional rehabilitation centers in specially equipped planes—all free of charge.

The epidemic peaked in July. Hospital admissions dropped steadily. By late August it was over. School opened on time in San Angelo, amidst the heartbreaking reminder of empty desks and chairs.

The year 1949 was a bad one for polio, and the worst was still ahead. Close to 40,000 cases were reported in the United States, one for every 3,775 people. San Angelo saw 420 cases, one for every 124 inhabitants, of whom 84 were permanently paralyzed and 28 died. It was one of the most severe polio outbreaks ever recorded. But its characteristics were familiar.[9]

The San Angelo epidemic arrived in the hotter months, preying mostly on children. It involved a town that had not experienced a major polio outbreak in recent years, a town undergoing rapid exposure to contact from outside. It appeared to hit tidy, stable neighborhoods even harder than those marked by poverty and squalor, an observation at odds with conventional wisdom linking cleanliness to good health. And it occurred on American soil.

The geography was revealing. Although poliomyelitis—or infantile paralysis—appeared throughout the world, the worst outbreaks of the twentieth century were reported in Western Europe, Canada, Australia, and, especially, the United States. Already fearful of a disease whose victims ranged from anonymous children to President Franklin Delano Roosevelt, Americans were primed to see polio as an indigenous plague with an indigenous solution—a problem to be solved, like so many others, through a combination of ingenuity, voluntarism, determination, and money. One of the most common mantras of the post–World War II era, repeated by fund raisers, politicians, advertisers, and journalists, was the bold (and ultimately) truthful, promise, "we will conquer polio."

THE DISEASE REACHED ITS PEAK at the height of the cold war, when a national crisis often took the form of a crusade. And this particular crisis, an epidemic targeting defenseless children, grew to dramatic proportions in an increasingly suburban, family-oriented society preaching ever-higher standards of protection for the young. How ironic, how *unfair*, that polio seemed to target the world's most advanced nation, where new wonder drugs like penicillin were readily available and consumers—mainly housewives—worked overtime to eliminate odors and germs.

No disease drew as much attention, or struck the same terror, as polio. And for good reason. Polio hit without warning. There was no way of telling who would get it and who would be spared. It killed some of its victims and marked others for life, leaving behind vivid reminders for all to see: wheelchairs, crutches, leg braces, breathing devices, deformed limbs. In truth, polio was never the raging epidemic portrayed in the media, not even at its height in the 1940s and 1950s. Ten times as many children would be killed in accidents in these years, and three times as many would die of cancer. Polio's special status was due, in large part, to the efforts of a remarkable group, the National Foundation for Infantile Paralysis, which employed the latest techniques in advertising, fund raising, and motivational research to turn a horrific but relatively uncommon disease into the most feared affliction of its time.[10]

This dread did not begin with the National Foundation. A growing pattern of epidemics—the worst occurring in 1916—had already drawn scattered notice in the press. The genius of the National Foundation lay in its ability to single out polio for special attention, making it seem more ominous and more curable than other diseases. Its strategy would revolutionize the way charities raised money, recruited volunteers, organized local chapters to care for local people, and penetrated the mysterious world of medical research. In doing so, the foundation created a new model for giving in modern America, the concept of philanthropy as consumerism, with donors promised the ultimate personal reward: protection against the disease.

This philanthropy, in turn, funded a furious competition for a vaccine. Millions of foundation-raised dollars were spent to set up virology programs and polio units across the United States. In the process, valuable new tools were introduced, such as the payment of indirect research costs to universities and the funding of long-term grants. At Johns Hopkins, Yale, and Michigan, at Pittsburgh and Cincinnati, scientists strove to unravel the mysteries of polio. How did it enter and travel through the body? How many different types of the virus were there? Why did polio primarily attack children and strike in hot weather? Why had it changed in recent years from a sporadic to an epidemic disease? Why did it thrive in the United States?

The vaccine quest had three main competitors: Albert Sabin, a long-time polio researcher at the University of Cincinnati; Jonas Salk, a relative newcomer at the University of Pittsburgh; and Hilary Koprowski, a scientist in private industry at Lederle Laboratories. All three were ambitious, competitive men who got caught up in the growing clamor for a cure. All were Jewish, two having emigrated from Eastern Europe. All were lavishly financed: Sabin and Salk by the National Foundation, Koprowski by Lederle's parent company, American Cyanamid. All faced ticklish moral questions about the safety of their vaccines as well as the role and scope of human testing.

Sabin and Koprowski championed a live-virus vaccine designed to trigger a natural infection strong enough to generate lasting antibodies against polio, yet too weak to cause a serious case of the disease. Salk favored a killed-virus version intended to stimulate the immune system to produce the desired antibodies without creating a natural infection. Most polio researchers backed the former strategy, contending that a live virus would provide better immunity against polio and lead to its complete eradication over time. The National Foundation remained officially neutral, though its leaders privately supported the simpler killed-virus vaccine, believing it could be marketed more quickly and with fewer health risks to the public. Speed and safety appeared to be on Salk's side.

Acting mostly on its own, with little government support or oversight, the National Foundation conducted the largest medical experiment in American history—the so-called Salk Vaccine Field Trials of 1954, involving almost two million elementary school children throughout the country. Never before had a public health experiment been subject to such intense media scrutiny. When the trials proved largely successful, Jonas Salk's life changed forever. He became an instant hero, a celebrity-scientist whose white lab coat and self-effacing demeanor symbolized the concrete benefits of medical research.

His competitors didn't give up the race; they simply chose a new course. Having done what he could to undermine the 1954 Salk trials, Albert Sabin would wind up testing his own vaccine inside the Soviet Union—a remarkable story of scientific cooperation and intrigue in the midst of the cold war. Hilary Koprowski would continue his experiments in Ireland, Eastern Europe, and Africa, with results—and consequences—that reverberate eerily to this day.

The Salk trials would have a profound impact on the federal government's role in the testing and licensing of future drugs and vaccines. And the prospect of vaccinating children en masse, free of charge, would lead to a furious debate among doctors about the perils of "socialized medicine." On a personal level, the enormous public adulation for Salk would seriously damage his standing in the cloistered world of scientific research. Some colleagues would accuse him of undermining his discipline by allowing "outsiders"—foundation bureaucrats—to dictate the pace and direction of his work. Others would question the actual value of his vaccine. It is revealing that while Salk was awarded his nation's two highest civilian honors—the Congressional Gold Medal in 1955 and the Presidential Medal of Freedom in 1977—he was denied admission to the elite National Academy of Sciences for the reason, it was said, that he had made no "basic scientific discovery." As Albert Sabin, a long-time academy member, sneered: "You could go into the kitchen and do what he did."[11]

The feud between Salk and Sabin would outlive them both. There is still an ongoing debate over which man produced the better vaccine and which vaccine should be used today. What is certain, however, is that the polio crusade that consumed them remains one of the most significant and culturally revealing triumphs in American medical history.

1

The First Epidemics

POLIO HAS BEEN CALLED many things since it was first described in the medical literature several hundred years ago. What doctors once referred to as "debility of the lower extremities," "Heine-Medin's disease," or "infantile paralysis" eventually became "poliomyelitis," a combination of the Greek words "polios" (gray) and "myelos" (marrow), and the Latin suffix "itis," describing inflammation. As the disease gained prominence following World War II, reporters and headline writers balked at the odd-sounding, thirteen-letter name. They trimmed it to "polio" to save space, and the abbreviation stuck.[1]

Polio is an enteric (intestinal) infection, spread from person to person through contact with fecal waste: unwashed hands, shared objects, contaminated food and water. The agent is a virus, a microbe long known to researchers but not actually *seen* until the invention of the electron microscope in the late 1930s. "Viruses represent life stripped to the bare essentials," a biologist has noted. "They are the smallest and simplest infectious agents identified to date." Unable to survive on their own, they must invade a living cell and take over its machinery in order to reproduce.[2]

Poliovirus enters the body through the mouth, travels down the digestive tract, and is excreted in the stools. Though some multiplication occurs in the lymph nodes of the throat and tonsils, the main breeding ground for this virus is farther along, in the small intestine. Most often, the infection it produces is slight, or inapparent, with minor symptoms such as headache and nausea or with no symptoms at all. In a small number of cases—estimated to be one in a hundred—the virus invades the brain stem and the central nervous system through the bloodstream, destroying the nerve cells, or motor neurons, that stimulate the muscle fibers to contract.

The extent and permanence of the resulting paralysis are difficult to predict. Some infected nerve cells will fight off the poliovirus while others will die. Furthermore, the surviving nerve cells are capable of taking on more work by enlarging themselves and sprouting new connections to the orphaned muscle fibers. At its worst polio causes irreversible paralysis, most often in the legs. The majority of deaths occur when the breathing muscles are immobilized, a condition known as bulbar polio, in which the brain stem (or bulb) is badly damaged.[3]

Over the years, researchers have learned much about this disease. They discovered that everyone harboring poliovirus is a carrier, no matter how slight the infection; that the immune system responds by generating antibodies which provide future protection; that there are three distinct antigenic types of poliovirus, Type I being the most common and virulent; and that immunity to one type does not provide immunity to the others. All of these findings have led to the production of safe and effective polio vaccines.

But there is much about the disease that remains a mystery. One of the ironies of the great polio crusade waged in the middle of the twentieth century is that its crowning achievement—the successful vaccines of Jonas Salk and Albert Sabin—helped close the door to future research. Public interest quickly faded. Questions and problems that had swirled about this once-terrifying disease now seemed beside the point, almost arcane. Why was polio among the most seasonal of afflictions, with thirty-five times as many cases in August as in April? What made children so susceptible to the virus, especially boys? Why did polio become epidemic in the twentieth century, a time when other infectious diseases were being brought under control? And why did the most serious outbreaks occur in the advanced "sanitary" nations of the West?

HISTORICALLY, POLIO HAS GONE THROUGH three general phases: endemic, epidemic, and postvaccine. Though poliovirus has long been present in the environment, the disease, for many centuries, caused little concern. Unlike influenza, smallpox, and bubonic plague, it triggered no great pandemics or epidemics around the globe. From ancient times forward, poliovirus survived in endemic form, circulating freely in dreadful sanitary conditions and passing harmlessly from one host to the next. The outcome, for almost everyone, was a mild infection followed by a lifetime of immunity.

As a result, the early records of polio refer to individual cases, not to major outbreaks. The first one, ostensibly, comes from Egypt around 1500 BC. On an upright stone tablet is the figure of a young man, probably a priest, with a withered right leg. He is using a cane to balance himself. Those who have studied the engraving call it "a probable case of infantile paralysis." In truth, this is little more than a guess.[4]

The ancient world's most renowned physicians, the Greek Hippocrates and the Roman Galen, both refer to polio-like deformities in their writings about clubfoot. But the number of cases they cite is very small. Sporadic references to paralyzed children appear in the Middle Ages, with more detailed accounts emerging by the seventeenth and eighteenth centuries. Among the afflicted was Sir Walter Scott. "I showed every sign of health and strength until I was eighteen months old," he wrote.

> One night, I have been often told, I showed great reluctance to be caught and put to bed. . . . It was the last time I was to show much personal agility. In the morning I was discovered to be affected with [a] fever. . . . It held me three days. On the fourth . . . I had lost the power of my right leg. . . .
> The impatience of a child soon inclined me to struggle with my infirmity. . . . Although the limb affected was much shrunk and contracted, my general health . . . was much strengthened by being frequently in the open air and . . . I who in a city [would have] probably been condemned to helpless and hopeless decrepitude, was now a healthy, high-spirited, and, my lameness apart, a sturdy child.[5]

By the mid-1800s, pediatricians were finding small clusters of infantile paralysis in Western Europe and the United States. A village near the French coast, a British town in Nottinghamshire, a rural parish in Louisiana, a farm community north of Stockholm—all reported a dozen or more serious cases in a short span of time. On the surface, these outbreaks appeared to have little in common, aside from the age of the victims (young) and the season of occurrence (summer). Yet all of them had erupted in remote, sparsely populated areas, where the physical isolation can affect one's immunity to disease.

An old virus was about to surface, in a frightening new way.

THE FIRST RECORDED polio epidemic in the United States occurred in the Otter Valley, near Rutland, Vermont, in 1894. It might well have gone unnoticed had it not been for the heroic efforts of Charles Caverly, a young country doctor with a strong interest in public health. Caverly ran down every case—123 in all—listing sex, age, symptoms, apparent cause, and final result (fifty were permanently paralyzed and eighteen died).

A majority of the victims were male, a finding that would mark future polio epidemics. Eighty-four cases were under six years of age. Most began the same way, with a headache, fever, nausea, fatigue, and a stiff neck.

The cause of this spreading sickness clearly baffled Caverly. He had no idea what had brought it to the Otter Valley or how it had spread. But logic told him it wasn't particularly contagious, because few families had more than one case of the disease. So Caverly played his hunches, listing causes that might lower a child's resistance, such as "chilling the body when heated" and "playing too hard on a hot day." The latter, he thought, might explain the greater incidence of polio among boys.

Caverly's work was impressive. He showed, most obviously, that polio could produce an epidemic. And, without fully understanding the implications, he emphasized two key points. First, the term "infantile paralysis" was misleading, since most of the victims were children, not infants, and several were adults. Second, there was likely an abortive or nonparalytic form of the disease in which the victim displayed minor symptoms but recovered quickly. Polio, he sensed, was more widespread than anyone imagined.[6]

In 1905 the disease swept through parts of Sweden, with twelve hundred reported cases. As in Vermont, it came during the summer, hit isolated areas hardest, and claimed mostly juvenile victims. The lead investigator was Ivar Wickman, a Stockholm pediatrician who had just published a thick book about polio based on a series of smaller outbreaks in his country.

Wickman was most interested in the transmission of the disease. How did it spread? With the skill of a medical detective, he traced the routes that carried the "polio germ" from town to town along rural roads and railroad lines, and from child to child through contact at local schools. Polio was clearly contagious, Wickman believed, and the carriers included people who barely knew they were ill. It didn't matter whether the case was mild or paralytic. Both could spread the disease, giving it real epidemic potential.[7]

But the *cause* of polio—the microbial agent—remained a mystery. Viruses were still invisible in this era, beyond the reach of the strongest microscopes. Scientists used the term "filterable viruses" to describe these microorganisms because, unlike bacteria, they were small enough to pass through the porcelain filters then in laboratory use. A handful already had been identified, including the viruses of smallpox, rabies, and foot-and-mouth disease. But no one knew how a virus reproduced, or created an infection, or differed from other organisms, except for its size.

Getting this information would not be easy. How did one study a particle that had not yet been cultured and had never been seen? A giant step was taken in 1908 by Karl Landsteiner, an ingenious researcher who would one day win a Nobel Prize for his discovery of the different human blood types, A, B, AB, and O. At his laboratory in Vienna, Landsteiner produced an emulsion from the spinal cord of a boy who had just died of polio. He passed the liquid through a porcelain filter, injected the contents into the stomachs of two rhesus monkeys, and waited to observe the result. It didn't take long; the monkeys proved to be wonderfully susceptible hosts. Both succumbed to polio, their spinal cords showing much the same damage that had occurred in the little boy. The poliovirus had been isolated.[8]

Landsteiner's work opened a new chapter in the polio story, the beginning of serious laboratory research. It also marked the spectacular progress being made in the field of bacteriology, where scientists like Paul Ehrlich, Robert Koch, and Louis Pasteur had identified—and in some cases neutralized—the organisms responsible for malaria, tuberculosis, diphtheria, typhoid, and syphilis. Never before had there been cause for such optimism in the terrifying struggle against infectious diseases.[9]

VIRTUALLY ALL of these recent breakthroughs had occurred on European soil, where the pursuit of medical research had wide popular support. In France contributions from an adoring public had created the Pasteur Institute. British philanthropists had honored Joseph Lister, the father of antiseptic surgery, by building a research institute in his name. The German government had financed the laboratories of Paul Ehrlich and Robert Koch. In Russia the tsar had generously sponsored the Institute for Experimental Medicine.[10]

Nothing comparable had happened in the United States. There were no research institutes of distinction, and the nation's medical schools were in sorry shape. Most, in truth, were profit-turning diploma mills staffed by local doctors looking to supplement their meager pay. Few required a college degree; fewer still were equipped with adequate laboratories. In 1900 Americans looking toward a career in medical research often traveled to Europe for their training. Few opportunities awaited them when they returned home.[11]

The situation was both dangerous and embarrassing. America had grown dramatically since the end of the Civil War, becoming a world leader in engineering, transportation, industrial technology, and factory production. It had also seen the rise of a new capitalist class—captains of industry to some, robber barons to others—holding individual fortunes almost too enormous to comprehend. The largest belonged to John D. Rockefeller, the founder of Standard Oil.

Rockefeller regarded his success as a triumph for the American virtues of thrift, hard work, and rugged competition. In an era that celebrated social Darwinism as a civic virtue, he personified the survival of the fittest. Yet Rockefeller was also a religious man who donated faithfully to Baptist causes, despised vulgar displays of wealth, and viewed himself as a vehicle for distributing a share of the world's riches to the less fortunate. The dilemma he faced was how to square his Christian duty with his belief in the evolutionary struggle. "It is a great problem to learn how to give," he lamented, "without weakening the moral backbone of the beneficiary."[12]

An acceptable solution was offered by Frederick T. Gates, Rockefeller's close friend and business advisor. Having recently convinced the oil tycoon to generously fund the University of Chicago in order to raise "moral standards" in higher education, Gates now bombarded him with warnings about the primitive state of affairs in the nation's laboratories and medical schools. What America needed, he told Rockefeller, was an institute based on top European models like the Pasteur Institute.

The timing was ideal. Rockefeller had recently come under withering assault from muckraking journalists for his cutthroat practices at Standard Oil. His public image needed some buffing; a project of this sort would certainly help. Other financial giants, including J. Pierpont Morgan and Collis P. Huntington, had begun to support medical education, and rumor had it that steel king Andrew Carnegie, a noted philanthropist, was planning to build an institute for scientific research in Washington, D.C.[13]

There were family reasons as well. In 1900 Rockefeller's first grandson, 3-year-old John Rockefeller McCormick, contracted scarlet fever, a disease with no known treatment or cure. A distraught Rockefeller offered one prominent doctor half a million dollars to save the child, who died within weeks of taking ill. After that, medical research became Rockefeller's consuming philanthropy, the ideal cause for a man who hoped to uplift society without blunting its competitive edge.[14]

The Rockefeller Institute opened its doors in New York City in 1902. Like the great European centers of that era, it aimed to create a pure research environment in which the best minds could do their best work free of petty worries and distractions. The salaries would be high, the laboratories perfectly equipped, the teaching duties minimal. For those fortunate enough to get the call, a gleaming world of privilege awaited, unlike anything they had ever known. "At the Rockefeller you did not smell the animals," a scientist recalled. "They were brought to you from a beautiful animal house in the bowels of the Institute" by a servant who also "washed the glassware and cooked the culture medium." Nothing was overlooked. The laboratory was the shrine.[15]

No one would do more to shape this environment than Simon Flexner, the institute's first director. Born in 1863, the son of German-Jewish immigrants, Flexner had emerged from humble surroundings, much like Rockefeller himself, to become a leader in the sparsely populated world of American medical research. It hadn't been easy. An eighth-grade dropout, completely self-taught, he discovered the world of science while clerking in a local drugstore. Needing a diploma to advance his career, Flexner enrolled at the University of Louisville Medical School—a marginal enterprise in 1887, even by the dismal standards of that era. His entire training consisted of two short lecture courses. He never saw a patient or dissected a cadaver. "I cannot say I was particularly helped by the school," Flexner recalled. "What it did for me was to give me the M.D. degree."

He had no desire to practice medicine. With help from his brother, Abraham—who would go on to a distinguished career as an educator—Flexner entered the graduate program in pathology at Johns Hopkins, then a relatively new university in Baltimore; built on the German model, it stressed laboratory work and original research. He seemed wildly out of place at Johns Hopkins, his son recalled—a little Jewish

man "dressed in crude provincial clothes, speaking in uneducated ac-
cents, this self-educated druggist." But his brilliance caught the eye of
William Henry Welch, the acknowledged "dean of American medicine,"
who tutored him, socially and scientifically, with great success. After
earning a faculty appointment at Johns Hopkins, Flexner left in 1898 to
become a professor of pathology at the University of Pennsylvania, the
nation's oldest medical school. He had just turned thirty-five.[16]

The new position didn't much appeal to him, despite its prestige.
The surroundings were more traditional than at Johns Hopkins, the
faculty more conservative, the anti-Semitism more severe. Flexner remained the quintessential outsider—the rare bird who hadn't attended
Penn's medical school, and one of only two Jews on the entire faculty
(the other being an expert on Semitic languages). When the Rockefeller
Institute came calling in 1902, offering him its directorship, Flexner
jumped at the chance. His starting salary, guaranteed to trump any
competing professorship, was a whopping $10,000 a year.

There were those, of course, who saw this new institute as a frivo-
lous pursuit. The value of basic research was still suspect in the United
States. Laboratory work seemed a poor substitute for simple bedside
observation. But Flexner quickly trumped this thinking with a breakthrough that fused the esoteric world of the institute to the real world
of suffering and disease. It came during a deadly epidemic of cerebrospinal meningitis in the winter of 1905.

The cause was already known. European researchers in the 1880s had
isolated a bacterium that inflamed the membranes of the spinal cord and
the brain. A serum had even been developed from the blood of inoculated horses, though it didn't do much good. In New York City that
winter, three-quarters of the four thousand meningitis victims had died,
including many who received the so-called horse injection.

Flexner was familiar with the disease, having studied an earlier epidemic during his time at Johns Hopkins. Working now with cultures
obtained from autopsies in New York City, he was able to infect lab
monkeys with relative ease. What he learned was that the horse serum
worked better when injected directly into the spinal cord, "the seat of
the disease."[17]

The discovery saved lives, providing the best defense against cerebrospinal meningitis in an era before sulfa drugs and antibiotics. It also
put the Rockefeller Institute on the map. Knowing a sure thing when
he saw it, the founder responded to this publicity bonanza—"Cure Is

Found For Meningitis With John D's Aid," read one headline—by generously padding the endowment. Even his rivals were impressed. Asked a short time later to fund a medical building, Andrew Carnegie refused. "That is Mr. Rockefeller's specialty," he said. "Go see him."[18]

When considering the diseases to be given priority, Flexner put polio near the top of the list. There were good reasons for doing so. His institute already had the resources to attract the world's top medical researchers and to equip a first-class polio lab. Flexner was confident that the disease could be vanquished quickly. It reminded him of cerebrospinal meningitis: an infectious agent, penetrating the central nervous system, to be tamed by a vaccine.

There also was some urgency to his quest. Polio was spreading. It had begun to reach the margins of public concern. New York City reported 2,000 cases in the summer of 1907. Similar outbreaks were noted in Massachusetts, Minnesota, Nebraska, Ohio, and Wisconsin between 1910 and 1914. Dr. Caverly faced a new epidemic in Vermont, far worse than the one of sixteen years before. "This disease," he warned, "has increased with alarming rapidity." From the field, polio seemed as baffling as ever. When examining the key variables—nationality, prior diseases, population density, sewer facilities, water supply, condition of premises, domestic animals kept—health officials could find nothing to connect the victims beyond their age. They saw no evidence that polio struck hardest in crowded, filthy neighborhoods, like so many other diseases. Indeed, officials in Ohio hinted that the reverse might be true. "The most ideal domestic environment does not shield from this infection," they wrote. "If anything, the so-called middle classes [seem to] suffer the most."[19]

Increasingly, the public looked to Flexner for help. With the press now portraying him as the nation's foremost "polio expert," he was flooded with letters seeking advice. One, from the mayor of Bastrop, Louisiana, put it well: "I have read . . . about the experiments your institute has been making with this disease and I am going to ask you on behalf of the thousands of children in this section who are threatened to give us something about your experience. Is there a cure? If so, can you tell us about the treatment? How the disease spreads? How it can be prevented?"[20]

These questions, it turned out, would consume Flexner for the rest of his career.

FLEXNER'S EARLY EXPERIMENTS were impressive. Using the spinal tissue of human victims, Flexner quickly replicated Landsteiner's finding that polio was caused by a filterable virus. He then took a huge step forward. Where Landsteiner had been successful in infecting two monkeys with human poliovirus, Flexner was able to pass the infection from one monkey to the next—which meant that the disease could be carefully studied in lab animals for the first time.

Monkeys do not make ideal subjects. They come from great distances, often in deplorable condition. They're costly and hard to handle. To be bitten by a lab monkey is a terrifying, and not uncommon, event. "I learned for the first time what neurogenic shock is," said Dorothy Horstmann, a pioneer in polio research, recalling a bloody encounter with a "pretty big cynomolgous" who grabbed her thumb, gashed it, and wouldn't let go. "I didn't black out, but I came very close to it."[21]

Polio, moreover, is a human disease. Animals cannot get it naturally; it has to be induced. In the early years of polio research, the monkey—cranky and expensive—was the only animal known to be susceptible to this virus. And the Rockefeller Institute was one of the few places with the resources available to import and care for large numbers of them. A rhesus monkey in those days sold for around seven dollars, more than the daily pay of the typical research scientist.[22]

In the long run, monkeys would prove invaluable to the polio story. More than 100,000 would be sacrificed in the fifty-year quest for a vaccine. In the short run, however, serious trouble arose. It began with an innocent mistake by Flexner, although no one knew it at the time. And it ended with a "discovery" that would slow the progress of polio research to a crawl.

Flexner was determined to find the portal of entry for poliovirus, a key piece of the puzzle. Learning how it got inside the body, and from there to the central nervous system, was essential in preparing a defense. Flexner began by feeding poliovirus to the monkeys by mouth; none took sick. Then he swabbed their nasal passages with the virus and watched them fall quickly to the disease. The message seemed clear: poliovirus entered through the nose and traveled along nerve pathways through the brain and into the spinal cord.

The implications were enormous. If Flexner was correct, then poliovirus did not go down the alimentary tract, nor did it circulate in the blood. His finding—if true—raised serious problems in fighting the disease. The most obvious weapon against polio would be a vaccine that stimulated the immune system to produce antibodies in the blood. But what good would it do against a virus that reached the central nervous system without ever entering the bloodstream? Where, exactly, was this battle to be fought?

Flexner wasn't sure. Over time, he would lose faith in the promise of a vaccine, working instead on ways to guard the nasal passages with some sort of chemical blockade" (see pp. 125–26). For the moment, however, optimism prevailed. In 1911 the *New York Times* gushed that polio would soon go the way of smallpox, typhus, and other vanquished plagues. Its impeccable—if single—source was Flexner himself. "We have already discovered how to prevent infantile paralysis," he noted. "The achievement of a cure, I may conservatively say, is not now far distant."[23]

Whatever led Flexner to make this wild prediction he never revealed. Perhaps the giant strides being made against other infectious diseases in recent years clouded his judgment. Or perhaps the growing strength of the antivivisectionist lobby, which had begun to target Flexner's use of monkeys in his medical research, encouraged him to show more progress than had actually occurred. Either way, his statement became a model of the false optimism that would dominate polio studies over the next forty years.

Research would later show that poliovirus entered through the mouth. What had led Flexner astray? For one thing, he unluckily chose the wrong monkey for his experiments. *Macaca mulatta* (rhesus monkey) is one of the rare primates that cannot contract polio through oral feeding. The virus simply does not replicate in its digestive tract. Indeed, the only sure way to infect this species is to shoot poliovirus directly to its brain or spinal cord, as Flexner had done. In the judgment of Tom Rivers, the father of modern virology, progress on a polio vaccine "was held up purely by chance because a big man like Flexner was using the rhesus monkey." Had he tried another species (the cynomolgous monkey or the chimpanzee), "the chances are," said Rivers, "that we might have had a vaccine that much sooner."[24]

This error, in turn, led to others. By passing poliovirus repeatedly through the brains and spinal columns of his monkeys, Flexner produced a strain—known as MV or mixed virus—that was highly neurotropic, able to multiply *only* in nervous tissue. This made the conquest of polio even more problematic since animal nervous tissue can provoke a serious allergic reaction in humans, making it a dangerous medium for growing the poliovirus needed for a workable vaccine. Given Flexner's prominence, MV quickly became the strain of choice in the polio field, leading researchers down yet another blind alley.

Such mistakes were part of a larger pattern. Flexner was a researcher who disdained the clinical side of medicine. Though the Rockefeller Institute was then composed of two divisions, laboratories and hospital, Flexner saw the latter as little more than a "testing ground" for the ideas and projects generated in the former. "The approach that led [him] astray," wrote one prominent researcher, "was concentration on laboratory experiments in monkeys, to the complete exclusion of studies involving patients." This reliance on an animal model for the development of polio would have serious consequences for the treatment of human beings.[25]

Flexner's tenure at the Rockefeller Institute covered more than forty years. In that time—as the institute director until 1935 and a staff member until his death in 1946—he hired and supervised the men and women who would revolutionize the field of virology. Herald Cox, Karl Landsteiner, Max Theiler, Thomas Francis, Isabel Morgan, Peter Olitsky, Tom Rivers, Albert Sabin—the list goes on. All of them acknowledged the vital role that Flexner played in developing their careers. And many of them, no doubt, identified with the acid portrait of him drawn by the novelist Sinclair Lewis in *Arrowsmith*—Flexner in the guise of the imperious Dr. A. DeWitt Tubbs, director of the all-powerful McGurk Institute, who prevented idealistic scientists from pursuing their dreams. At the Rockefeller, Flexner's word was the law.[26]

IN JUNE OF 1916, a few miles and yet a world away from the gates of Flexner's gleaming institute, a health crisis was reported in a thickly populated immigrant area of Brooklyn known as Pigtown. According to the newspapers, frightened Italian parents had approached local doctors and priests, "complaining that their child could not hold a bottle or that the leg seemed limp . . . and there had been a little loss of appetite and some restlessness." When the first deaths were confirmed a few days later, the Health Department had rushed dozens of investigators to Pigtown for a house-to-house inspection. The diagnosis was polio.[27]

New York City was no stranger to epidemic disease. Smallpox, cholera, typhus, yellow fever, diphtheria, tuberculosis—each had taken its deadly toll over the years. Until the late nineteenth century, New York

City had a higher mortality rate than London or Paris, Boston or Philadelphia, making it one of the most dangerous places in the western world. In the 1870s, 20 percent of the babies born there did not live to see their first birthday. And among those lucky enough to reach adulthood, one-quarter died before the age of thirty.[28]

Foreigners shouldered much of the blame. New York's population had exploded in the 1800s, as waves of impoverished immigrants—first from Ireland, then from central and southern Europe—overwhelmed the city's housing stock, social services, and sanitation facilities. Living in wretched, overcrowded conditions, they became synonymous with sickness and filth. In the 1840s, the Irish were accused of bringing cholera to New York City; fifty years later, the Jews were suspected of spreading tuberculosis, also known as "the tailor's disease." Each time an epidemic appeared, native New Yorkers looked reflexively toward the immigrant slums.[29]

Still, this outbreak was unexpected. Mortality rates had dropped dramatically since the 1870s, the result of better sanitation, a healthier diet, and stunning breakthroughs in research. In a remarkable 1910 report, signaling a watershed in American medicine, the New York City Health Department listed cancer and heart disease as the most serious threats to future generations, replacing standard killers like smallpox, tuberculosis, and diphtheria. "Without exception," it noted, the area "in which a reduction of mortality has been most effected belongs to the class of infectious diseases."[30]

The news from Pigtown rekindled old fears. Widely viewed by Americans as the lowest of the low—vicious, ignorant, and unclean—Italians were the logical scapegoats for the spread of a mysterious new plague. "Steerage passengers from a Naples boat show a depressing frequency of low foreheads, open mouths, weak chins, poor features, skew faces, small or knobby crania, and backless heads," wrote the prominent American sociologist E. A. Ross in 1914. "Such people lack the power to take rational care of themselves; hence their death rate in New York is twice the general death rate and thrice that of the Germans." Although quarantine officers at Ellis Island insisted there was no evidence of infantile paralysis among entering immigrants, rumors flew that foreigners had imported "deadly germs" from the port cities of southern Europe. "Since May 15," warned the New York Times, "90 immigrant Italians, including 24 children under the age of 10 [have] gone to live in Brooklyn, where the outbreak [first] appeared."[31]

What could be done? Despite the optimistic predictions of Flexner, no magic bullet for polio had yet been found. Producing a vaccine would prove far harder than anyone had imagined. And that left public health officials in an awkward position, scrambling to combat an infection they barely understood.

Their responses emphasized traditional methods of control. Other epidemic diseases like cholera and typhoid fever had been tamed by better sanitation, attacking the filth that spread their deadly germs. In most places, this involved the regulation of sewage, the purification of water, and the pasteurization of milk. It included public health campaigns to educate people about quarantining the sick and keeping their dwellings clean. Implicit in these reforms, of course, was the assumption that immigrants were the primary carriers of infectious disease.[32]

For Pigtown residents, this bias was both a blessing and a curse. Street cleaners suddenly appeared in their neighborhood, trash was picked up, windows were screened, and stray animals carted away. "72,000 Cats Killed in Paralysis Fear," read one of that summer's more remarkable headlines. At the same time, however, a selective quarantine was enforced. Assuming that germs traveled only in one direction—from the slum areas outward—health officers scoured the city's Italian neighborhoods, posting signs on "contaminated" buildings, closing theaters to minors, hospitalizing sick children, and canceling the three-day festival of Our Lady of Mount Carmel, a hugely popular event. According to press reports, local resistance to these measures included "death threats" from the much-feared Italian Black Hand: "If you report any more of our babies to the Board of Health, we will kill you. . . . Keep off our streets and don't report our homes and we will do you no harm." The note, said one newspaper, was written in blood.[33]

By early July, as the epidemic worsened, all children leaving New York City were required by the Health Department to get a "travel certificate" proving they were "polio-free." The surrounding communities were not impressed. Many closed their doors to outsiders. From Hoboken to Hastings-on-Hudson, heavily armed policemen patrolled the roads and rail stations in search of fleeing New Yorkers, the *Times* reported, "with instructions to turn back every van, car, cart, and . . . instruct all comers that they would not be permitted under any circumstances to take up residence in [their] city."[34]

The disease continued to spread. By August polio outbreaks were reported in New Jersey, Connecticut, Pennsylvania, and upstate New

York. Among the towns under siege was elegant Hyde Park, the home of Franklin Delano Roosevelt, then a young assistant secretary of the navy. From Washington that summer, Roosevelt instructed his wife, Eleanor, to keep their five children at the summer residence on Campobello Island, off the Canadian coast, until the epidemic had passed. That fall, a U.S. Navy destroyer brought the family home, landing at Roosevelt's private dock on the Hudson River.

The epidemic lasted through October, claiming 27,000 American lives. New York City alone reported 8,900 cases and 2,400 deaths, 80 percent being children under five. Normally, this would have been cause for alarm. But Americans were looking elsewhere in 1916, consumed by news of unimaginable slaughter in Europe. That very summer, a huge Anglo-French offensive in the Somme against dug-in German forces had left a half-million dead. Polio was of marginal interest beyond parts of the Northeast, barely visible to a people bitterly debating their own participation in this war.

Those who studied the outbreak, however, had reason for concern. Why hadn't the quarantine and the sanitation measures been more effective in controlling its spread? Why were rural and affluent neighborhoods hit with equal, if not greater, force than the teeming urban slums? The latter question was more intriguing because it placed cultural issues at the heart of the debate. Almost everyone assumed that poor living conditions—filth, poverty, overcrowding, and ignorance— were responsible for breeding epidemic disease. Yet polio did not appear to fit this mold. In New York City, for example, public health officials found the epidemic to be most prevalent on Staten Island, which had the lowest population density and the best sanitary conditions of the city's five boroughs. Another study showed that recent immigrants living in the most congested parts of Brooklyn and Manhattan had a lower incidence of the disease than native-born Americans living in rural areas of upstate New York. The same held true for New Jersey and Pennsylvania, where the "wealthy" and "exclusive" neighborhoods were especially hard hit. "In all homes where polio exists," a Philadelphia newspaper claimed, "children have been declared well nourished and cared for."[35]

How could such findings be explained? Most people believed that polio had been brought into the better neighborhoods by immigrant carriers who worked as cooks, maids, and chauffeurs; by disease-bearing insects that had traveled up from the slums; or by innocent middle-class folk who rode the city subways "reeking with billions of germs caused by the filthy foreign element constantly using them." To some public health experts, however, the 1916 epidemic suggested a very different reality, at odds with current wisdom and common sense. Was it possible, they wondered, that those who lived in crowded, unsanitary conditions had been naturally immunized by exposure to poliovirus at an early age? Was it possible, in fact, that squalor actually *protected* a child from this disease?[36]

The answers to these and other troubling questions about polio would take years to unfold. The "menace for the future," warned a federal official, "is very real."[37]

2

Warm Springs

—

F. D. ROOSEVELT ILL
OF POLIOMYELITIS
Brought on Special Railroad Car from Campobello,
Bay of Fundy, to Hospital Here
Recovering, Doctor Says

T HIS FRONT PAGE STORY on September 16, 1921, must have startled
the readers of the *New York Times*. Polio was still a new disease, and the
only major epidemic, five years before, had been said to target immigrant children from the slums. How, then, could it possibly victimize a
man like Franklin D. Roosevelt: thirty-nine years old, robust and athletic, with a long pedigree and a cherished family name?

In retrospect, the events surrounding his illness are not as random
as they first appeared. The summer of 1921 had been a terribly stress-
ful time for FDR. Already worn down from his unsuccessful campaign
for vice president on the Democratic ticket the previous year, he suddenly found himself under attack from a hostile Republican Congress
for his role in a sex scandal that had occurred in 1919, when he was an
assistant secretary of the navy. The details were explosive, involving a
secret plan, supposedly endorsed by Roosevelt, to gather evidence of
homosexual behavior at a naval training center by using undercover
agents to entrap young sailors. Though Roosevelt denied any detailed
knowledge of these operations, he had been forced to return to Washington in the stifling summer heat of 1921 to clear his name. The episode ended badly, leaving him bitter and depressed. "Lay Naval Scandal
to F.D. Roosevelt: Details Are Unprintable," said the *Times*.[1]

Before departing for his summer home on Campobello Island, Roosevelt had stopped off to attend a Boy Scout jamboree near the family estate in Hyde Park. A poignant photo shows him marching alongside dozens of uniformed children. It is the last one ever taken of FDR walking unassisted. From there, he had sailed with friends to Campobello, a trip marked by rough waters and fog. "I thought he looked tired when he left," wrote his secretary, Missy LeHand.[2]

Campobello Island sits in the Bay of Fundy, off the southern coast of New Brunswick, Canada, not far from Maine. The Roosevelt home— fifteen rooms on ten rocky water-front acres—had been given to Franklin and Eleanor as a wedding present by his mother. By the time he arrived on August 7, 1921, his family had been there for a month. Determined to bury his troubles, he roared from one activity to the next—swimming, boating, and drinking into the night.

The next day began, as usual, with a family sail. On the way home, Roosevelt noticed a brush fire on a nearby island and spent several hours putting it out. Back on Campobello, the children challenged him to a race. "He accepted with alacrity," recalled Anna Roosevelt, the eldest, then fifteen. "This entailed a two mile dog-trot across the island, a swim across a long and narrow fresh water lake, a dip in the freezing waters of the Bay of Fundy, then a reversal of this process until we reached home." FDR spent the late afternoon in a wet bathing suit, reading newspapers and answering his mail. By then, a strange feeling had come over him—a mixture of numbness, deep muscle ache, and frightening chills. "I'd never felt quite that way before," he remembered.[3]

Exhausted and unsteady, Roosevelt went upstairs to change. "In a little while," said Eleanor, "he began to complain [of illness] and decided he would not eat supper with us, but would go to bed and get thoroughly warm." He woke up the next morning in pain, running a fever, and dragging his left leg. "I managed to move about to shave," he recalled. "I tried to persuade myself that the trouble with my leg was muscular."[4]

The local doctor stopped by for a look. His comforting diagnosis— a "bug" compounded by physical exhaustion—made perfect sense. Even the most severe polio cases can be mistaken for run-of-the-mill influenza, until paralysis sets in. For Roosevelt, however, a downward spiral had begun. His pain grew worse, the fever lingered, and numbness spread to both legs. His skin was so sensitive that he couldn't tolerate the feel of his pajamas or even the rustle of a breeze. He felt the silent panic, he later admitted, of someone very close to death. "I don't know what's the matter with me," he kept repeating. "I just don't know."[5]

A second doctor was summoned: William Keen, an elderly Philadelphia surgeon who happened to be vacationing in nearby Bar Harbor, Maine. Keen, at least, understood that some sort of paralytic injury had occurred, the result, he thought, of a "clot of blood from a [bladder infection that] had lodged in the lower spinal cord temporarily removing the power to move though not to feel." The prognosis looked good, he told Eleanor; her husband should recover fully in a matter of weeks. Keen recommended deep massage and exercise in order to stimulate the weakened muscles. His bill for $600—"rather high," the family thought—arrived a few days later.[6]

By week's end, FDR had lost all movement below his waist. Eleanor attempted to massage his legs, as the doctor had instructed, but the pain was unbearable. A relative wrote her, urging yet another consultation. Though "a fine old chap," he said, Keen "is not a connoisseur [of] this malady," and "it would be very unwise to trust his diagnosis." A specialist soon arrived at Campobello: Robert Lovett, a professor of orthopedic surgery at Harvard and the Children's Hospital of Boston. His recent book, *The Treatment of Infantile Paralysis*, was considered then and remains today one of the classics in the field.[7]

Lovett had no trouble making the diagnosis: poliomyelitis. He was cautiously optimistic about the patient's future. "I told them very frankly," he said, "that no one could tell where they stood, that the case was evidently not of the severest type, that complete recovery or partial recovery . . . was possible."[8]

Lovett was a pioneer in the field of orthopedic recovery. He believed in a gradual aftercare program for polio patients, starting with weeks of bed rest, warm baths, and the mildest forms of stretching to prevent muscle contraction. To his thinking, Keen's advice had been dangerously off-base, adding needless pain and further damaging the overtired muscles. Lovett urged Roosevelt to return to New York as soon as his condition had stabilized, so that that proper rehabilitation could begin.[9]

Though a number of servants were on duty at Campobello, the great bulk of nursing care fell to Eleanor Roosevelt, who rarely left her husband's side. It was exhausting, at times nauseating, as the paralysis spread temporarily to the bladder and the bowels. Moving a cot into his room, she bathed him, catheterized him, gave him enemas, administered painkillers, and carefully turned him in bed. Alarmed that his disease might spread to the five children, she allowed them no closer than his sickroom door, where they could peek in to wave hello. "Mother told us not to talk about polio, as so many people were scared of it," Anna Roosevelt recalled. "But rumor travels fast; we found out that many of our friends had been told by their friends not to go near the Roosevelt children as 'they might have polio.'"[10]

Indeed, fears were raised about allowing James, the oldest son, to return to Groton that fall. Though Dr. Lovett assured the headmaster the boy was not contagious, Eleanor had to agree that James "wears clothing which he did not wear at Campobello, that he puts on fresh underclothing, and that he takes a bath and washes his hair immediately before leaving."[11]

WAS FRANKLIN ROOSEVELT a uniquely vulnerable target? The answer, most probably, is yes. Carefully sheltered as a youth, tutored in relative isolation, he had avoided the common childhood illnesses until his arrival at boarding school as a teen. From that point forward, his medical history resembled an encyclopedia of contagious diseases. The list included typhoid fever, swollen sinuses, infected tonsils, stomach problems, and endless sore throats, some of which forced him to bed for weeks. During the Spanish influenza pandemic of 1918, he took sick on an ocean liner, "spent the journey in his bunk, shivering and semicoherent," and wound up with a case of double pneumonia that almost took his life.[12]

In 1921, his body weakened by stress and exhaustion, FDR attended a large gathering of young people in midsummer, when polio is most likely to occur. He followed that with a manic spurt of activity at Campobello, including a swim in the Bay of Fundy, which he later described as "water so cold it seemed paralyzing." By the time he was properly diagnosed, he had undergone a series of excruciating leg massages that may well have increased the severity of the disease.

For Roosevelt everything came together at once. There is strong evidence today that stress can hamper the immune system, that physical exertion after the onset of polio can worsen the paralysis, and that "chilling" can further weaken a worn-down body's resistance to disease. Add in Roosevelt's medical history and his ill-timed visit with the

Boy Scouts, and the picture is grim. Though no one is predestined to contract polio, he surely ran a higher risk.[13]

A recent article has raised the possibility that FDR did not have polio, but rather Guillain-Barré syndrome, a disease characterized "by progressive symmetrical paralysis and loss of reflexes, usually beginning in the legs." The authors note that there is a strong case to be made for FDR's polio, since it was then prevalent in the Northeast, it struck him in the summer months, it appeared after intensive exercise, and it was accompanied by a fever (unlike Guillain-Barré). However, they argue that very few people of FDR's age contracted polio in those years, and that a number of his symptoms closely matched Guillain-Barré. As one of the authors put it: "We feel from the clinical evidence, which is all that exists, that's it's more likely he had Guillain-Barré syndrome. . . . We did not examine him. He had very fine physicians who were experts in their field who did."

What is certain, however, is that FDR believed he had polio, as did his family, his doctors, other polio victims, and the American public. Without him, the great polio crusade would never have been launched.[14]

THERE WAS ANOTHER FACTOR AS WELL. The era in which FDR came of age was marked by an almost religious zeal, particularly within the United States, to sanitize the environment in the hope of conquering disease. Sometimes this crusade paid off; at other times it didn't. In the case of polio, it may have brought a sleeping giant to life.

Most Americans today have a passion for cleanliness. Their sensitivity to germs and odor and grime, their obsession with well-scrubbed bodies and spotless surroundings, is an essential part of their modern character, a way to judge the larger world and be judged in return. What is easy to forget in such a deeply antiseptic culture is that life in the United States was not always this way. Chasing dirt didn't come naturally, nor did it come early.

Americans are fond of quoting John Wesley and Benjamin Franklin about cleanliness being next to godliness. In truth, the words "American" and "cleanliness" rarely graced the same sentence before the twentieth century. In 1900 toothbrushes were still rare in the United States, deodorants and shampoos almost unheard of. Few people bathed more than once a week or rinsed their hair more than once a month. Fewer still washed their hands before eating or after using a toilet. Spitting was almost universal. Travelers shared beds and chamber pots with complete strangers. Most houses, lacking screens, attracted swarms of insects in warm weather. Water supplies were unfiltered, and food was poorly refrigerated, if at all. Cities reeked from the stench of garbage, horse droppings, slaughterhouses, tanneries, and open sewers.[15]

But change did come to the United States, triggered by remarkable advances in science, technology, and commerce. By the 1870s researchers had begun to link unseen agents to *specific* maladies like typhoid, cholera, tuberculosis, and gonorrhea. Known as the "germ theory of disease," it taught people to accept the rather odd notion that they shared their communities, their homes, even their bodies with an invisible, often dangerous, world of microorganisms. They learned that neighbors could carry these deadly germs without showing the slightest symptoms—Typhoid Mary being the most infamous example. The message was clear: what you *don't* see can make you very sick.[16]

The germ theory combined with the rapid growth of cities in the late nineteenth century to fuel a growing concern with cleanliness and health. Reformers championed new public measures, such as the vaccination of schoolchildren, the medical inspection of immigrants, and the passage of pure food and drug laws. Innovations in plumbing led to more indoor bathrooms and safer water supplies. A jump in literacy quadrupled the number of magazines, which focused increasingly on the dangers posed by germs. A sampling of articles from this era includes "The Perilous Barber Shop," "Disease From Public Laundries," and "The Most Dangerous Animal in the World" (the housefly). One expert urged Americans to fumigate their homes each time a guest departed. Another recommended the spraying of cyanide, a risky procedure that involved "running rapidly from room to room and instantly closing the door."[17]

In the early 1900s, a movement erupted to treat paper money as a health hazard. "The popular opinion today," a journalist noted, "is that [it] is very filthy and extremely dangerous to handle." When a rumor spread that "borrowed volumes" were carriers of dangerous disease, the New York Public Library vowed to spray its books with chemicals until "not a live germ can be found." In the words of *Popular Science Monthly*, "The hostile microbe is in fact everywhere—within and without us, seeking, we might say, what it might devour."[18]

Americans thus came to believe that cleanliness was good, that proper hygiene would keep them healthy and alive. "Men shaved their beards and women shortened their skirts to eliminate potentially germ-catching appendages," wrote one medical historian. More homes contained "the white china toilet, the vacuum cleaner, and the refrigerator." People were taught to cover their coughs and sneezes. "Hotels began to supply individual cakes of soap and to use extra-long sheets so that sleepers might fold them back over potentially germ-ridden blankets. Churches adopted individual communion cups, and cities installed sanitary water fountains."[19]

These changes went hand in hand with the explosion of the consumer economy and the growing sophistication of mass advertising campaigns. By the 1920s, the old formula of simply alerting people to the presence of a new product had given way to the more aggressive process of actively shaping the public's wants and needs. Not surprisingly, advertisers played upon the fears of an increasingly germ-avoidant population, creating fresh anxieties about odors, blemishes, and disease.

One of the biggest success stories of this era was the marketing of cellophane, invented by Du Pont in 1908. Once a modest-selling industrial product, it became an overnight sensation, a household staple, following an ad campaign in women's magazines that portrayed it as the consumer's ultimate defense against microbes: "Strange Hands, Inquisitive Hands. Dirty Hands. Touching, feeling, examining the things you buy in stores. Your sure protection . . . is tough, clear, germ-proof Cellophane."[20]

Other advertisers followed suit. Paper companies used germ fears to push toilet tissue and disposable cups (the latter to avoid "salivary exchange"). In one of the bolder marketing ploys of the 1920s, the Lambert Pharmacal Company of St. Louis took an old disinfectant named Listerine (after the nineteenth-century British surgeon Joseph Lister) and turned it into a cure for "halitosis," defined in Lambert's new ad campaign as "the *unforgivable* social offense." Though the product remained the same, its yearly earnings jumped from $115,000 to more than $8,000,000. Before long, "halitosis" had entered dictionary as "stale or foul-smelling breath."[21]

These new ads cleverly mixed social fears with medical concerns. Listerine not only protected one against the consequences of bad breath—"Always the bridesmaid, Never the bride"—it also destroyed a host of sinister-sounding microbes, such as *Streptococcus hemolyticus*, *Staphylococcus aureus*, and *Bacillus typhosus*. This winning strategy led Lever Brothers to market its new LifeBuoy Health Soap as a potent germ killer with a pleasing smell—the answer, indeed, to America's latest social affliction: B.O. In 1927, the nation's leading soap manufacturers combined to form the Cleanliness Institute, a propaganda outlet aimed at children in particular. Lavishly funded, the institute worked with school districts to impose a "soap-and-water" curriculum for students at each grade level—how many baths to take, when to wash their hands and to change their underwear, why dirty toilets posed a health danger. "The object should be not merely to make children clean," said the Institute, "but to make them love to be clean."[22]

It seemed to work. A national survey of consumer needs in the 1930s showed that soap, a product of limited appeal only two decades before, now ranked third (just behind bread and butter, but ahead of coffee and sugar) on the list of the so-called essentials of life. Americans had come to trust the culture of cleanliness; and why not? Epidemic disease was on the decline. Cholera, diphtheria, typhus, tuberculosis, yellow fever—all had been wiped out or minimized in recent years with the aid of better hygiene and medical research.

What Americans could not foresee was that their antiseptic revolution brought risks as well as rewards. As the nation cleaned up, new problems arose. There was now a smaller chance that people would come into contact with dangerous microbes early in life, when the infection was milder and maternal antibodies offered temporary protection. In the case of polio, the result would be more frequent outbreaks and a wider range of victims. Franklin Roosevelt was no longer alone.

IN LATE SEPTEMBER, the Roosevelt family left Campobello Island for New York City. The trip was carefully planned to conceal Franklin's helpless condition. Reporters were kept at a safe distance as he was moved by stretcher from a chartered boat to a private railroad car. "Every jolt was painful," Eleanor recalled. What the press saw, from the open train window, was a beaming FDR, propped up in bed with pillows, his trademark cigarette holder in place, petting his favorite dog. The accounts were generally upbeat. While noting that Roosevelt did, indeed, have "infantile paralysis," they described him as "smiling," "feeling more comfortable," and, above all, "recovering." "He definitely will not be crippled," said one of his medical advisors. "No one need have any fear of any permanent injury from this attack."[23]

These stories were revealing. They marked the start of a conscious campaign by Roosevelt and his inner circle to shield a massive disability from public view. Some of it no doubt reflected the upper-class stoicism that had been drilled into him from birth, the art of suffering in silence, smiling through the pain. And some of it revealed the embarrassment of a powerful adult laid low by a condition associated with helpless children. "I am telling everybody who asks that you have a very severe rheumatic attack from 'excess bathing,'" a close relative assured FDR in 1921. "It is too silly for you to have an 'infantile' disease."[24]

Mostly, however, it was meant to remove the enormous stigma attached to a handicap of this sort. To be crippled in this era was viewed by many as a moral failing, a sign of inner weakness, a character flaw requiring the afflicted person's removal from normal society—and, in some cases, the limb's removal as well. ("When a leg is completely useless—i.e., when it cannot be swung forward and backward—it is better to amputate it through the thigh," said a leading medical textbook of the time.) Those lacking the proper resources were packed off to grim institutions, with names like the Children's Home for Incurables, so as not to burden others with a sight better left unseen.[25]

Roosevelt's wealth and status shielded him from the worst of it. Yet many who knew him assumed that his political career was over. "He is only 39," confided one family friend to another, "both too old and too young for such a fell germ to disable him. He had a brilliant career as assistant [secretary] of the Navy under Wilson and then a few brief weeks of crowded glory and excitement when nominated by the Democrats for the Vice-Presidency. Now he is a cripple—will he ever be anything else?"[26]

He could always spend his days as the sheltered invalid that his mother and some other family members envisioned for him. The harder road lay in returning to the public sphere, where life was less forgiving. Roosevelt might well summon the needed courage and will power, but these traits by themselves would not be enough. For him to succeed in the larger world, his polio would have to be disguised. It was there, but not really: an affliction, perhaps, but not a handicap; a disease, in short, with no disabling features.

This behavior was hardly unique. Public figures, including a number of American presidents, had routinely concealed their medical problems while in office. George Washington nearly died of pneumonia in 1790. "We have been very near losing the President," his secretary of state, Thomas Jefferson, admitted to a friend. Grover Cleveland underwent a life-threatening operation in 1893 to remove a huge cancerous lesion from his jaw; the White House described it as a minor dental problem involving an infected tooth. "My God," the groggy Cleveland remarked upon awakening from the anesthesia, "they nearly killed me." When Woodrow Wilson suffered a major stroke in 1919, nothing remotely truthful was revealed about his condition until after he had left office the following year.[27]

Roosevelt's task would be more difficult, given the visible and permanent nature of his condition. As a result, he became a master of concealment, especially after reentering the political world. He reached a gentleman's agreement with the press not to be photographed in a wheelchair or a helpless position. He hid his leg braces under long capes and blankets. The Secret Service prepared for his speaking appearances by constructing portable ramps and putting hand grips on the podium. The staging was so elaborate, wrote one presidential scholar, that it "rivaled the legitimate theater in its handling of the scenery and props." Some believe that the "bubble" around the modern presidency can be traced back directly to FDR.[28]

The ruse was largely successful. Few Americans would ever know the struggle it took for Roosevelt to get to his feet, to speak while standing, or to move from place to place. According to Hugh Gallagher, himself a polio survivor, "among the thousands of political cartoons and caricatures of FDR, not one shows the man physically impaired. In fact, many of them have him as a man of action—running, jumping, doing things." Gallagher called it "FDR's splendid deception."[29]

Roosevelt returned to work in the fall of 1922. "I too have had a wretched time," he told a sick friend in a rare acknowledgment of his misfortune. "[After being] in bed for six months, I have been getting around with great difficulty, as my legs were pretty well knocked out. They are coming back, however, slowly but surely, and though I still wear braces on them, I am physically in splendid shape."[30]

In truth, they were barely responding at all. His arms, shoulders, and upper back had gained extraordinary strength and definition as a result of endless exercise designed to get him up and moving, but his once-powerful leg muscles had mostly withered away. He now used hip-to-ankle braces, made of steel and leather, simply to lurch a few paces on the arm of an attendant, and even then he needed a cane.

His disability had at least one positive feature. It allowed him to jettison his law practice, mainly trusts and estates, which bored him terribly, by claiming he could no longer navigate the steep front steps

of the firm's office building in Manhattan. This move, though personally satisfying, carried some financial risk. Roosevelt could still count
on substantial income from his family trust and a sinecure at a major
bonding firm, but his lifestyle remained as lavish as before. He had
several houses, a yacht, a personal staff, five children to educate, and a
string of bad investments to overcome, including a warehouse meant
to store lobsters until the price rose (it didn't) and an air passenger
service that relied on helium-filled dirigibles.

During one of his infrequent visits to the bonding firm at 120 Broadway, Roosevelt crossed paths with Basil O'Connor, a young lawyer who
worked in the building. The two had met at least once before. O'Connor's
older brother, John, a member of New York City's Tammany Hall political machine, had introduced them at the Democratic National Convention in 1920. As legend has it—and there are witnesses who swear by
the story—a more fateful meeting occurred in the lobby of 120 Broadway two years later, when Roosevelt, on the arm of his chauffeur, slipped
on the polished marble and crashed heavily to the floor. Basil O'Connor
was among those who helped him to his feet.[31]

A partnership was born. O'Connor, thirty-two, was looking for ways
to drum up business; FDR's name and connections would surely help.
Roosevelt, meanwhile, was hoping to start a law firm "with my name at
the head instead of at the tail." He wanted a position that was visible
enough for him to remain in the public eye, yet flexible enough for
him to continue his exhausting struggle against polio. The new firm
was called Roosevelt and O'Connor, with the former providing general legal advice and the latter doing the actual work.

At first glance, the two men had little in common. O'Connor was a
rags-to-riches type, raised in the Catholic working-class town of
Taunton, Massachusetts, the son of a tinsmith. Short and slightly built,
with none of Roosevelt's easygoing charm, he had made his way through
Dartmouth by playing violin in a dance band. When the mainline campus fraternities were slow to accept him, he started his own chapter of
Sigma Phi Epsilon, serving for three years as its president. A champion
debater, voted Most Likely to Succeed, O'Connor moved on to Harvard
Law School, where new obstacles were surmounted. He studied so hard
that he went blind for a while—a problem that required medical treatment but failed to slow him down. He graduated on time, near the top
of his class, by having fellow students read him the assignments.[32]

Following law school, O'Connor clerked in a Boston firm before setting out on his own. His specialty became the oil business, forging ties between producers and refiners. His small office suite at 120 Broadway never seemed to close. He routinely put in 14-hour days, using two secretaries in equal shifts. What marked him—then and later—was an intimidating sense of purpose, light on personal charm. "If Roosevelt was the young prince," said one observer, "O'Connor was the perfect vassal."[33]

Together, they would turn the conquest of polio into a national crusade.

IN THE SUMMER OF 1924, Roosevelt received a letter from George Foster Peabody, a Georgia native, about a local man who had overcome a severe case of polio. Roosevelt and Peabody were long-time friends. They had gone to Harvard together and staked out high-profile careers in politics and business. Best known for his devotion to charitable causes—the list ranged from southern Negro colleges to the bohemian artist colony Yaddo—Peabody had been a major donor to FDR's 1920 vice-presidential campaign.[34]

The local man in question, Lewis Joseph, had contracted polio at about the same time as FDR. That, however, was where the similarity ended. Joseph was a younger man, in his twenties, and his paralysis had been less severe. Swimming in warm, soothing waters, he said, had restored the damaged muscles in his legs. His lower body was strong. He could walk again with the aid of a cane.[35]

Roosevelt was intrigued. His progress could not compare with Joseph's, despite three years of intensive therapy. He had seen every specialist, done every exercise, considered every "miracle cure" from electrical stimulation to an oxygen tent that spurred muscle growth through "increased atmospheric pressure." Like other polio patients, moreover, Roosevelt was fascinated by hydrotherapy, the use of water to treat disability and disease.

The method was as old as medicine itself. Hippocrates had employed it to treat a wide range of muscle and joint diseases in ancient Greece. By the nineteenth century, Americans were flocking to warm-water springs and mineral spas for healing and relaxation; the most popular venues were Saratoga Springs in New York, Hot Springs in Arkansas, and White Sulphur Springs in West Virginia. On the advice of Dr. Lovett, Roosevelt had already begun to swim and exercise in the heated pool of Vincent Astor, his Hudson Valley friend. "The water put me where I am," Roosevelt told a family servant, "and the water has to bring me back."[36]

Peabody's letter to FDR had not told the entire story. Peabody was part owner of a struggling Georgia resort—the very one, it turned out, where Louis Joseph had waged his triumphant struggle against polio. By 1924, the place was failing badly. Its main building, the Meriwether Inn, was a ramshackle Victorian structure composed of forty-six mostly vacant rooms. There were fifteen private cabins scattered about, all in need of repair. What made the property distinctive was the water that bubbled up from below, high in mineral content and consistently 88 degrees. Marketed properly, it had real potential as a health spa—a Saratoga Springs with good weather and southern charm. A visit by Franklin Roosevelt, properly publicized, would certainly help move things along.

Warm Springs, Georgia, had seen better days. Set in the pine forests of rural Meriwether County, about 75 miles southwest of Atlanta, the land had first belonged to the Creek Indians who, legend had it, gave safe passage to those in need of the healing waters. In the antebellum era, influential southerners like John C. Calhoun and Henry Clay had come by stagecoach, seeking remedies for dyspepsia, rheumatism, and chronic diseases of the liver, kidney, and bladder. Though tourism naturally declined during the Civil War and Reconstruction, Warm Springs made a comeback in the 1890s when the Georgia Midland Railroad came through town. The Meriwether Inn opened in that decade, a thousand-acre spread complete with tennis courts, spas for men and women, and a huge spring-fed swimming pool.[37]

The prosperity didn't last. Bad management put the Meriwether in serious debt. Meanwhile, a new invention, the automobile, allowed tourists to travel greater distances to better known resorts. The grounds "became overgrown," a visitor recalled. "Underbrush climbed higher on the roadway leading to the old Warm Springs resort, and by 1919 . . . all was genteel ruin."[38]

FDR didn't much care about the aesthetics. Seeking a cure for polio, he arrived at the tiny Bullochsville (soon to be renamed Warm Springs) train station in October of 1924, accompanied by Eleanor, Missy LeHand, and Irvin McDuffie, his African American valet. The immediate surroundings—unpaved roads, tumble-down shacks, "white" and "colored" signs everywhere—did little to deflate him. "Really beautiful country," he said.

Eleanor thought otherwise. There was little about Warm Springs that appealed to her beyond Franklin's optimistic dream of recovery. The Meriwether Inn was a dump. Their personal cottage was so flimsy, she recalled, that one "could look through the cracks and see daylight." Rural southern life seemed "hard and poor and ugly." The racism was appalling, and the natives, though friendly, were far too primitive for her tastes. "I can remember driving one day . . . to buy some chickens," she wrote in her autobiography, "and my perfect horror when I learned I had to take them home alive, instead of killed and dressed. . . . In Warm Springs they ran around our yard, until the cook wrung their necks amid much squawking and put them in the pot. Somehow I didn't enjoy eating them!"[39]

Eleanor left quickly. Franklin and the others stayed on for several more weeks. Though the resort had closed for the winter, the pool remained open. Anxious to get started, Roosevelt met with Louis Joseph, a slender young man who walked slowly, deliberately, with the aid of a cane. "No braces at all?" asked Roosevelt. "Not any more," said Joseph, who gave his famous guest a full account of the Warm Springs experience, complete with the program he had used to gain back the use of his legs.[40]

The spring contained no magic elixir. What made it special was its consistent warmth and high mineral content (calcium and magnesium) that increased the water's buoyancy. As a result, polio patients could stay in the pool for longer periods while balancing themselves with relative ease. Roosevelt could *feel* the heat soothing his muscles and the minerals lifting his weight. "How marvelous," he yelled. "I don't think I'll ever get out."[41]

Joseph made a suggestion. "Why don't you try using your legs? The water is different. You float so easily." Standing shoulder deep, Roosevelt tried to elevate his right leg, the stronger one, while grasping the pool's edge. A slight movement occurred; the leg stirred briefly—a tribute to both the patient's willpower and the water's natural lift. Roosevelt was ecstatic. His doctors had warned him that further improvement was unlikely. If progress didn't occur in the first six months, they said, there was little hope for the future. But Louis Joseph had already proved this theory wrong, and FDR hoped do the same. Within weeks, he was boasting, "I walk around in water 4-feet deep without braces or crutches almost as well as if I had nothing the matter with my legs."[42]

The initial visit to Georgia would mark the high point of Roosevelt's optimism about polio. He would never give up his dream of walking—yet he would never again feel as certain of recovery as he had at that moment, when anything seemed possible. Having found what he believed to be the perfect spot for rehabilitation, Roosevelt left Warm Springs with a powerful but ill-formed vision of its future. "I am going to have a long talk with Mr. George Foster Peabody," he wrote his mother. "I feel that a great 'cure' for infantile paralysis and kindred diseases could well be established here."[43]

DURING HIS VISIT, Roosevelt had spent several days with a reporter from the *Atlanta Journal*, who planned to write a human interest story about a celebrity's courageous struggle with a devastating disease. The fact that a positive spin might also benefit the Georgia economy was not lost on the newspaper. Appearing in its Sunday supplement and syndicated nationally under the title "Franklin Roosevelt Will Swim to Health," the story portrayed Warm Springs as a Mecca for the disabled, filled with sunshine, healing, and hope.

> He swims, dives, uses the swinging rings and horizontal bars over the water and finally crawls on the concrete pier for a sun bath that lasts another hour. Then he dresses, rests a bit on the delightfully shady porch and spends the afternoon [motoring] over the countryside in which he is intensely interested.

To Franklin Roosevelt, the story concluded, "everything in Warm Springs is 'Great' or 'Fine' or 'Wonderful.' That is the spirit that has carried him to remarkable heights for a man just past his fortieth year, and it is the spirit that is going to restore him to his pristine health and vigor, for political and financial battles and successes in the years to come."[44]

The response was predictable. When Roosevelt returned to the Meriwether Inn a few months later, he found six polio patients—known as polios—on the grounds, with dozens more on the way. This was a problem; the inn had no facilities for these people, and the regular guests were appalled. Some found the patients unsightly; others feared "catching" their disease. "The regular guests [would] stare as if observing freaks," said one polio. "An organized request was made that [we] be barred completely from the inn and grounds."[45]

Roosevelt did his best to keep the two groups apart. He moved the polios into vacant cottages, got them a dining room in the hotel basement, and oversaw construction of a small pool tucked away from public view. Meanwhile, he informed Peabody of his interest in buying the entire property, a deal strongly opposed by Eleanor Roosevelt and O'Connor. Both thought it a high-risk venture and told him so, deeply wounding FDR's pride. He "feels . . . that he's trying to do a big thing which may be a financial success & a medical and philanthropic opportunity for infantile [paralysis] & that all of us have raised our eyebrows & thrown cold water on it," Eleanor wrote a friend. "There is nothing to do but to make him feel one is interested & to try to keep [the negative points] before him."[46]

For FDR, however, there was no turning back. He signed the real estate contract in April 1926. "I had a nice visit from [the Peabodys]," he told his mother, "and it looks as if I bought Warm Springs." He had—the inn, the cottages, the springs, and the surrounding acres—at a cost of $200,000, about two-thirds of his personal fortune, and twice the price that Peabody had paid for the property a few years before. Eleanor did not interfere; she knew how much it meant to her husband's morale. As one biographer noted: "For the first time in his life, Franklin had become fully engaged in something that promised to benefit others as well as himself."[47]

On the advice of Basil O'Connor, Roosevelt turned the property into a nonprofit institution, the Georgia Warm Springs Foundation, which allowed it to receive tax-free gifts and charitable grants. From that point forward, its progress would be one of the great passions of his life. He made dozens of visits and built a home on the grounds, known later as "the little White House," where he would die of a stroke on April 12, 1945. He loved Warm Springs so dearly that Eleanor believed he would have become its full-time manager had he not been elected New York's governor in 1928.[48]

It was the one place where Roosevelt could truly be himself, surrounded by those who lived and suffered as he did, and dreamed the same dreams. There was nothing to hide from the polios, no reason to deceive. To them he was simply "Dr. Roosevelt," rolling his wheelchair through the grounds, crawling around on his knees, sunning his frail legs without embarrassment. His correspondence from these years is dotted with remarkable acts of kindness toward fellow patients, from detailed medical advice to notes of encouragement. In 1925, his physician asked him to "consider letting me take some [of your] blood to make serum to treat acute cases of infantile paralysis," adding: "I shall perfectly understand if you don't want to do this." Roosevelt replied: "Sure you can bleed me. You have not bled me as much as some doctors I know, so you are entitled to the opportunity. . . . How many cocktails does one need after the bloodletting to restore the circulation?"[49]

Patients flocked to Warm Springs from across the United States— 106 in 1927, 151 in 1928, and 218 in 1929. The benefits they received went well beyond physical therapy. As one observer put it: "Warm Springs provided an opportunity to meet people, undertake joint activities, make friends, date, fall in love. . . . New patients were welcomed into the group. Their handicap did not isolate them from the norm; it *was* the norm."[50]

There were problems, however. For one thing, the $42 weekly rate for polios did not begin to cover the foundation's operating expenses, much less its grand plans for expansion. For another, Roosevelt's obsession with Warm Springs had begun to squeeze out other parts of his life. "Between 1925 and 1928, Franklin would spend more than half his time—116 of 208 weeks—away from home," a biographer noted, "struggling to find a way to regain his feet. Eleanor was with him just four of those 116 weeks, and his mother was with him for two."[51]

Basil O'Connor saw less of him as well. His time with Roosevelt in these years was spent mostly at Warm Springs, an exhausting twenty-four-hour train ride from New York City. At one point, O'Connor sent a note to his absent law partner begging him to make an occasional appearance at 120 Broadway. It would show "that you really have a law firm and are active in it," he wrote, adding: "This is really a very busy office and I am sure your acquaintances would be quite impressed with the reality of it." Ever careful, O'Connor scribbled in the margin: "Don't gather from this that I am dissatisfied in any way."[52]

Interestingly, however, this period of convalescence had a beneficial effect on FDR's political career. It allowed him to maintain a safe distance from the vicious squabbles then plaguing the Democratic Party, and it kept him from seeking the White House at a time when the Republican Party was at the height of its popularity. Instead, Roosevelt used his spare time to crank out letters to the Democratic faithful, giving advice and support, and maintaining his reputation in a neutral, statesmanlike way. Meanwhile, Eleanor became the "public" Roosevelt, standing in for her husband and exerting her own independence as a champion of social causes.[53]

In 1928, FDR's moment arrived. The Democratic presidential nominee that year, Governor Al Smith of New York, faced an uphill—some said hopeless—campaign. Republican candidates had won landslide victories in the previous two elections, and the party's current nominee, Herbert Hoover, was a widely respected business leader and public servant. The nation was at peace, the economy seemed strong, and Smith, a Roman Catholic, faced a certain backlash among voters on religious grounds. Knowing that he couldn't possibly win the national election without also carrying his home state of New York, Smith needed a magnetic figure to run for governor on the Democratic ticket—namely FDR.

Roosevelt was reluctant to enter the campaign. The timing was poor. Smith was almost sure to lose in 1928, and he could easily take others down with him. Why risk a defeat? Furthermore, Roosevelt did not want to interrupt his physical therapy or his commitment to Warm Springs. His own timetable had him returning to politics in 1932, when his legs would be stronger and the Georgia foundation more secure.

The pressure, though, was relentless. Public pleas from Democratic leaders were accompanied by private pledges of financial support. When Roosevelt said he needed time off to continue his rehabilitation, he was told that others would cover his gubernatorial duties should he win. When he complained that most of his assets were tied up in the Warm Springs Foundation, he received a personal check for $250,000, compliments of John J. Raskob, the multimillionaire chairman of the Democratic National Committee. Roosevelt's resistance dwindled. He agreed to run.[54]

The campaign was short but vigorous. Nominated in early October to oppose Albert Ottinger, the state's attorney general, Roosevelt spent the remaining four weeks in search of votes. The Republican strategy was simple: play up national prosperity on the one hand and Roosevelt's disability on the other. According to the GOP, a desperate Al Smith had forced a noble but crippled friend to reenter the political arena against the advice of his doctors—and perhaps at the risk of his life. Republican newspapers had a field day, describing FDR's campaign as "pathetic," "pitiless," "unfair to Mr. Roosevelt," and "equally unfair to the people of the State." Al Smith's response would become a part of American political folklore. "A governor does not have to be an acrobat," he said. "We do not elect him for his ability to do a double backflip or a handspring. The work of the governorship is brainwork [and] there is no doubt of [Franklin Roosevelt's] ability to do it."[55]

Campaigning was another matter. For FDR, the key issue was not his health or his stamina but rather the logistics involved in getting from one stop to the next. Everything was new, an experiment, a process of trial and error. A steel bar was built into his touring car so he could rise to a standing position and lock his leg braces in place. At rallies, he would walk the last few feet to the podium on the arm of a handler, swinging his hips with the aid of a cane, sweating profusely from the effort, and bantering with the crowd. When stairs or tight spaces were involved, and he had to be carried, Roosevelt bore it with typical aplomb. By election day, he had made more speeches and campaign stops than his opponent. "Herkimer, Fonda, Gloversville, Amsterdam . . . Schenectady . . . and now . . . Troy," he told the cheering crowd. "Too bad about this unfortunate sick man, isn't it?"

FDR won a razor-thin victory for governor in 1928. Smith, meanwhile, was buried in the national Republican landslide, losing New York State as well. When Roosevelt arrived with his chauffeur to vote on election day, he was surrounded by the press. "No movies of me getting out of the machine, boys," he called out, and the photographers dutifully obeyed.[56]

The "splendid deception" was firmly in place. His comeback was under way.

3

"Cripples' Money"

IN THE FALL OF 1929, THE STOCK MARKET CRASHED. On October 24—"Black Thursday"—a selling panic hit Wall Street. In the next two weeks, the index of common stocks fell by 40 percent, with investor losses totaling more than $26 billion. Though the crash of 1929 did not cause the Great Depression of the 1930s, it did reveal serious weaknesses in the nation's economy. The great bull market was over. Hard times lay ahead.

In the world of politics, this reversal provided new hope for important Democrats like FDR. Having taken full credit for a decade of roaring prosperity, Republicans were now being held responsible for the worst economic collapse of modern times. There was no single moment that marked the onset of the Great Depression, just a numbing downward slide. Unemployment jumped from 1.5 million in 1929 to 8 million by 1931. Banks failed everywhere and food prices collapsed, forcing farmers from their land. By 1932 more than thirty million Americans were living in family units with no income at all. Towns and cities saw the new symbols of hardship and poverty: apple peddlers on street corners, hobo villages filled to overflowing, breadlines snaking for blocks.

Millions blamed Republican president Herbert Hoover for getting America into the Depression and—worse—for failing to get America out. His name was reviled. The cardboard shantytowns of the homeless became Hoovervilles; an empty pocket turned inside out was now "a Hoover flag." A popular joke of the era had Hoover asking Treasury Secretary Andrew Mellon for a nickel to phone a friend. "Here's a dime," said Mellon. "Call *all* your friends." Journalist Russell Baker remembered an aunt telling him: "People were starving because of Herbert Hoover. My mother was out of work because of Herbert Hoover. Men were killing themselves because of Herbert Hoover, and their fatherless children were being packed away to orphanages . . . because of Herbert Hoover."[1]

Roosevelt was a natural choice to oppose Hoover in 1932. His family name was political magic, and he had done well governing New York State in perilous times. He was an effective campaigner, as shown by his surprising triumph in 1928 and landslide reelection two years later. When he won the Democratic presidential nomination in 1932, the hard part seemed over. Herbert Hoover had already defeated himself.

As before, a key issue was Roosevelt's health. Would he be able to withstand a grueling *national* campaign? Could he effectively govern a country demanding aggressive leadership as almost never before? Anticipating such questions, Roosevelt had allowed himself to be examined by a group of doctors, whose positive findings were published in a national magazine. But the issue hadn't died. A piece in *Time* quoted a source close to the New York political scene as saying, "This candidate, while mentally qualified for the presidency, is utterly unfit physically."

Politics aside, such comments left deep wounds. Upon hearing a rare press report that he had fallen down during a 1932 campaign appearance, FDR replied: "The losing my balance and toppling is not true. As you know I wear a leg brace to lock the knee and on one occasion when I was speaking, the brace broke with the result that I went half way down." (In fact, Roosevelt wore braces on both legs, in addition to using crutches and canes.) "Frankly," he fumed, "I cannot see the importance of all this nonsense when I am in perfect health and get through three times as much work in the average day as three ordinary men."[2]

Such bravado had its price. In 1932, with the presidential campaign heating up, the Roosevelts were invited to the White House for a ceremony honoring the nation's governors. The couple arrived early to allow extra time for Franklin to get from the limousine to the reception room. As luck would have it, Hoover was running late that day. According to one account, "The governors were kept waiting, and FDR was forced to stand on his braces, gripping Eleanor's arm tightly as his only support. He chatted manfully with the other reception guests, but it was a painful business and the sweat ran from his forehead. Twice, White House ushers offered FDR a seat; both times he refused, unwilling to appear handicapped and weak, seated while all others were standing." The Roosevelts saw the delay as a purposeful slight, intended to humiliate FDR, but this is unlikely. It wasn't Hoover's style, and he didn't raise the health issue during the 1932 campaign. Years later Hoover wrote: "I greatly admired the courage with which [Roosevelt] fought his way back to active life and with which he overcame the handicap which had come to him." He added: "I considered that it was a great mistake that his friends insisted upon trying to hide his infirmity, as manifestly it had not affected his physical or mental abilities." In truth, of course, it was FDR himself who did the insisting.[3]

In any event, Roosevelt's disability was of little interest to the voters. The overwhelming concerns in that election year were the Great Depression and the misery it had caused. With Hoover downcast and discouraged, FDR's jaunty optimism proved an enormous advantage, the ideal tonic for a nation also struggling to get back on its feet. On election night, as his landslide victory became apparent, Roosevelt shared a rare private doubt with his son James before going to bed. "All my life I have been afraid of only one thing—fire," said the president-elect. "Tonight I think I am afraid of something else." When James asked what it was, his father replied: "I'm afraid I may not have the strength to do this job."[4]

Once in the White House, Roosevelt became a potent symbol for polio victims and their families. Like most Americans, they viewed him through the lens that he himself had created: as an inspiring figure who had overcome an illness, not as a cripple with a permanent disability. And like most Americans, they had found a leader to confide in, someone who understood their isolation and their pain. "Every time I hear your voice on the radio and read about your attitude toward physical handicaps—that they don't amount to a 'hill of beans'—I am strengthened and my courage is renewed," wrote the mother of a young boy in leg braces. "Your life is, in a way, an answer to my prayers."[5]

Public perceptions of the physically disabled had begun to change. Older views of the cripple as a hopeless burden on family and society, best hidden in an upstairs bedroom or a dreary institution, had given way to more positive notions of recovery, thanks in large part to the example of FDR. Press accounts increasingly portrayed polio victims in one of two ways: either as struggling successfully to defeat their handicap, or, in the most severe cases, as graciously accepting their fate. Stories appeared in magazines like *Good Housekeeping* and the *Saturday Evening Post* documenting the struggles of those who had overcome the physical effects of the disease through hard work and "the right mental attitude." Implicit in these tales was the growing sense of polio as a *temporary* illness, affording its victims the chance to gain back what had been lost.[6]

In counterpoint were the stories of those who had achieved a moral victory over polio by not allowing it to depress them or steal their zest for life. There was "cheerful" Catherine, who had "cheated death in the paralysis plague of 1916" and now "laughs at hard luck" despite a body so frail she had "contracted pneumonia eight times." And gritty Joyce, "a true Spartan who smiles her troubles away." And "vivacious" Christine, who "has never danced or even known what it is to walk," but "is happy to be home, delighted that she can paint and draw and sew and earn a dollar now and then so that she is not too much of a burden to her mother."[7]

Roosevelt received hundreds of letters from fellow polios seeking his reassurance and advice. Unlike the magazine stories, there was little cheer or optimism in their words. Many wrote him about the shame attached to being a cripple. A teenager asked what to do "since I can't play a good game of ball . . . and they say I'm a sissy." A wife worried about her husband, who walked with a limp and was ridiculed "in such a cruel way." A college student expressed the humiliation she felt at the stares of "interested strangers." A mother begged the president to write a few encouraging lines to her son, who "couldn't even hold his food down because . . . he has now developed a decided disgust for the disease and its effects."[8]

Others told him of their economic fears. Employers frowned on hiring the disabled in the best of times; the Great Depression had made a bad situation that much worse. Roosevelt heard from those who couldn't find a job ("With the competition as great as it is today, the physically superior have the advantage"), and from those too discouraged to look ("The world has no place for a cripple"). He heard from the wives and parents of polios who had lost their homes and farms and could no longer keep up with the medical bills. As one father told FDR: "We had a nice little piece of money once, ready to build and furnish and pay cash. Then my boy took sick with infantile and we spent the whole thing, but I never begrudged one penny."[9]

The 1930s were a time when politicians, even presidents, still answered much of their own mail. FDR replied to these polios, urging them to heed their doctors and to never give up. His letters, brief and formulaic, were relentlessly upbeat. "You are making a brave fight," he would say, and "with this fine courage and determination you are bound to win." Some have criticized Roosevelt for offering little more than false hope and glib homilies to people who deserved to know the truth. Yet, according to a disabled scholar who studied hundreds of these letters: "Writing to the president became a way to share some of the power of his office and to put aside, for the moment at least, the crippling stigma of polio. The shared experience of polio validated the writer's own struggle with deformity and limitation. A letter from Roosevelt changed nothing, and changed everything. However briefly, the recipient was distinguished for what he had, not for what was missing."[10]

WHEN ROOSEVELT REENTERED POLITICS in 1928, he needed someone to replace him at the Warm Springs Foundation. The man he chose, his Wall Street law partner Basil O'Connor, was not exactly thrilled to be asked. In truth, O'Connor hadn't the slightest interest in helping any "cripple" other than FDR. "My decision," he recalled, "had no more emotional significance than taking over several file folders of unfinished business for a colleague who had embarked on a new project that would keep him overly busy."[11]

O'Connor, in turn, hired Keith Morgan, a fast-talking insurance salesman who had made a fortune in the booming bull market of the 1920s. Morgan's job, as spelled out in a personal meeting with FDR, was to "sell" the concept of Warm Springs "to a lot of wealthy people who've never heard of it." This seemed like a good idea since private philanthropy was still the province of the very rich. But Morgan came on board in 1929, the year the stock market crashed. All of a sudden there were fewer rich people with a lot less to give.

With the Depression, Warm Springs almost went under. Contributions plummeted from $369,000 in 1929 to $30,000 by 1932. There was no money to pay the bills; new patients had to be turned away. In desperation, Morgan sought out a friend who had made a reputation as a rising star in the rapidly expanding field of public relations. His name was Carl Byoir.[12]

The son of Jewish immigrants, raised in Iowa, Byoir lived by the motto, "A successful salesman is an attention getter." In college, he had made a handsome profit selling yearbook advertising. At Columbia Law School, he had created a company, the House of Childhood, that offered franchises for a learning system developed by an Italian woman named Maria Montessori. (Byoir is credited with popularizing Montessori schools in the United States.) After that, he went to work for the Hearst chain, quickly reversing the decline of its flagship magazine, *Cosmopolitan*, by giving cash prizes to distributors who sold the most copies. When America went to war in 1917, Byoir joined the Committee on Public Information (CPI), which had the onerous task of selling Woodrow Wilson's war aims to a divided nation. Known for its relentless boosterism, the CPI became a training ground for a pioneering generation of public relations men, including Byoir's future partner, the legendary Edward Bernays.

These wartime contacts propelled Byoir to the top of his field. In the early 1920s, he handled the public relations that helped establish the new Republic of Czechoslovakia, and followed that with a successful campaign to win U.S. recognition for Lithuania. To promote the sale of Blondex hair products, Byoir created the enduring image of the sexy "platinum blonde." His most successful, and controversial, effort came in the late 1920s, when he worked with the corrupt dictator Geraldo Machado to increase American tourism to Cuba. "Carl Byoir may not have moved mountains," said one observer, "but he definitely made a career of motivating people to do it for him."[13]

One of Byoir's most important clients was Henry L. Doherty, founder of the Cities Service Corporation, the largest distributor of natural gas and electricity in the United States. Known as a master of strong-arm tactics, Doherty had hired Byoir to soften his ruthless public image. A well-publicized philanthropic gesture seemed a good place to start. When Byoir suggested a private meeting with Keith Morgan, Doherty jumped at the chance. There were rumors that the Federal Trade Commission would soon be looking into his sale of Cities Service stock on the eve of the great crash. Having a friend in the White House, he thought, might do him some good.

Doherty agreed to finance a fund-raising campaign for the Warm Springs Foundation. At a brainstorming session, Byoir suggested a nationwide party to celebrate Roosevelt's birthday. The first problem was getting the president to agree. Using his name could easily backfire. Some would see it is as a partisan move, allowing Democrats to pose as the protectors of crippled children. Others would question the participation of an industrial pirate like Henry Doherty. For Roosevelt, however, these were minor concerns. What mattered most to him was keeping Warm Springs in the black. "If my birthday will be of any help, take it," he told Morgan. The party was on.[14]

Byoir set up shop in Manhattan's Waldorf-Astoria, which provided him a suite of offices free of charge. He had less than two months to prepare; the event was scheduled for January 29, 1934. From a public relations standpoint, Byoir had to connect an immensely popular president to a rare and mysterious "children's disease." The concept, as he saw it, was to extend the optimism of the early New Deal into the realm of philanthropy, allowing people to celebrate a leader who cared about the less fortunate and embraced the promise of better times ahead. The slogan "We Dance So that Others Might Walk" seemed to mirror the nation's hopeful mood.

As a former journalist, Byoir sent letters to newspaper publishers across the country, asking each to find a civic leader "who would feel honored in being appointed Director of the Birthday Ball in your city." Specific rules were attached: "The Director will formulate the local committee, select the ballroom, direct the arrangements and manage the expenditures, so that from the sale of each ticket the National Committee will receive one dollar for the [Warm Springs] endowment fund."[15]

Byoir kept a close eye on the responses. Those slow to reply got a second letter inquiring about the delay. "Time is exceeding short," it said. "Kindly wire us collect no later than December 28th and let us know what we may expect." A week later, Byoir fired off telegrams to the remaining stragglers:

PRACTICALLY EVERY CITY AND TOWN IN THE UNITED STATES IS GIVING A BIRTHDAY BALL IN HONOR OF THE PRESIDENT TO CARRY ON A NATIONAL BATTLE AGAINST INFANTILE PARALYSIS, WHICH EVERY YEAR CRIPPLES THOUSANDS OF CHILDREN. YOUR CITY IS ONE OF THE VERY FEW NOT YET ORGANIZED. IN VIEW OF THE SHORTNESS OF TIME, WILL YOU WIRE ME PERSONALLY?[16]

By January more than three thousand local birthday ball committees had been established, a triumph by most yardsticks but a disappointment to Byoir. Expecting twice that number, he turned to those most likely to support the cause—local Democratic Party officials and patronage appointees (including Basil O'Connor's brother James, the postmaster of Bangor, Maine). "No question about it. Our approach in those days was 90 percent political," said a birthday ball planner. "It had to be. We had to work with our friends."[17]

To rally the troops, Byoir barnstormed the country with Wiley Post, the popular one-eyed pilot who had just set the speed record—7 days, 19 hours—for circumnavigating the globe. At each stop, Byoir held a press conference, lined up local Democrats, and spelled out the plan. For small towns, he suggested square dances, church suppers, and card parties. For large cities, he recommended union halls for the working classes and black-tie banquets for the financial elite. He got newspapers to run free advertising, phone companies to remind their subscribers to attend, and department stores to run window displays of the shoes, clothing, and hats to be worn at each event.[18]

The night of January 29 was a smashing success. More than 6,000 parties were staged, from Puget Sound in Washington State to the southern tip of the Florida Keys. Skiers in Berlin, New Hampshire, formed a huge "R" for Roosevelt with exploding red flares. Fifty-two white doves were released in Grafton, West Virginia, to mark the president's age. Schools and businesses closed early in Chicago, where dances were held in lodge halls, fight clubs, local taverns, church basements, and the major Loop hotels. Ticket sales were so brisk in Philadelphia that the premier event had to be moved to the 10,000-seat Convention Hall. From Browning, Montana, came word of a tribal dance on the Blackfoot Reservation.

Nothing outdid the scene at the Waldorf-Astoria, where 5,000 people, crammed into four adjoining ballrooms, watched 52 debutantes in white evening gowns mount a multitiered birthday cake, 28-feet in diameter, as George M. Cohan, surrounded "by detachments of the Army, the Navy, and the Marines," performed a "special ballad" he had written for the occasion, titled "What a Man." As Cohan finished, at precisely 11:30 P.M., the president's voice was heard over a nationwide radio hookup from the Oval Office. "This," he said, "is the happiest birthday I have ever known."[19]

It took several months to total the contributions and pay the bills. At a White House ceremony on May 9, 1934, a committee led by O'Connor and Byoir handed the president a check for $1,016,443. O'Connor had expected a profit of perhaps $100,000; Byoir knew better. When FDR turned to him and said, "Carl, I'll bet you a good tie that you can't top this figure next year," Byoir took the wager. He saw even bigger days ahead.[20]

There had long been charities in the United States associated with specific diseases, the most successful being the National Tuberculosis Association, which invented the Christmas Seal in 1907.

Put this stamp, with message bright,
On all the mail you send.
Every penny helps the fight,
The dread White Plague to end.[21]

Yet in the realm of American philanthropy, the watershed event had been the nation's entry into World War I. Overnight, the act of giving became a patriotic duty. All people, not just the very rich, were expected to buy Liberty Bonds and support the American Red Cross, a quasi-government operation that raised a "spectacular, precedent-shattering" $114 million in 1917 alone, using professional fund raisers and public relation experts to tie its activities directly to the war.[22]

The 1920s saw further growth. Churches and colleges hired professionals—many of them veterans of the CPI like Byoir—to raise money for great cathedrals such as St. John the Divine in New York City and to bolster the endowments at Harvard and Yale. The concept of the Community Chest took root, with civic groups and charities now appealing for donations under one umbrella. Studies in this era showed that large gifts from the wealthy ($100 or more) still provided the lion's share of the funding, but that small gifts were dramatically on the rise. In 1920 the various Community Chest drives, known for attracting modest donors, raised a total of $19 million. By 1929 that figure had more than tripled.[23]

The Great Depression changed everything. Charitable contributions dried up. Gifts to higher education fell from $92 million in 1929 to $23 million by 1933. Donations to Community Chests reached $101 million in 1932 and dropped steadily thereafter. Basil O'Connor got a whiff of the problem when he tried to solicit money from a group of philanthropists following the market crash. He couldn't get a face-to-face meeting, much less a donation. One industrialist wrote him: "I haven't $1,000, Doc, and if I did I think there are many cases (at home) that could use a little money very nicely."[24]

That's what made Byoir's work so impressive. The birthday balls had employed the latest techniques in advertising and public relations to turn traditional philanthropy on its head. Large gifts were hard to come by in the 1930s; the secret lay in small donations. Who wouldn't contribute *something* to see a crippled child walk again? The key was to reach millions through the modern media—people who had never given to a charity before, or who, in truth, had never been asked.

Byoir's campaign was relentlessly upbeat. Avoiding the scare tactics that would mark future polio fund drives, it reflected the optimism of a leader who assured his flock that times would improve, that a united people could surmount any obstacle, that "the only thing we have to fear is fear itself." As the *Baltimore Sun* noted, the birthday balls were "a revolutionary event . . . indicative of the profound social change that has affected this country since the New Deal began."[25]

Each year brought something new, a gimmick to spur public interest and support. In 1935, with the Warm Springs Foundation back on solid footing, O'Connor announced that 70 percent of the birthday ball revenues would remain in the local communities for the care and treatment of polio victims. The following year, Metro-Goldwyn-Mayer sent three of its biggest stars, Jean Harlow, Ginger Rogers, and Robert Taylor, to glamorize the Washington festivities, opening a celebrity pipeline that would mark fund raising for decades to come.[26]

There was a problem, however, with linking philanthropy to FDR. The president was both a popular and a polarizing figure, despised by conservatives of both major parties. His failed attempts to "pack" the U.S. Supreme Court in 1937 and purge "reactionaries" from Democratic ranks a year later had created a political firestorm. Some opponents refused to support a charity so intimately connected to a man they despised. "I am willing to contribute to the [polio campaign] on any day but Roosevelt's birthday," said the wife of a Republican leader, in what had become an all-too-common refrain. "I consider January 30 to be a sad day in the history of the United States."[27]

Others went further, accusing Roosevelt of milking the charity for financial gain. Stories appeared with titles such as "Cripples' Money: Who Gets the Proceeds of the Presidential Birthday Balls" (the answer alleged in such articles was FDR himself). "Warm Springs is located in my state," said Georgia Governor Eugene Talmadge, a long-time Roosevelt hater. "The place is not a charitable institution. I have made several efforts to get pitiful little children who had infantile paralysis in this hospital, and have never succeeded."[28]

These charges stung. Revenues from the birthday balls slowly declined. In 1937 Carl Byoir resigned his unpaid position, furious, it was said, over the president's disastrous court-packing scheme. A new strategy was in order, with FDR remaining the inspiration for the polio battle but no longer its guiding force. It was time to depoliticize the crusade.

In 1938 Roosevelt announced the formation of a nonpartisan group to be called the National Foundation for Infantile Paralysis. Its major aims, he said, were to find the cure for polio while providing the best treatment for those already afflicted. Standing next to the president that day was Basil O'Connor, FDR's hand-picked director, who vowed to move the new foundation down an independent path. "I am," said O'Connor, "very confident of our future."

THE NATIONAL FOUNDATION became the gold standard for private charities, the largest voluntary health organization of all time. Its success in raising money, generating publicity, caring for patients, and sponsoring medical research would serve to redefine the role—and the methods—of private philanthropy in the United States. Most of the credit would go to Basil O'Connor, and much of it was deserved. A master organizer, relentless and opportunistic, he would use the model created by Morgan and Byoir to turn polio into the country's number one health threat, uniquely dangerous on the one hand, eminently beatable on the other. Defeating this disease would become a top national priority, America's greatest medical crusade.

O'Connor lost no time. After renting office space in Manhattan, he composed an organization chart that included a vice president for "medical affairs," another for "public relations," and a third for "field services" that included "fund raising" and "chapter development." His main problem was money. There were huge start-up expenses to cover, in addition to the ambitious long-range plans. "This is going to [take] more than a one-day party," said O'Connor. "I don't know how much it's going to take, but it's going to take millions."[29]

Within the public relations department was a separate unit for radio and motion pictures. Hoping to line up celebrities, the foundation turned west toward Hollywood, then, as now, a bastion of liberal Democratic support. Heading the list was Eddie Cantor, the hyperanimated veteran of vaudeville, blackface comedy, silent movies, and the *Ziegfeld Follies* who had introduced numerous popular songs to American audiences, including "Dinah," "If You Knew Susie," and "Makin' Whoopee." Known as Banjo Eyes for his bulging orbs, Cantor was said to be the nation's highest paid performer, starring in big-budget musicals like *Kid Millions* and *Ali Baba Goes to Town*, while hosting a popular national radio program, the *Chase & Sanborn Hour*, each Sunday night.

Born on the Lower East Side of Manhattan, Cantor had a deep interest in politics, campaigning for Al Smith in 1928 and serving as president of the Screen Actors' Guild in the 1930s. But his greatest allegiance was to Franklin Roosevelt, whom he viewed in almost reverential terms. "He was certainly closer to F.D.R. than any entertainer had ever been to a president," wrote Cantor's most recent biographer, tracing a friendship that began when Cantor was in vaudeville and Roosevelt was a healthy young politician with an apparently golden future.[30]

Cantor was an ideal match for the National Foundation—a devoted husband and parent whose sentimental ramblings about his wife, Ida, and their five girls were the most popular parts of his act. Listening to him on radio was akin to swapping stories with a favorite uncle. "He made himself 'a member of the family' to millions of Americans," said one observer, "in a way that no performer had ever sought to be."[31]

At a strategy session with Hollywood friends in 1938, Cantor suggested a slogan for the National Foundation's 1938 fund-raising campaign. "We could call it the March of Dimes," he said, mimicking the popular newsreel feature, *March of Time*, that was shown in movie theaters just before the main feature came on. "We could ask the people to send their dimes directly to the President at the White House."[32]

It seemed like a dreadful idea, a reversal of the National Foundation's plan to distance Roosevelt from the polio crusade. Had it come from anyone else, it surely would have been ignored. But this was Eddie Cantor: a celebrity, a friend of the president, and a master at gauging public taste. As Basil O'Connor recalled, there was nothing else to do but inform the president and "see if [he'd] stand for it." To most everyone's surprise, his reply was, "Go ahead."[33]

Cantor went first, using his radio show to launch the project. "The March of Dimes," he said, "will enable all persons, even the children, to show our president we are with him in this battle." The Lone Ranger made own appeal, followed by Jack Benny, Bing Crosby, Rudy Vallee, Edgar Bergen—the list went on. Ira T. Smith, who ran the White House mail room, had been alerted to expect a modest increase in volume. "Two days later," he recalled, "the roof fell in—on me. We had been handling about 5,000 letters a day at that time. We got 30,000 on the day the March of Dimes began. We got 50,000 the next day. We got 150,000 the third day. We kept on getting incredible numbers, and the Government of the United States darned near stopped functioning because we couldn't clear away enough dimes."[34]

Stacks of mail piled up in the halls. Loose change littered desks and floors. When counting proved impossible, the coins were shoveled on to large scales for weighing and trucked over to the Treasury Department. The end result showed 2,680,000 dimes, in addition to thousands of dollars in checks and small bills. "It was days before we began to restore some kind of routine," Smith added, "and it was four months before we had cleaned up the debris."[35]

From that point forward, the National Foundation's fund-raising arm would be called the March of Dimes, with the dime itself becoming the emblem of the fight against polio. While Cantor's scheme of flooding the White House with mail was not repeated, the concept of collecting dimes to protect the health of children would remain a potent symbol for the nation, culminating in the release of the Roosevelt dime in January 1946 to mark the late president's sixty-fourth birthday. The timing was hardly coincidental. "It is desired," said Leland Howard, director of the U.S. Mint, "that the new dimes be produced at the beginning of the calendar year in sufficient quantity to use them in the infantile paralysis drive."[36]

IN PREVIOUS YEARS, a small percentage of the President's Birthday Ball money had been used for polio research. An advisory medical committee had been formed, run by Paul de Kruif, a science writer with a somewhat checkered career. Holding a Ph.D. in bacteriology from the University of Michigan, de Kruif had worked briefly at the Rockefeller Institute before being fired by Simon Flexner in 1922 for penning anonymous magazine pieces critical of the progress of medical research in the United States. Four years later, de Kruif published *Microbe Hunters*, a recounting of the dramatic discoveries of microbiologists from Antony Leeuwenhoek and Lazzaro Spallanzani to Paul Ehrlich and Walter Reed. The book, still in print today, is considered one of the classics in its field. Translated into more than a dozen languages, the basis for two Hollywood movies and a Broadway play, it is said to have inspired a generation of biological scientists, including Albert Sabin and Jonas Salk. In the 1930s, Tom Rivers recalled, "Paul de Kruif was probably the world's leading writer in the field of medicine and science, and I suspect it was this preeminence which brought him [to] the advisory committee of the Birthday Ball Commission."[37]

De Kruif fancied himself a man of action. He also held a deep grudge against Simon Flexner from their days together at the Rockefeller Institute.

What could be more satisfying to de Kruif than to discover the very thing that had eluded Flexner and his Rockefeller colleagues for the past twenty-five years, the cure for polio? With funding at his disposal, de Kruif approved more than a dozen research grants, the largest one going to William H. Park, a professor of bacteriology at New York University Medical School. Park was one of the few American scientists with a reputation to match Flexner's. Even better, the two men were bitter rivals, with a long history of bad blood.[38]

In 1934, with Park's endorsement, New York University hired a young Canadian researcher named Maurice Brodie, who was then working on a killed-virus polio vaccine. Like others in the field, Brodie had obtained the virus from its only available source: the ground-up nerve tissue of infected monkeys. To it, he had added a formaldehyde agent (known as formalin) in the hope of inactivating the virus without destroying its ability to produce antibodies against the disease.

In some ways, Brodie was ahead of his time. His killed-virus experiments would become the model for the later success of Jonas Salk. In 1934, however, *any* attempt to produce a polio vaccine was dangerously premature. Far too little was known about the disease itself. Brodie had no idea that there might be more than one type of poliovirus. He was oblivious to the risks of injecting animal nerve tissue into human beings. And he had at best a primitive knowledge of the delicate chemistry involved in properly "cooking" (or inactivating) a live virus with formaldehyde.

What Brodie did have was the enthusiastic backing of Park. And this alone gave him access to the funding and the professional attention that propelled him to instant stardom—and eventual disgrace. Brodie began by inoculating twenty monkeys with his vaccine. The results were encouraging. Several of the monkeys produced antibodies to the killed poliovirus, and none contracted the disease. Following medical tradition, Park and Brodie next tested the vaccine on themselves. There were no problems beyond some muscle discomfort near the injection site. Then a dozen children were vaccinated, all supposedly "volunteered by their parents." In 1935 Park and Brodie published their results in the prestigious *Journal of the American Medical Association* (*JAMA*), informing the scientific community that human testing of their vaccine was, in fact, well under way. "Experiments in monkeys," they wrote, "indicated that immunity could be developed by the injection of virus treated with solution of formaldehyde and that the vaccine was non-infective. Inoculation of this material into several human volunteers having shown that it was probably safe for human administration, it was used in children."[39]

"Probably safe?" "Used in children?" These words, so chilling today, were hailed as progress by a public just awakening to the threat of polio. Park had impeccable credentials, after all. And Brodie seemed like the second coming of Louis Pasteur. Indeed, the news that children had been injected without incident led health officials in states then experiencing minor polio outbreaks to invite Park and Brodie to test their vaccine on a much larger scale. These trials, said the *Literary Digest*, "are expected to settle the question of whether the new vaccine is useful. . . . [We already know] it can not possibly give the disease to children; the experiment consequently is perfectly safe."[40]

It didn't turn out that way. The trials were conducted so haphazardly that no accurate data could be drawn. Officials at the scene did not believe that the Park-Brodie vaccine had prevented polio. Some, in fact, suspected that the reverse was true: the vaccine had *triggered* the disease in a handful of cases. Meanwhile, researchers at the Rockefeller Institute were unable to reproduce the results that Park and Brodie had reported in *JAMA*. Their vaccine, a virologist recalled, "was made in the most incredible sloppy manner."[41]

Why had Park and Brodie moved so quickly to test it on children? One scientist blamed Park, the senior partner, claiming "he was never one to let grass grow under his feet." Another blamed Brodie, who had done the actual work, for taking advantage of Park's "failing" mental health. What all could agree on, however, was that both men were under intense pressure to get their vaccine out before a competitor named John A. Kolmer could beat them to the punch. Kolmer, a Philadelphia pathologist, was working furiously on his own polio vaccine in 1935, using a live virus, weakened by chemicals, to create immunity through a mild natural infection in the body. Some called it "a witch's brew."[42]

Kolmer was a prolific writer, best known for his textbooks on laboratory techniques. His funding came from a consortium of Philadelphia hospitals and medical schools. He had no connection to the President's Birthday Ball Commission, which turned out to be a blessing for O'Connor and FDR. Kolmer began testing his vaccine at virtually the same time as Park and Brodie. After a few simple experiments on monkeys, he vaccinated himself, his two sons, and twenty-three other children—all, he claimed, "with the written consent of their parents."

Kolmer moved on to other youngsters, more than 10,000 in all. The results were alarming. At least a dozen cases of paralytic polio were attributed to his vaccine, nine of them fatal. At a medical convention in 1935, James Leake of the U.S. Public Health Service came close to accusing Kolmer of committing murder. According to one participant, Kolmer stood up and replied: "Gentlemen, this is one time I wish the floor would open up and swallow me." He sat down without saying another word.[43]

Kolmer wasn't alone. "The vaccines were dead," said a prominent virologist, "and so were careers." But some suffered more than others. For the aging Park, who retired shortly after, the vaccine fiasco was little more than a blip on an otherwise distinguished resume. He died in 1939, honored by his colleagues and his students and best remembered for his role in eradicating diphtheria. For Maurice Brodie, however, it was the end of the line. Young and vulnerable, he became the prime scapegoat for these vaccine failures, the lightning rod for criticism from all sides. Fired from his job at New York University, he moved from one minor position to the next, sinking further into obscurity. Brodie, too, died in 1939. The official cause was a heart attack, though rumors flew that he had committed suicide or succumbed to polio as a result of taking his own vaccine. He was thirty-six years old.[44]

The vaccine race between Park-Brodie and Kolmer was more significant than observers in 1935 possibly could have imagined. On one level, of course, it had severely dampened expectations about the prospects of a safe and effective polio vaccine. On another level, however, it had fueled the curiosity of researchers about what had to be learned before proceeding again. In a primitive way, the vaccine race of 1935 offered a preview of the competition two decades later between Jonas Salk and Albert Sabin—the former with his killed-virus polio vaccine, the latter with his live-virus vaccine. The key difference between 1935 and 1955—the difference between deadly failure and stunning success— would rest on the enormous body of scientific information accumulated in these intervening years.

DE KRUIF WOULD SOON BE GONE. When the National Foundation was formed in 1938, Basil O'Connor began to look elsewhere for medical advice. Determined to avoid another Park-Brodie fiasco, he asked Thomas Rivers, director of the Rockefeller Institute Hospital, to head up a committee on scientific research, telling him (as Rivers recalled):

"I'm only a layman . . . but I think maybe we haven't been building our case from the ground up. Perhaps we've been trying to get a conviction with insufficient evidence. How about drawing up a list of research priorities, so that we can emphasize first things first and try to get somewhere for a change?"[45]

Rivers seemed perfect for the job. Those in the relatively new field of virology saw him as the dean of the field, its greatest living pioneer. John Enders, a Nobel Prize winner, once toasted Rivers by saying: "We the members of the church salute the apostolic father." Born on a Georgia farm in 1888, Rivers had something of a storybook life. After graduating first in his class at Emory University and entering Johns Hopkins Medical School, he was diagnosed with a fatal form of muscular dystrophy. Returning home, Rivers "kind of got fed up waiting to die." He took a job in a hospital in Panama, where, with little supervision, he "performed 85 major operations, 150 autopsies, and learned how to work the . . . primitive x-ray machine. He even pulled teeth."[46]

Somehow, unexplainedly, his condition stabilized. Rivers returned to Johns Hopkins, graduated at the top of his class, and took a position at the Rockefeller Institute, where he helped promote the idea that viruses belong to a unique group of disease-causing agents, distinct from ordinary bacteria. His edited volumes *Filterable Viruses* and *Viral and Rickettsial Infections of Man* became the standard works in the field.

Rivers could be difficult. Colleagues described him as "pugnacious" and "irascible," a man who did not look kindly upon opposing points of view. He prided himself on being "a roughneck" who said what he thought and loved a good fight. As a son of the rural South, he had trouble adjusting to a profession in which urban Jews were emerging as a powerful force. "In Rivers' world," said one writer, "everyone was a boy of some sort—an old boy, a smart boy, a good old boy, or a Jewboy." But such prejudices did not cloud his judgment where talent was concerned. Indeed, what made Rivers so valuable to Basil O'Connor was his ability to recruit the cream of the academic laboratories for the gathering polio crusade.[47]

Rivers had little use for De Kruif's approach, which had focused on finding the "magic bullet"—the drug, vaccine, or vitamin— that would quickly tame the disease. To his mind, one had to identify the major gaps in scientific knowledge before considering the issues of prevention and a cure. In 1938 Rivers presented his agenda to the Scientific Research Committee. Listed in order of importance, it included such fundamentals as the pathology of polio (first), the portal of entry and exit (second), and the mode of human transmission (fifth). At the bottom of the list, in eleventh place, was the "production of a good vaccine."[48]

The Rivers agenda laid the groundwork for the future. Priority would be given to basic research. Funding would be decided by "specialists" in the field. Implicit in this strategy was the belief that polio would not be conquered overnight. There was no magic bullet. The process would chew up time and money, and public impatience would have to be soothed with small victories along the way.

With Rivers in charge, the advisory committee funded individual grant proposals by promising researchers like Albert Sabin of Cincinnati ("how poliovirus enters the body") and Paul Clark of Wisconsin ("nutrition and diet in relation to all infectious diseases"). But the largest grants were used to establish public health programs and virus laboratories at Yale and Johns Hopkins and Michigan, where researchers worked together in so-called polio groups. The Yale and Michigan units would focus primarily on the epidemiology of polio, its movement from person to person and place to place; the roles played by flies and sewage, contaminated water and food. The Hopkins unit would concentrate on the pathology of polio, the way in which it spread through the body and affected the central nervous system. All three groups would add superb young talent to the research mix; all would lay the groundwork for the polio vaccines to come. One can imagine the excitement of Howard Howe, an assistant professor of medicine at Hopkins, as he wrote to offer his friend David Bodian a place on the faculty, compliments of a hefty new grant. "Basil has made us a proposition," Howe reported. "[He] promises to put $300,000 in the bank in the next year to be used over a five-year period and indicated that the Foundation will commit itself to a similar grant at the end of the five year period if it is still alive, kicking, or anything else."[49]

The battle had been joined.

4

"And They Shall Walk"

WHEN FRED SNITE JR. CAME DOWN WITH POLIO in 1936, he had just turned twenty-five. From a wealthy Chicago family, a devout Catholic and a graduate of Notre Dame, Snite had joined his parents on a dream vacation that spring, a trip around the world. Upon reaching Peiping (now Beijing), he felt feverish and dizzy. His stomach ached. He suspected food poisoning, perhaps a bad cold, or the flu. The next morning, his right arm went limp. Rushed to Rockefeller Memorial Hospital, named for its prime benefactor, Snite was barely able to breathe. His paralysis had spread quickly, involving the muscles of his legs, throat, and chest. "I assure you, Mr. Snite," the administrator in charge told the young man's father, "that nowhere else in the world could your son receive better care."[1]

This was no idle boast. The hospital, known as the Johns Hopkins of the Orient, was staffed with top doctors from the West. Snite's personal physician was a graduate of Harvard Medical School. Most amazing—and fortuitous—the hospital possessed the only iron lung in China. "In 1936," an expert noted, "there were 222 [of them] in the entire world. The machine in Peiping was the eighth one ever made," an enormous steel box weighing 1,200 pounds. It was primitive, but it worked. "Swish, swosh, bing, bang! The machine filled the hospital room with its welcome racket." The patient survived.[2]

The modern iron lung, invented in 1928 by Philip Drinker, a medical engineer at Harvard, was an airtight iron tank designed to exert a push-pull motion on the chest through alternating pressure that forced the diaphragm to expand and contract. The idea was to assist patients in the acute phase of polio, those who needed help in the short run but were fully expected to breathe again on their own. It was meant to bring people back to health, not to keep hopelessly damaged bodies alive. The intent, said Drinker, was to "give all patients with respiratory paralysis [the] opportunity to recover normal breathing by maintaining artificial respiration over a period of hours, or even days." No one had seriously pondered the long-term implications of this lifesaving technology for a society just beginning to grapple with the impact of a frightening new disease.[3]

Fred Snite provided a glimpse into that future. Fourteen months after his attack, without ever leaving his iron lung, he began the dangerous trek from Beijing to Chicago, described in press reports as "one of the most outstanding medical odysseys of modern times." He traveled from the hospital to the railroad station in a "generator-equipped ambulance," where he was hoisted into "a specially rigged baggage car" for the 900-mile trip across the plains of China to the port of Shanghai. At each stop, large crowds gathered to see Snite—nicknamed Crazy Foreign Devil—packed inside the metal contraption with only his head sticking through. In Shanghai, the Snites boarded the ocean liner *President Coolidge* with "a staff of 25 doctors, nurses, and medical attendants" for the long trip home. "My most valuable possession is in [a] steel respirator," Fred Snite Sr. explained. "I told him that all of my dollars might as well be wooden if not devoted to saving his life."[4]

What would happen to young Fred Snite? The answer was anybody's guess. *Newsweek* assumed that a gradual healing would take place, allowing "the prisoner [to] one day step from his iron cage." *Time* was pessimistic, thinking Snite would steal "a few more years of life before his unusable muscles and joints become too frail to support his will to live." No one expected him to stay inside his respirator indefinitely. It seemed impossible, unbearable, unimaginable for this to drag on without end.[5]

But that's precisely what occurred. The months turned into years. Snite endured. A portable respirator, strapped to his chest, allowed him to spend short stretches outside his iron lung. Public interest grew. The press followed him to Lourdes in 1939, where—accompanied by a doctor, five nurses, two orderlies, a physiotherapist, and a mechanic to service his machine—Snite bathed in the frigid, healing waters. "If it's God's will that I be cured, I will be; if not, I won't," Snipe told reporters. "I figure I have a right to ask only one thing: the strength to face up to it."[6]

Physically, there was nothing more to be done. "To Frederick after Lourdes," said a priest who knew him well, "came the miracle of resignation." Snite remained in his iron lung, on his back, unable to brush his teeth, comb his hair, shave himself, or wipe his nose. He had lost the ability to cough, so his throat had to be regularly suctioned. He had to be fed in rhythm with the respirator, which caused his chest to rise and fall every four seconds, 21,600 times a day.

But that was only part of the story—the lesser part. What kept Snipe in the public eye was his determination to lead an otherwise "normal" life. He became a tournament-tough bridge player, reading the cards in a rear view mirror placed above his head. He traveled to race tracks and college football games in a trailer equipped with a spare iron lung. "His arrival at Notre Dame stadium was one of the events of the afternoon," a friend recalled. "Enter the visiting team, polite cheers. Enter the home team, loud cheers. Enter Frederick, pandemonium." The Notre Dame faithful, remembering the Four Horseman of Coach Knute Rockne's fabled 1920s backfield, dubbed Snite "the Fifth Horseman," an accolade he cherished. "He was a legend at Notre Dame," said a Fighting Irish publication, "one of [our] all-time great competitors."[7]

In 1939 Snite married Teresa Larkin, a woman he had known before he got polio. The news caused a national sensation—"Man in Iron Lung Weds." The Snites had three children, each birth duly noted in the press. Over time, his health troubles mounted: stomach ulcers, kidney stones, heart problems, bone degeneration—all took their toll. When he died in 1954, at age forty-three, the cause was listed as heart and lung failure from the "prolonged use of respirator." (Or, as his long-time nurse put it, "eighteen years in that hunk of steel!") His passing, said *Time*, had "ended perhaps the most famed fight an American has ever made to stay alive and to enjoy life against terrible odds."[8]

Snite was not a typical patient, of course. Few adults contracted polio in this era. Even fewer experienced a paralysis of the breathing muscles that required an iron lung. And fewer still had the resources that marked his particular case. All told, Snite's father estimated that he spent more than a million dollars to meet his son's various medical needs.

Typical or not, Fred Snite became a powerful voice for polio survivors in this era—someone, unlike FDR, who welcomed, even encouraged, the public's fascination with his disease. He made regular appearances for the National Foundation, calling himself "the Boiler Kid," and representing all polios with the slogan: "I know their need."

On one level, Snite symbolized the amazing triumph of "spirit over body." On another level, however, he showed just how complicated and expensive it was to keep that body functioning and alive. Was it possible to treat Snite's relentless optimism as anything more than a façade? How could it be otherwise for people trapped inside this private version of hell? "The misery of their existence," recalled the director of a foundation-run respirator center, "often led those attending them to wonder if the 'iron lung' was indeed the blessing to mankind which its inventor intended it to be. . . . Little wonder that [the patient] begins to think he would be better off dead, and that for all practical purposes he *is* dead."[9]

Snite, of course, did not need the assistance—or pity—of the National Foundation; his circumstances were unique. Yet his compelling story meshed perfectly with the foundation's egalitarian ethos, its promise to provide the best possible care to all polio patients regardless of expense. A wealthy young man had seen his life dramatically extended. Didn't others deserve the same chance as well?

For Basil O'Connor, the answer surely was yes. He had built his foundation on "the corporate model," in order, he claimed, to assure quality care for all. Unlike the typical charity, in which local units retained a large measure of autonomy, major decisions at the National Foundation for Infantile Paralysis (NFIP) were left to O'Connor and the cohort of staffers and experts he personally chose. All plans flowed downward to an army of salaried workers and unpaid supporters at the grass-roots level, split into two distinct groups: those in the local foundation chapters and those in the March of Dimes. The first group, smaller but more dedicated to the goals of the national organization, saw to the year-round needs of polio patients in its region. The second group, the fund-raising arm, was composed of thousands of volunteers, mostly women, who came together for a few hours each year to collect money for the March of Dimes. Half of that total went to the national office; the other half stayed in the community where it was raised.[10]

In 1939, when the first foundation chapter was established in Coshocton, Ohio, most polio survivors languished in their homes. How many? Estimates varied from 100,000 to five times that number. More than 15,000 new cases were reported in 1931, but only 1,700 in 1938, the year the foundation was created. What seemed clear, of course, was that the *total* number of people disabled by polio was rising, with most forced to struggle on their own. The average hospital in this era was ill equipped to treat the disease, and the cost was prohibitive. At a time when less than ten percent of the nation's families had any form of health insurance, the expense of boarding a polio patient (about $900 a year) actually exceeded the average annual wage ($875).

The local chapter became the branch office of the National Foundation, its eyes and ears on the ground. How many people required assistance? What were their needs? Were area hospitals equipped to deal with polio epidemics and patient aftercare? How much did local doctors and nurses really know about the disease?

The answers were often depressing. There was no polio infrastructure to speak of at this time—no federal money for research or rehabilitation; no government agency beyond the bare-bones U.S. Public Health Service to provide the slightest measure of guidance or support. Almost everything would have to be built from the ground up, with the National Foundation doing the lion's share of the work.

This would prove enormously expensive. In the years between 1938 and 1955, the foundation would spend $233 million on patient care—about two-thirds of its total budget—with most of it going to pay individual medical bills. True to their word, foundation officials set no means test for those requiring help. The goal was to serve the entire community, not to function as a charity for the poor. "*While we expect a family to do what it reasonably can do financially,*" the national office told its local chapters, "we do not insist that it prove itself totally indigent to obtain needed care. If it is evident that the high cost of polio care would result in undue hardship, force the family to sell a car [or] mortgage its home or otherwise drastically lower its standard of living, the Chapter should offer to pay for all or that portion of the cost than cannot be reasonably met." In the end, more than eighty percent of the nation's polio patients would receive significant foundation aid.[11]

Some, however, got more than others. While O'Connor was fond of saying that "no victim of infantile paralysis, regardless of age, race, creed or color, shall go without care for lack of money," the fact remained that race did, indeed, play a role. In the era of Jim Crow, the National Foundation did not dare challenge the prevailing color line of the South. When Eleanor Roosevelt suggested that a cabin be built for "Negro polio victims" on the grounds at Warm Springs, she was told that "such a thing would not be desirable in Georgia." Socially, it would cause racial unrest. Medically, it would do no good. Blacks were widely believed to be "less susceptible" than whites to polio, and therefore less in need of care.[12]

Something had to be done, however. Ignoring the Negro South could be a public relations nightmare for the foundation as well as for FDR, who had begun to bring black voters, traditionally Republican, into the Democratic fold. In 1939, at Roosevelt's direction, O'Connor solved the problem by announcing that the foundation would give the all-black Tuskegee Institute in rural Alabama a grant of $172,000 to build an Infantile Paralysis Center "for the colored race." When it opened two years later, Roosevelt was there to deliver the keynote address. "Tuskegee is a perfect setting," the president said. "Everything here combines to make this particular location ideal."[13]

Founded by Booker T. Washington in 1881, Tuskegee already housed a hospital and nursing school. Furthermore, the institute's most celebrated faculty member, George Washington Carver, known to millions as the Peanut Man, was working on a cure for polio that included the massaging of damaged muscles with peanut oil. While most researchers dismissed the idea as quackery, Roosevelt, ever the politician, took a soothing approach. "I do use peanut oil from time to time," he wrote Carver, "and I am sure that it helps."[14]

The Tuskegee polio unit was state-of-the-art—a three-story building with a gymnasium, a brace-fitting room, and a 20,000-gallon treatment tank. The staff included nurses and therapists and "one of only two Negro orthopedic surgeons in the entire country." Most important, Tuskegee trained dozens of health care professionals to work with polio patients—white and black—in segregated facilities across the South.[15]

The foundation pumped more than a million dollars into Tuskegee in the 1940s, portraying these grants as proof of its concern for all polio victims, regardless of race. At the same time, however, foundation officials seemed to accept the notion that polio was a lesser problem for blacks. In 1946 Harry Weaver, the director of research, asked a prominent grantee for guidance on the subject, adding: "Perhaps I am being rather stupid but I have been under the impression that most people believed that there was less poliomyelitis among Negroes than whites. I would be very interested in hearing from you in this regard."[16]

Weaver was hardly alone. The belief that blacks did not get polio in large numbers went back to the 1916 epidemic in New York City, when a public official announced that "Negro children are more or less immune and the virus attaches itself more often to blondes than brunettes." Though New York's health commissioner, Haven Emerson, quickly debunked this statement, noting that the incidence of polio "among colored people is not essentially different from its incidence among other racial groups in this city," the idea that blacks were largely resistant to the disease took on a life of its own. Weaver's interest in the subject may have been heightened by a 1946 government survey of selected American households showing higher rates of polio among white than among blacks. What he may not have seen was a disclaimer buried deep in the survey that read: "There is the possibility, however, that reports from the colored were not as complete or in other aspects were not comparable with those of whites."[17]

The response to Weaver's query was enlightening. There were no hard data to support the racial angle, said Thomas Francis, a pioneer in polio research. "In Charleston in 1939 the rates for whites was 114/100,000 and for colored 147/100,000. . . . In Ft. Worth in 1943 the incidence by race was exactly the same as the distribution of population. In Tennessee in 1945, this was essentially the same." If anything, Francis noted, the figures were biased *against* blacks, since "there has been a tendency in the past not to seek out colored cases as well as white."

Weaver was thankful—and relieved. "I am passing your letter on to [others here]," he replied, "who will, I know, be interested in it."[18]

THE MONEY THAT FUELED the National Foundation came from its annual fund-raising drive, the whirlwind of events surrounding Franklin Roosevelt's birthday. The basic strategy remained in place: rely on small donations from the masses, giving millions of ordinary people a stake in the crusade. The main addition in these years was the recruitment of a volunteer army—the March of Dimes—to solicit contributions. The job was simple yet rewarding. The volunteer attended a meeting or two each January, followed by the fund-raising event. The hard work was done by others—the bureaucrats in New York City, the officers of the local foundation chapters, the nurses and therapists who devoted their lives to polio aftercare, the researchers who searched for the cure.

Fund raising now spread beyond the one-night birthday balls. In 1939 the national office suggested a "Mile O'Dimes" campaign, with towns competing to produce the "longest line" of coins. (The gimmick, said Keith Morgan, raised "some $200,000 of what we like to call 'new money.'") The following year, O'Connor convinced the Hollywood studio heads to show a short film about polio in their theater chains as a "March of Dimes mother" passed a collection box through the crowd. The most memorable of these shorts, produced by the foundation's publicity department, was called *The Crippler*. It began, a journalist noted, with "a dark cloud spreading over playground and farm, mansion and tenement, a cloud that takes the shape of a hunched and sinister figure who cackles over his many victims. The fearful shadow of the Crippler is finally dispelled by a National Foundation volunteer, played by a very young actress later known as Nancy Reagan, but the overall effect of the film was to terrify a great many people into making contributions." In 1941, the March of Dimes took in $435,000 from movie collection boxes alone.[19]

Then came Pearl Harbor. As the nation mobilized for war, Americans again heard the patriotic calls to buy Liberty Bonds and support the Red Cross. O'Connor didn't quite know how to proceed. Should the foundation suspend its fund-raising drive? Barely nine thousand cases of polio had been reported in 1941. Would an aggressive March of Dimes campaign be seen as selfish pleading in the midst of a global catastrophe? Might it simply be ignored?

The foundation hoped to keep its crusade alive, and so, too, did FDR. In a pointed note to O'Connor, the president opposed "any interruption" as "extremely inadvisable," adding: "The fight being waged against infantile paralysis . . . is an essential part of the struggle in which we are all engaged. Nothing is closer to my heart than the health of our boys and girls and young men and women. To me it is one of the front lines of our National Defense."[20]

This statement—in truth, solicited by O'Connor—gave the foundation just what it needed: a presidential endorsement of the polio crusade as a complement to America's wartime aims. Using the politically neutral slogan "Polio Wears No Party Label," the March of Dimes branched out dramatically in these years. At FDR's urging, Hollywood lent its full weight to the flagging birthday balls. One studio promised a West Coast extravaganza, with "Judy Garland singing 'The Trolley Song,' Sinatra 'I Wonder Who's Kissing Her Now,' and Crosby one of those old-fashioned Illustrated Picture glide songs." Another agreed to send Jack Benny, Ann Sheridan ("America's sweetheart"), and a "galaxy of stars" to liven up the East Coast events. Still another suggested that silent-screen star and former "America's sweetheart" Mary Pickford be made the honorary director of "women volunteers" at the March of Dimes. Roosevelt liked the idea. Pickford got the job.[21]

Though the birthday balls recovered much of their luster, the leading source of revenue was now the movie collection box. The National Foundation kept very close tabs—theater by theater, region by region, studio by studio. A confidential memo noted: "Incomplete reports from Loews Theaters shows approximately $530,000 in [1945] as against $444,000 in 1944 . . . RKO Theaters collected about $232,000, a substantial increase over their 1944 total of $199,000." The numbers kept rising. In 1938 annual contributions to the March of Dimes amounted to $1.8 million. By 1945 that figure had reached $19 million, the most ever raised by a charity other than the American Red Cross. Forty percent—almost $8 million—came from local movie houses.[22]

But something else was at work in these years. The number of reported polio cases had begun to rise as well—from 9,000 in 1941 to more than 19,000 in 1944, the largest total since the great polio epidemic of 1916. No one could quite explain why. Some suspected that returning soldiers had brought the poliovirus home with them. Others thought that the great domestic migrations of the war—from farms to defense plants—had exposed millions of vulnerable people to dangerous new germs. Still others wondered if the growing American fetish with cleanliness, so essential in controlling other infections, had somehow played a role. "Infantile paralysis is not primarily a disease of the slums, the malnourished or the underprivileged," a foundation study concluded in 1942. If anything, the reverse was more likely true.[23]

It took a while for the public to notice. All eyes were focused on the needs and casualties of war. But the foundation's relentless publicity coupled with the growing number of polio victims, began to slowly make an impact. In 1944 a series of full-blown epidemics gave Americans a brief but terrifying glimpse of the future. Polio swept through defenseless communities with devastating effect. The worst one, near the town of Hickory, North Carolina, would provide the first real test for Basil O'Connor and the National Foundation.

IT BEGAN IN EARLY JUNE, as allied troops prepared to storm the beaches at Normandy. A boy in western North Carolina took sick with a fever and a stiff neck. He was rushed to Memorial Hospital in Charlotte and diagnosed with polio. Other cases followed—so many that the isolation ward soon ran out of beds. Feverish children, delivered by car or wagon or ambulance, were packed into army tents on the front lawn. Surrounding hospitals were overwhelmed. "Like a tidal wave the plague swept through the Catawba River Valley," *Life* magazine reported. "Youngsters with painful, useless limbs, some unable to swallow or scarcely able to breathe, they came from mining villages up in the hills, mill towns in the valley, from outlying farms and urban centers."[24]

Their stories had a common thread. Addie Flowers, then fourteen, recalled the awful pain she felt in her back as polio took hold. Within hours, her arms and legs were paralyzed. She couldn't sit up or feed herself. "It was terrifying," she said. "I thought I was going to die." Nine-year-old Alice Dalton went to bed complaining of a headache and stiffness in her neck. She awakened to use the chamber pot and crashed hard to the floor. "Mama, come help me," she cried. "I fell and I can't get up. . . . My legs won't work." Both girls were rushed to the hospital; both houses were quarantined. A health worker told the Daltons: "All of Alice's toys and books have to be burned. Get you a good fire going in one of those tall trash cans out back. Burn everything!"[25]

Panic swept the region. Public events were canceled. Swimming pools, movie theaters, and libraries were closed. People drove through the sweltering summer heat of Hickory with their car windows rolled up. Trains sped by without stopping. Health officials in neighboring states warned North Carolina residents to stay away. A list of "polio pointers" appeared in newspapers and mailboxes and store windows: "Avoid overtiring and extreme fatigue [and] sudden chilling such as would come from a plunge into extremely cold water on a very hot day . . . Pay careful attention to personal cleanliness . . . Use the purest milk and water . . . Keep flies away from food . . . Do not swim in polluted water . . . Avoid unnecessary contact with [other children] . . . Don't visit in epidemic areas."[26]

Hickory, a furniture-making town of 15,000, was dubbed Polio City by the press. "Outsiders looked toward [us] as they would a leper's colony, shunned our people as they would lepers," a native recalled. The towns-people turned to the National Foundation, which had just organized a chapter in Catawba County. When word reached New York City, Basil O'Connor took personal charge. He viewed the crisis as both a humanitarian challenge and a public relations bonanza—a chance to confront a surging epidemic head-on. Hickory would provide the stage.

The foundation agreed to equip and staff a makeshift polio hospital, to be built by local residents on the grounds of a nearby summer camp.

The plan was risky. It called for the people of Hickory to accept polio victims from across the state, bringing even more "germs" into a community already devastated by the disease. Epidemics produce few heroes. Indeed, as the local newspaper admitted: "Had grownups been stricken and not [our] children, everybody from the mayor to the street-sweeper likely would have fled town."[27]

A call went out for volunteers. Hundreds showed up, "hiding the fear," said one, "that had [us] quaking in our boots." Merchants donated building material made scarce by wartime rationing. Carpenters, plumbers, and electricians brought their own tools to the site. Floodlights were installed to allow round-the-clock construction. The telephone company installed a switchboard. Families loaned their electric washing machines and vacuum cleaners. Carloads of toys appeared. Farmers trucked in meat and vegetables. County convicts cleared brush and dug water mains, watched by shotgun-toting guards. The governor paroled thirty-two female prisoners to help with the domestic chores.

It was up and running in 54 hours: a "rough pine board hospital" containing an admissions center, a kitchen, and a laundry; a laboratory and an operating room; isolation wards, dormitories, and a therapy wing. Orthopedic nurses arrived from the University of Minnesota, and physical therapists from Johns Hopkins. Most had been trained through grants provided by the National Foundation. The Yale Polio Unit sent a team of epidemiologists to find the source of the outbreak. It tested the water and sewage, trapped flies and insects, took blood samples—but couldn't find the cause. Iron lungs, hydrotherapy tanks, and medical supplies were flown in from regional equipment depots set up by the Foundation in recent months. A doctor in Hickory recalled the numbing procession of vehicles to the hospital on its first night of operation. "It was opening the door of ambulance after ambulance," he said. "One mother rose from her crouching position over her child and put a finger to her lips. 'Sh-h-h,' she whispered. He has been sleeping since we left Charlotte.' The child was dead."[28]

Like most polio epidemics, the one in North Carolina faded with the cooling winds of fall. Before closing its doors, the makeshift hospital had treated 454 patients, including 71 from Catawba County alone. Two-thirds of those admitted that summer were said to have "recovered completely." All told, the foundation spent about $400,000 during the epidemic and a far greater sum on the aftercare of the survivors.

The publicity, of course, was priceless. "The Miracle of Hickory" became a staple in future fund-raising efforts, breathlessly described as the medical equivalent of war. Photographs of smiling victims were distributed nationwide. The caption read: "These are some of the Children your Dimes and Dollars Helped."

> Youngest polio victim of the North Carolina epidemic, baby Kenneth was just seven months old when infantile paralysis crippled his back and legs. Rushed to the hospital, the baby responded rapidly to treatment and three months later was home again, fully recovered.
>
> Jerry, not quite two years old, was just learning to walk. His first efforts were interrupted by an attack of polio that crippled his back and legs, but prompt hospitalization and treatment enabled Jerry to make a fast recovery.
>
> This is three-year-old Judy. Admitted to the hospital with painful involvement of the neck, back, and legs, expert care helped Judy to a rapid and complete recovery.[29]

Here were the first poster children, the modern-day faces of polio: young, fair-skinned, determined, recovering, and *special*. As one North Carolina newspaper said: "If your child is beautiful, lively, personable, active, vivacious, attractive, cute, a leader, or above average in intelligence, then he or she [was] in greater danger of polio. There are but a very few dull, unattractive patients [here]." The reason, it appeared, was that bright, attractive children tended to be more active and involved. "They have a more competitive attitude toward their playmates, and therefore will swim harder in the pool, run harder on the playground [and] become more exhausted. And where fatigue goes, old man polio stalks pretty close behind, getting his victims where he can from the group that gets run down, worn out, too tired for safety."[30]

This theory, widely believed in the Catawba Valley, would spread like wildfire in the coming years. What parent of a polio victim wouldn't want to believe it was true. And what parent anywhere wouldn't feel more vulnerable after reading a description like this? Where did it come from? The locals seemed to know. It originated, they said, with "the experts that the National Foundation for Infantile Paralysis . . . sent to North Carolina."[31]

AMONG THE MOST VIVID recollections of those who spent time at the makeshift polio hospital in Hickory is the odd, musty odor that wafted through the wards. "I cannot remember any of the doctors or nurses," said one Hickory patient, fifty years later, but "to this day, a wet wool smell takes me back. I remember how hot the packs were. I always considered them as torture!"[32]

"It was really funny how every survivor had the memory of the smell of the hot wet wool from the hot packs," said another. "It is a smell that you will never forget." Some recalled the hot pack treatment in meticulous detail.

> I was measured—neck, shoulders, lower arms, hands, mid-section, upper and lower legs, and feet. Then three sets of wrappings were cut out to meet my measurements. . . . One set . . . was made from Army blankets; one set, from some kind of . . . plastic; and a third from cotton blanketing. . . . The Army blankets would be placed in a pressure cooker. They would be steamed until hot, very hot. . . .
>
> The woolen pack would be wrapped piece by piece and covered by plastic. Then the cotton blanket would be pinned on to hold everything together. . . . The packs stayed on for an hour, at which time they were removed and another set . . . placed on our bodies. . . .
>
> There were two other strong feelings or sensations related to hot packs. One was itching . . . the other was smell.[33]

The hot packs were the trademark of Sister Elizabeth Kenny, the most popular, and controversial, physical therapist of that time. Born in New South Wales, Australia, in 1880, Kenny had spent her early career as a bush nurse in a particularly remote part of the outback known as Never, Never (because, legend had it, travelers vowed "never, never" to return). On one such tour, she came across a little girl whose body was painfully twisted and paralyzed. Kenny telegraphed her observations to a surgeon, who replied: "Infantile paralysis. No known treatment. Do the best you can with the symptoms presenting themselves."[34]

Kenny lacked formal training. She was not a graduate of nursing school, despite her later claims to the contrary. What she did have was a remarkably keen sense of human anatomy, gleaned from years of personal observation. Her instincts told her that the key to treating these symptoms was to force the affected areas to relax. She saw infantile paralysis as a spasm of the muscles, rather than a disease of the nerves. And she returned from the outback with a powerful story, claiming to have cured six crippled children by applying homemade hot packs—strips of wool dipped in boiling water—to their damaged limbs and then "reeducating" the loosened muscles to function again.[35]

Her method triggered a predictable response. The medical establishment in Australia was hostile, but desperate patients flocked to her side. Following years of controversy, a blue-ribbon panel was formed to study her results. Its 1938 report, condemning Kenny's work as sloppy and unscientific, led her to depart Australia for the United States, where, she believed, her unorthodox medical thinking would find a welcome home. The American doctor, she said, "possesses a combination of conservatism and that other quality which has put [that country] in the forefront in almost every department of science—that is, an eagerness to know what it is really all about."[36]

The timing seemed perfect. Polio aftercare was still at a very primitive stage. In 1916, a path-breaking book written by Robert Lovett, who would later care for Franklin Roosevelt, had recommended complete bed rest during the acute (or immediate) stage of the disease, followed by warm baths, exercise, and massage. In the following years, a handful of American orthopedists had suggested a course of treatment quite similar to the one that Kenny would soon be calling her own. Their voices were ignored. By the 1930s, a new approach had taken hold—a ghastly process, worthy, in retrospect, of a Dr. Frankenstein, that called for immobilizing the patient with wooden splints and plaster body casts in order to keep the muscles and joints from being pulled out of shape. "One thing *was* evident," a polio expert recalled. "It was going to take a vigorous personality to show that the prevailing system of rigid and prolonged fixation of paralyzed limbs was not having the desired effect, and could be harmful."[37]

A vigorous personality, indeed. Elizabeth Kenny was a phenomenon—the term "Sister" came from her service in the Commonwealth Nursing Corps—who collected friends and critics, it was said, the way others collected stamps and coins. "The woman suggests vast resources, the stubbornness of the innately shrewd mind, a fierce pride, and a sharp tongue," a reporter noted. "In appearance, she is a human tornado—big and unwieldy with bristling white hair, flushed face, and a grim, set mouth." Kenny wore big-brim flowered hats, her trademark, which made her look "about seven feet tall . . . huge," a patient recalled. A tireless self-promoter, she crafted a larger-than-life image to match her imposing size. During World War I, she boasted, "I spent more time on dark ships in danger zones than any other woman in the world." Coming to America at the age of fifty-nine, she lopped off six years, and sometimes more, in her interviews with the press. "Honesty was not her strongest suit," a critic observed. "She claimed to be a nursing sister when she had no basic nursing training. . . . She did not improve matters when she claimed to have been invited to work at a number of British hospitals, which was not true. She even invented a college education for herself in *Who's Who in America*."[38]

Her reception was mixed, to say the least. Armed with testimonials from patients who swore by her treatment, Kenny went to see Basil O'Connor in New York City. "He listened for three hours," wrote Kenny's biographer, Victor Cohn, "but she was told, finally, that the Foundation conducted no research or treatment, that it merely made grants to institutions that did." Worse, when O'Connor asked Tom Rivers, the foundation's top medical advisor, to sit down with Kenny for a few minutes that day, Rivers flatly refused. The woman knew almost nothing about polio, he said, and personally, he "couldn't stand her."[39]

Rivers wasn't alone. Kenny got a similar brush-off from Morris Fishbein, the imperious editor of the *Journal of the American Medical Association*. "She came in wearing that hat that made her look like Admiral Nelson," he scoffed. "She *looked like* a screwball." Kenny moved on to the Mayo Clinic, where she received a more civil reception. A doctor told her of a polio outbreak in nearby Minneapolis, suggesting she go there to volunteer. With her options all but exhausted, Kenny took his advice. In Minneapolis, she found several orthopedists willing to entrust their patients to her care. The early results were heartening. "What we saw was almost unbelievable," the mayor of Minneapolis recalled. "The polio ward, once a place of tomb-like silence, was now filled with laughter! One look, and we knew this granite-faced woman had something good."[40]

Kenny had brought some humanity to a field in desperate need of it. Polio did not damage the body's motor neurons, she believed. Instead, it caused a series of painful muscle spasms that badly distorted the torso. Since the disease was muscular, rather than nerve-related, immobilizing the patient for long periods was the worst possible thing to do. Splints and casts were more likely to cause deformities than to prevent them. But hot packs and gentle exercise could relieve these spasms, freeing patients to reeducate their "alienated" muscles much as one might reeducate a victim of amnesia, using both the mind and the body to *visualize* and then practice the movements that once had been a normal part of everyday life. "Whether or not she knew of animal experiments that proved it," said a doctor who supported her methods, "she had realized that constant, graded exercise gets results if there was no irreversible paralysis. Until this time, a kid with polio might be put in splints at age three, and kept in them for two years, until mentally the child ignored the limb. If you could show patients that they had a considerable degree of recovery in the unused limb, you could frequently cause them to walk, to throw away their crutches, and dramatically recover."[41]

To many, Sister Kenny's old theories about the nature of polio were far less important than her clinical shrewdness in treating the disease. Those who saw her in action were often converted on the spot. An onlooker recalled:

> A little girl who had lost the use of one of her anterior thigh muscles solemnly informed Sister that she had spoken crossly to her *quadriceps femoris* for being so lazy, and she was sure it would do better today.
> "Well, it has been very ill," Sister smiled. "But it is time we put it back to work, isn't it . . . ?"
> Sister Kenny explained her charges' startling proficiency in Latin: "In the last analysis, it is the patient who must reopen the nerve path between the mind and affected muscle. It is a much easier task if [she] has a speaking acquaintance with [her] anatomy."[42]

It was hard to argue with success. Many of those she treated, including children labeled "hopeless" by others, showed notable gains. Exactly how many and for what reasons became matters of bitter dispute. Kenny insisted that 80 percent of her patients recovered without paralysis, as opposed to only 10 to 15 percent of those who underwent orthodox treatment, a claim she never tried to prove. "I came to America to teach my method—not to enter a research experiment," she declared. Yet, few could doubt that her system worked better than the alternative, or that her devotion to these youngsters was anything less than complete. In the words of a Minneapolis doctor, "If one of my children had polio, I would want him to have the Kenny treatment."[43]

Word spread quickly. Newspapers and magazines portrayed Kenny as a tireless crusader, fighting a one-woman war against a closed-minded medical elite. The more ridicule she endured—the lowly female nurse versus the exalted male doctors—the more her legend seemed to grow. The *Saturday Evening Post* hailed her as the "Healer from the Outback." *Reader's Digest* headlined its story: "Sister Kenny vs. the Medical Old Guard." She's "a strong-minded woman who has no time for politics," it said, "but does possess an unfortunate faculty for treading heavily on sensitive toes." *Life* magazine called her "the most publicly controversial figure in the medical world today." A Gallup poll of the "ten most admired living people" ranked Kenny ninth. Her 1943 autobiography, modestly titled *And They Shall Walk* (from Isaiah 40:15), became an instant best seller. Hollywood made an adoring movie of her life, starring Rosalind Russell (whose young son had been treated by Kenny for a "spastic muscle" in his leg). The plot, according to one reviewer, contained the following truths: "1) that all acute cases of [polio] treated by Sister Kenny recover completely and rapidly; 2) that she can enable seven out of ten children wearing orthopedic appliances to cast aside all such braces . . . 3) that, if treated by orthopedists, '88 out of every 100' patients will always be crippled; 4) that all but a few orthopedists are opposed to Sister Kenny and have nothing to do with her treatment."[44]

This ground swell put Basil O'Connor on the spot. The good work of Sister Kenny would not only have to be recognized but funded as well. She was a bona-fide celebrity, adored by millions who gave faithfully to the March of Dimes. The public clearly expected Kenny to receive foundation support, and Kenny did too. The problem was one of control. "Miss Kenny," wrote one foundation official, "will not cooperate with any individual whom she cannot dominate, nor will she become associated with any organization in which she is not supreme."[45]

The same, of course, could be said of O'Connor. What he truly disliked about Kenny was her abrasive independence, her refusal to defer to him or anyone else. He claimed she had "a Jehovah complex," which undoubtedly was true. "I have a message to give to the world, and I shall not be thwarted," she said. To Kenny's thinking, O'Connor was simply a means to an end—put on earth to fund her projects, ask no questions, and help the healing begin. "When O'Connor sneezes, he wants everyone to jump," she said. "But not me."[46]

Funding Sister Kenny, O'Connor recalled, was a disagreeable chore. Most polio specialists viewed her as a quack. Indeed, a committee of the American Medical Association in 1944 debunked her claims about recovery rates as "a deliberate misrepresentation of the facts," adding: "There is no evidence that the Kenny treatment prevents or decreases the amount of paralysis resulting from poliomyelitis." Even more troubling, from O'Connor's perspective, were the financial risks for the National Foundation, which had vowed to provide the best available polio care, regardless of cost. As one analyst explained: "Immobilization treatment had been simple and cheap: one nurse could watch many patients. The new Kenny method was far more complex [and expensive], but it was what people wanted." For worried parents, nothing else would do.[47]

Under intense public pressure, the foundation spent large sums in the early 1940s to fund a series of nine-week courses on the Kenny method and to pay the bills of those undergoing her treatment. For Kenny, however, this wasn't good enough. Charging that the courses were superficial and poorly taught, she demanded a two-year program of study, with herself in charge. In 1946 the foundation turned down her grant request for $840,000, claiming that her operation in Minneapolis, now known as the Elizabeth Kenny Institute, didn't merit such extravagant funding. Her response was predictable. The "O'Connor Foundation," she fumed, was "ignoring the cries of crippled children."[48]

But Kenny's days were numbered. The artful O'Connor had stolen her thunder. Crippled children couldn't wait two years for a handful of therapists to appear. They needed help *now*. What mattered was immediate access to the Kenny method—not whether Kenny personally ran the show.

She left the United States for Australia in 1951, a broken figure, and died the following year. The obituaries rightly hailed her as a pioneer whose common-sense methods had revolutionized the field of polio aftercare. Though some recalled her angry battles with the National Foundation, there was little sense of the challenge she had posed to its ironclad grip on the direction of the polio crusade. The last time Elizabeth Kenny saw Basil O'Connor was at an international polio conference in Europe a few months before her death. She hadn't been formally invited, and he refused to shake her hand. Given their history, it seemed a sad but fitting goodbye.[49]

5

Poster Children, Marching Mothers

On April 12, 1945, President Roosevelt died of a cerebral hemorrhage at "the little White House" in Warm Springs, Georgia. As his hearse left the grounds that day, the driver paused in front of Georgia Hall, the main building, to let the staff and patients pay their final respects. Hundreds turned out, many in wheelchairs and on stretchers, a sea of white in their starched garments and medical robes. "Visually, the companionship had never been so completely illustrated," a witness recalled. "Children waited quietly beside men of middle age. There was no restlessness." A musician emerged from the crowd to play the folk tune "Going Home" on his accordion, tears streaming down his face. Roosevelt was among friends.[1]

To millions of Americans, he was the only president they had known—or, at least, could remember. He had been in office for a dozen years, elected in 1932 and reelected three times thereafter. He had led the country through the Great Depression and World War II, the defining events of their lives. "He was the one American who knew, or seemed to know, where the world was going," wrote *Life* magazine. "The plans were all in his head."

His death sent tremors through the National Foundation. He was its founder, its spiritual source, and its magnet for raising funds. His passing put a quick end to the celebratory birthday balls that had brought in millions over the years. Worse, it loosened the bonds between the Foundation and the Hollywood studio moguls, whose interest in polio never went much beyond their personal devotion to FDR. In 1944 they had pledged their support in these words:

Resolved—That we of the Motion Picture Industry, assembled to discuss our March of Dimes drive, take this opportunity to extend greetings to the Honorable Franklin Delano Roosevelt whose inspiring leadership has done so much to advance this humanitarian cause.[2]

Things changed quickly. In 1946 the studios decided to end individual theater collections in favor of a flat contribution to the United Way, with the March of Dimes getting a modest check for $30,000. O'Connor was livid. The foundation had just lost its best fund-raising source. "It's a dirty trick," he fumed. "I believe that the theater patrons are glad and eager to give to the March of Dimes. . . . The refusal of the large chains to permit audience collection is therefore unexplainable." In truth, it was perfectly explainable. Franklin Roosevelt was dead.[3]

The loss of theater revenue was a tremendous blow. But even more troubling, in the long run, was the emergence of federated giving, or "one big charity," as exemplified by the United Way. In place of the $19 million it had raised on its own in 1945, the foundation might be forced to pool this money with other, less successful charities, all but destroying the March of Dimes.

O'Connor wasn't about to let this happen. Following World War II, he waged a relentless campaign against federated giving, painting its boosters as closet socialists bent on perverting the values that had made America great. "Independence of mind; freedom of choice; the right to act according to the best dictate's of one's conscience—these are the inalienable rights of every citizen," he said, modestly aligning himself with "the passengers on the Mayflower, the men who tossed the tea into Boston Harbor, the signers of the Declaration of Independence." By standing alone, the foundation had become the nation's most successful charity. By standing alone, it had riveted public attention on a devastating disease. By standing alone, it would prevail.

Polio was unique, O'Connor stressed. It left thousands of children disabled, some needing years of expensive treatment and care. It was the only epidemic disease still on the rise in America, a disease with no known prevention or cure. What other group but the National Foundation could send *immediate* aid when an outbreak occurred? Or see to it that every survivor's need was met? Or mobilize an army of scientists to unlock the secrets of polio and wipe it from the earth? "We will not desert our volunteers," O'Connor pledged. "We will not desert our men in white. We will not desert our worthy young graduate students.

And we will not place the welfare of a single patient at the mercy of the Health Monopolists, whose only slogan is 'convenience.'"[4]

Local chapters were soon bombarded with memos from the national office about the evils of joint fund raising and federated appeals, and warned, again and again, that those who challenged this sacred position would have their charters revoked. The mantra never changed:

> The March of Dimes will not be coerced into this camp.
> The March of Dimes stands alone as the Virus Polio stands alone.
> Virus polio recognizes no budgets.
> Therefore the March of Dimes cannot be budgeted.[5]

Roosevelt's death signaled a new direction for the March of Dimes. "The loss of theater revenue turned out to be a good thing," a foundation official recalled, "because it forced [us] to expand and diversify our fund-raising efforts." The plan was to focus more attention on the plight of crippled children as a way of getting parents—mothers, mainly—more involved in the crusade. Fighting polio would now be the responsibility of each American family. It would become part of the larger post-war mosaic of raising healthy youngsters, and protecting them, in an increasingly middle-class, child-centered culture.[6]

This was the baby boom era, a time of unprecedented prosperity and population growth in the United States. One of the most popular songs among returning World War II veterans was "I've Got to Make Up for Lost Time." Starting in 1946, the nation experienced a surge in marriages and birth rates, following record lows in the Great Depression. The number of children per family in the 1940s jumped from 2.6 to 3.2. Birth rates doubled for third children, and tripled for fourth children, as the country's population increased by a record 19 million in this decade. At a time when birth control information was rapidly expanding, America's growth rivaled not England's but rather India's.

Polio was on the rise, too. In 1946 the number of reported cases reached 25,000, almost matching the epidemic of 1916. From that point forward, the yearly toll would jump more often than it fell, reaching a high of 58,000 in 1952. For children and adolescents, polio now became the fastest growing infectious disease. Statistically, the chances of getting a serious case were small, the chances of being permanently disabled by it were very small, and the chances of dying from it were miniscule. Psychologically, however, the impact of polio was profound. Percentages didn't really matter when the victims were so visible and so young. There was no mistaking the sight of a child struggling in leg braces, or sitting in a wheelchair, or laid out flat in an iron lung. There was no escaping the damage that polio did, the random way in which it struck, or the gruesome truth that everyone was at risk.

Rarely, if ever, had Americans been exposed to so much information about a single disease. Most of it came from the National Foundation, which skillfully mixed the public's dread of polio into its larger message of inevitable triumph. The Public Relations Department, now thirty strong, churned out pamphlets and articles by the score. One could hardly pick up a women's magazine or visit a medical waiting room in the 1940s without spotting "A Message to Parents About Infantile Paralysis," or "How You Can Help in the Fight Against Polio," or "Doctor . . . What Can I Do?" Indeed, a hefty proportion of all journalistic pieces about polio in this era were commissioned, and sometimes ghostwritten, by foundation publicists in New York.[7]

In 1946 the March of Dimes introduced its first "official" polio poster child. The idea was controversial, spurring serious debate. How did one portray a polio victim? As cheerful and optimistic or frightened and sad? As moving confidently toward a full recovery or facing a cruelly uncertain future? Guided by the "Miracle of Hickory" campaign—the poignant photos of beaming children on the road back to health—the foundation chose option number one. The poster child would be "a vibrant model of the ideal polio survivor," wrote one historian: "well-dressed, well-groomed, full of vitality, needing only the support of the public to be complete. It was exploitative and manipulative, but the cause was worthy, and the campaign worked."[8]

The first poster child was six-year-old Donald Anderson, from a small town in Oregon, who had been diagnosed with polio in 1943. A local doctor described his symptoms this way: "slight stiffness of the neck, weakness of the left arm, exterior weakness of the right arm, extensive weakness of both thighs and abductor weakness of the right thigh." Upon reaching the Shriners' Hospital for Crippled Children in Portland, which had a polio ward funded by the National Foundation, the boy was in desperate shape, almost completely paralyzed. Following seven months of treatment, Donald had left the hospital wearing "a neck and arm brace and a stay support" for his back. He was able to walk.[9]

A March of Dimes volunteer had photographed Donald in the hospital polio ward, peering out from his crib. The picture caused a local sensation; his "wistful look" and "enormous eyes" seemed to capture the impact of polio upon the most innocent of lives. Even better, the boy clearly relished the spotlight. "Despite a lot of affectionate attention, he remains tractable," said a foundation memo. "He has a slight tendency to show off and, although he is obedient, he assumes a comically patronizing expression when parents or nurses order him about."[10]

By coincidence, the Andersons had just moved to Warm Springs, Oregon, a perfect tie to the memory of FDR. (The name was "strictly a misnomer, but good!" wrote a March of Dimes official, who claimed the town was "colder than the proverbial well-digger.") Because the family was poor—the father worked in a sawmill—it had not been charged for Donald's medical expenses. "Without the March of Dimes," the boy's mother admitted, "it would have been a tragic and heartbreaking experience to fight polio alone. Instead, we have a victorious ending to our story."[11]

The 1946 March of Dimes poster had Donald in two photographs—before and after. The first one showed him as a three year old in his hospital crib, bandaged and braced. The second one was recent, with Donald "striding briskly along, unsupported and radiating confidence." These words, from the accompanying publicity blurb, were not exactly true. Donald's progress had been steady but slow, and a full recovery was still very much in doubt. He now attended school, rode a bicycle, and played the normal childhood games. But an internal memo in 1948 rated his overall condition as only "somewhat improved," adding: "Donald receives daily physical therapy exercises. . . . He wears a back brace to support weak abdominals on right side. It still may be necessary to fuse part of his spine later to prevent deformity. . . . Parts of body [still] affected are right abdominal muscles, left arm, left side of neck and left side of trunk."[12]

For the National Foundation, of course, there was a greater story to tell. Donald Anderson, perilously close to death, had been saved and brought back to health by the contributions of ordinary Americans to the March of Dimes. Millions of people could see the fruits of their generosity through the progress of this precious little boy. "Donald is not a cripple. He mastered Polio," the March of Dimes boasted. The era of the poster child had arrived.[13]

"DO YOU WANT TO SPEND the rest of your life in an iron lung?" By the 1940s, these words, or some close approximation, had become a standard parental rebuke, explaining all one needed to know about the lurking dangers of polio. Children heard these words when they begged to go swimming or to play outside. They heard them when they balked at taking a nap or at washing their hands. They heard them when they jumped through a puddle or shared a friend's ice cream cone.[14]

Each June, like clockwork, came the photos of jam-packed polio wards and eerily deserted beaches. Newspapers kept running tallies of the victims—age, sex, type of paralysis—akin to baseball box scores. To help stem a local outbreak in 1946, the *Minneapolis Daily Times* ran a public service ad that read: "Hey, Gang! Have FUN at Home. Just Look at These Swell Games You Can Play in Your Own Neighborhood." Parents checked for every symptom: a sore throat, a fever, the chills, an aching limb. Some gave their children a daily "polio test." Did the neck swivel? Did the toes wiggle? Could the chin reach the chest?[15]

A researcher who studied the parents of polio victims found that many blamed themselves for not fully protecting their offspring. A "key assumption in the American value scheme," he wrote, is that "misfortune rarely touches those who take the proper precautionary measures." Since Americans had been warned about the need to fight germs, to practice good hygiene, to keep their children well rested and away from crowds, a case of polio could generate powerful feelings of guilt. Was the house clean enough? Should we have taken that family vacation? Why did I ever let my boy go to the movies? As one father put it: "I got caught. It was my fault. That's what goes through your mind. That's what you think. Your better judgment says, we can't control these things. We know we can't. But it's still there."[16]

Polio seemed to turn the postwar culture upside down. For this new generation of parents, a suburban home bursting with children was no longer just a dream. Everything was in place—mortgage money, tract housing, schools, parks, superhighways, even a flood of literature about the increasingly complex world of parenting. Never before had America's mothers and fathers been given so much public instruction regarding a role so long taken for granted. "For this first wave of parents nurtured on the advice of the pediatrician Benjamin Spock, having children became a self-conscious act, something to do well and to read about, think about, and talk about. . . ," a journalist recalled. "Into this buoyant postwar era came a fearsome disease to haunt their lives and to help spoil for those young parents the idealized notion of what family life would be. Polio was a crack in the fantasy."[17]

Actually, those who read Spock's best-selling *Common Sense Book of Baby and Child Care*, first published in 1945, should have been comforted by his advice. For Spock made it clear that the public's obsession with polio, while understandable, was clearly overblown. Serious cases were the exception, he pointed out. The "majority of children who catch it don't have any paralysis at any time. A fair number of those who are paralyzed for a while recover completely [and] most of those who don't recover completely improve considerably." Of course, Spock urged common sense in dealing with the disease. "There's no point being panicky or shutting your children away from all human contact," he advised. Stay calm; don't overreact. "If you were going to be that careful with [your child] the rest of his life, you wouldn't ever let him cross a street."[18]

Sound advice, no doubt, but few were listening. It was hard to accept these words when the headlines screamed, "Polio Scourge," "Polio Panic," and "Polio's Deadly Path." "Last week, it struck down a six-week-old boy in Chicago and a 62-year-old farmer in Kansas City," *Newsweek* reported during the summer outbreak of 1946, "the youngest and oldest victims ever from those cities." As a result, what seemed appropriate to Dr. Spock gave little comfort to his readers, who were frantic to protect their children but powerless to do so. That was now the dilemma facing America's parents: a feeling of personal helplessness in the midst of an apparently runaway epidemic, grimly chronicled in local newspapers and national magazines.[19]

There was an alternative, however. Since worry did no good and quarantine seemed fruitless, parents might best protect their children by helping others to discover a vaccine against polio and, perhaps, even a cure. This kind of research demanded big money. To raise it through small donations—the traditional path—would not be easy. The foundation needed to fund raise even more aggressively, building on the concepts of child protection and parental involvement, and backed up an army of devoted volunteers. "Our only shame," said Basil O'Connor, "is that we haven't done enough. But we are young; give us a little more time."[20]

Though both parents were encouraged to take their child-rearing roles seriously in modern America, women, as usual, were expected to do more. They were cast as the primary homemakers, given the lion's share of domestic responsibility, and seen as the front-line defenders of family health—a position heartily endorsed by, among others, the good Dr. Spock. It was hardly surprising, therefore, that the National Foundation focused on housewives and wage-earning mothers as the ideal foot soldiers of the polio crusade—women with a few hours to give and a good reason to get involved. An elaborate study of female volunteers in this era showed that those who joined the March of Dimes, as opposed to other philanthropies, were more likely to view their task as a parental obligation, a way of protecting their loved ones from the ravages of a child-based epidemic disease.[21]

Led by Elaine Whitelaw, a journalist-turned-fund raiser, the National Foundation created a Women's Division to recruit and marshal these volunteers. In 1945, with the lucrative movie house collections in jeopardy, Whitelaw introduced the first of several substitutes: the March of Dimes Fashion Show. Held at the Waldorf-Astoria on (or around) FDR's birthday, the "Fashion Vernissage" began a tradition that lasted more than three decades, expanding into one of the largest social events of the year. In a typical evening, Joan Fontaine, Grace Kelly, and Marilyn Monroe would model the latest hats, scarves, gloves, dresses, handbags, shoes, furs, and jewelry of designers such as George Kay of California, Lawrence of London, Lilly Daché, and Christian Dior. Stage sets would be designed by Salvador Dali and Alexander Calder, entertainment provided by Eartha Kitt, Ezio Pinza, and Gypsy Rose Lee. In 1950, Whitelaw recruited Helen Hayes, the "first lady of American theater," to host the event, which had now become a national phenomenon featured in *Life, Look, Town and Country, Woman's Home Companion, Harper's Bazaar, Good Housekeeping, Vogue, Mademoiselle*, and the *Ladies' Home Journal*.[22]

The choice of Helen Hayes was sadly appropriate. Her daughter Mary, an aspiring actress, had died from polio the year before, at the age of nineteen. Hayes added a regal presence to the event; Whitelaw managed the details. From choosing the entertainment to forming the patroness committee (Mrs. William Randolph Hearst Jr. and Gloria Vanderbilt, among others), to thanking Benson & Hedges for supplying the cigarettes and the House of Seagram for donating the vermouth, Whitelaw left nothing to chance. A script of one fashion show began: "Fanfare . . . Houselights Dim . . . Basil O'Connor Welcomes Crowd and Introduces Helen Hayes From Audience . . . Miss Hayes Moves to Poster Child . . . Picks Him Up . . . Miss Hayes And Child Go Down Runway . . . Applause."[23]

The concept spread quickly to other venues. In 1947 a March of Dimes volunteer wrote to Whitelaw: "Dear Elaine, I have some very bad news for you. We are going to promote a fashion show in Buffalo that will make your New York show look like a carnival." Wishful thinking, no doubt, but that show, and dozens more like it in Baltimore and Dallas, Chicago and San Francisco, raised millions of dollars for the cause.[24]

Whitelaw, in truth, was just warming up. In 1949 she got jeweler Harry Winston to sponsor a traveling exhibit of his extensive gem collection, which toured the country as "The Court of Jewels." For a small donation to the March of Dimes, people got a glimpse of the world's most precious stones—the Inquisition Necklace, the Star of the East, the Hope Diamond, and the Jonker Diamond. Whitelaw's unit put on giant parades, organized sewing bees that produced outsized "polio blankets" (the forerunner of the AIDS quilt), and staged the phone-bank telethons that became such an integral part of modern American philanthropy.[25]

The best idea, however, came from deep down within the ranks. In the late 1940s, several March of Dimes chapters had tried simple house-to-house solicitations, with encouraging results. Volunteers had raised funds quickly by knocking on the doors of the people least likely to turn them down—their neighbors and friends. In 1950 the local chapter in Maricopa County, Arizona, took this idea a step further. On January 16, at exactly 7:00 P.M., the city of Phoenix came alive. Sirens wailed, car horns sounded, and searchlights swept the sky. Women appeared carrying shopping bags and Mason jars. Their job was to canvass each neighborhood in the city, targeting private houses, apartments, even the downtown hotels. The mission lasted for an hour.

This was no alien invasion. Advertisements had been placed in newspapers and in store windows, on billboards and on radio. Sound trucks roamed the streets on the day of the event and children brought home flyers from school. The message was simple: "Turn On Your Porch Light! Help Fight Polio Tonight!"

There was an urgency to the plan. The Maricopa County March of Dimes had collected $68,000 in 1949, keeping half for local needs and sending half to the local office. It wasn't nearly enough. With polio on the rise, the chapter had spent $76,000 that year for medical bills, physical therapy, a hospital clinic, transportation, braces, crutches, and shoes. An emergency allotment from the National Foundation had covered some of the shortfall, but desperate times lay ahead. "THERE ARE NO

MORE FUNDS AVAILABLE," read an internal memo. "We must depend upon the coming March of Dimes [campaign] to pay the balance."[26]

Thus was born the Mothers' March on Polio. More than 2,300 volunteers walked the streets that January evening in 1950, collecting $44,890 from 42,228 donors—about a dollar per contribution. Every city neighborhood was covered. "Much public relations work was done with minority groups in Southwest Phoenix," said one report, "among Negro and Mexican mothers who had never before been asked to take an active part in a community-wide project." It seemed to work. "Families actually stood in front of their shacks or humble homes, holding candles, lanterns, and even matches to welcome marching mothers. . . . A total of $2,414.02 was collected from this less-chance area."[27]

Why was the idea so successful? One reason, chapter officials noted, was that it appealed to the movement's natural constituency. "When polio strikes, it hits the heart of the home," said one, "and the heart of the home is the mother." Another reason was simplicity. "The women were delighted with a plan that took a minimum amount of time and effort," a chapter official explained. "They attended but one organization meeting. They worked only one hour." In addition, they "didn't have to make a single call where they would meet resistance. There was no selling to do. Those who wanted to give welcomed [them] by turning on the porch light."[28]

The National Foundation took notice. Within weeks, it had announced plans for a countrywide Mothers' March in 1951, based on the Phoenix model but controlled from the top. The Public Relations Department produced a film for the local chapters, showing sacks of money being poured out on tables by smiling women volunteers. A firm male voice provided the instructions: "Remind people what's coming . . . Go after local advertisers . . . Strike and strike hard . . . Sell the public . . . Plant slogans everywhere . . . Mother is the star . . . It's only a one-day stunt, *so have no fear of overdoing it.*"[29]

There was little chance of that. The foundation sent each chapter a "plan book" worthy of a military campaign. There were sections on promotion, recruitment, leadership, mapping, and supplies. The organization chart included a community chairman (the general), district captains, section lieutenants, block wardens, and contact mothers (who did the actual collecting). Those living in houses without porch lights or electricity were told to leave a candle in the window. Those in apartments and hotels could place a shoe outside the door. There were different plan books for cities, suburbs, and rural areas, but a single rule for handling the funds:

> When the March is over, money will be counted at the block warden level. Each lieutenant delivers collection envelopes for her section to you, with a report of the total amount collected. You in turn fill out the report on the reverse side of this sheet and place all collection envelopes in the large bag provided. A police officer will be assigned to escort you to Mothers' March Headquarters.[30]

An observer who followed a "marching mother" on her one-hour mission was astonished by the response. "Perhaps three quarters of the houses had the porch light on," she reported, and people were excited to give. It made them feel good. One house was completely dark, except for the porch light. The volunteer knocked nervously, and an old woman appeared at the door. "I think this is what you want," she said, offering a dollar bill. "For a moment the void which separates the world of the blind from that of the seeing was temporarily bridged, and the [volunteer] learned what all blind people know as a matter of course: the blind only use lights to help others."[31]

The vast majority of these volunteers were middle- and upper-class women who did their canvassing very close to home. In truth—despite the Phoenix model—the March of Dimes showed little interest in mobilizing poorer neighborhoods, seen by some volunteers as dangerous and confusing: "Many working people live in multiple-family dwellings, or in houses without porch lights, or in houses which are not visible from the street." Furthermore, polio was increasingly viewed as a disease of the small towns and the neatly groomed suburbs, more likely to strike the children of the well-to-do.[32]

Still, millions joined the cause. The portrait of mothers marching against polio became one of the indelible images of postwar America. For an hour each year, on a January evening, these women formed the largest charitable army the country had ever known, serving as models for the later marches by mothers against nuclear testing and environmental pollution. What could be more natural than a mass movement based on the maternal protection of the young?[33]

The results were impressive. Between 1951 and 1955, the National Foundation would raise $250 million, more than twice the amount of the previous five years. Some of this could be attributed to the growing public excitement over the development of a polio vaccine. But those inside the foundation knew what had changed most. As a memo from the Fund Raising Department explained: "The March of Dimes continued to increase steadily through 1951 and 1952, and then with the introduction of the Mothers' March on a nation wide basis, the increase was sharp. . . . It has now become the single greatest activity in the entire March of Dimes."[34]

IF POLIO MOCKED THE DREAMS of middle-class culture, it mocked the gods of science even more. The first half of the twentieth century marked a golden age for western medicine. Rapid-fire discoveries had isolated a host of disease-carrying germs and then produced the remedy to destroy them. This biomedical process of cause and cure, begun with Paul Ehrlich's 1910 discovery that an arsenic compound could wipe out syphilis, gained dramatic momentum in the 1930s with the coming of sulfa-based drugs to treat bacterial infections. In 1941 two Oxford University scientists, Howard Florey and Ernst Boris Chain, refined Alexander Fleming's previous discovery of penicillin by purifying the compound, testing it successfully on humans, and encouraging pharmaceutical houses in England and the United States to mass produce it. Penicillin became the first true antibiotic, capable of obliterating a wide range of bacteria without also poisoning the human body. Widely hailed as "the most glamorous drug ever invented," it would soon be treating everything from deadly pneumonia to the common sore throat.[35]

Though penicillin quite naturally overshadowed other discoveries, it was hardly alone. In 1943 Selman Waksman, a Rutgers University biologist, and his graduate assistant, Albert Schatz, found that streptomyces, a soil-based microorganism, produced an antibiotic that could help control tuberculosis, one of history's deadliest infections. Called streptomycin, it proved extremely effective in clinical trials of TB patients, especially when used with other drugs. By the mid-1940s, antibiotic remedies were being pursued at universities, research institutes, and commercial laboratories throughout the world. For the first time, moreover, the U.S. government took an active role in biomedical research, with dramatic funding increases for the National Institutes of Health. Medical science now appeared within sight of a most improbable goal: a planet free of deadly infectious disease. "Will such a world exist?" a scientist asked. "We believe so."[36]

The signs certainly were there. Life expectancy in the United States had climbed from 49 years in 1900 to 68 years by 1950. According to the best estimates, 80 percent of this improvement "resulted from reduced mortality for those below 45, with the bulk [being] infants and children." And the main reason was the decline of former killers like pneumonia and tuberculosis, tamed by a combination of better diet, stricter personal hygiene, more aggressive public health measures, and the introduction of antibiotics. In 1900 infectious diseases had been the leading cause of death in the United States; by 1950 this was no longer true. In the new age of Kleenex and mouthwash, pasteurized milk and purified water, wonder drugs and antiseptic cleansers, the war against germs, it appeared, had turned into a rout.[37]

There were exceptions, of course, and polio topped the list. A cleaner environment had done nothing to stop its spread. The amazing antibiotics that wiped out bacteria were of no use against viral infections. As a result, Americans were still of two minds about polio—terrified of its impact, yet confident of its demise. The country had just survived an economic depression and won a two-front global war. Science and technology were riding high. The future spoke of atomic energy and television sets, of space travel and miracle cures. No medical problem seemed beyond the reach of the laboratory any more. Americans could play their part against polio by supporting the March of Dimes. Science would do the rest.

6

The Apprenticeship of Jonas Salk

IN THE SUMMER OF 1947, ten children took sick at a sleep-away camp in Pennsylvania. The symptoms were ominously familiar: fever, nausea, abdominal pain, sore throat, and muscle weakness. Fearing the worst, the camp owners contacted the National Foundation, which quickly dispatched one of its grantees, University of Michigan professor Thomas Francis Jr. to the scene.

Francis had studied polio outbreaks across the United States. In past years, he'd been to Illinois, Nebraska, Idaho, and the Rio Grande Valley of Texas. A skilled epidemiologist—some considered him the best in the world—he traveled in a mobile laboratory equipped with test tubes, syringes, flytraps, and dry-ice chests to preserve the specimens. His job was to determine how polio reached a given community and why it flourished there. It was, he admitted, a scientific guessing game.[1]

This one was particularly challenging. A children's summer camp brought every potential hazard into play: close contact, isolated surroundings, poor sanitation, flies and insects, contaminated food and water, frequent swimming, and physical exhaustion. Francis did what he could. Stool specimens and throat swabs confirmed the widespread presence of poliovirus in the camp. Ten more cases were noted, most of them mild. But a close inspection of the facilities turned up no obvious source. The camp was "unusually well run," he wrote, "and the sanitary conditions well devised. There was a chlorinated swimming pool; food was carefully prepared: the kitchen was clean." Though Francis listed two possible trouble spots—"the water system" and "the handling of milk"—he could find no solid explanation for what had transpired. Why had polio struck this particular camp? Why were a handful of children left paralyzed, when 250 others, living side by side in identical surroundings, were not? Francis couldn't say.[2]

He wasn't alone. In 1947—four full decades after the virus had been discovered—polio was still a mystery to scientists, and hope was wearing thin. "While I was in America recently," wrote the distinguished Australian virologist MacFarlane Burnet following World War II, "I had a good opportunity to meet most of the men actively engaged on research in poliomyelitis and to discuss the present state of knowledge with them. The general impression I gained was a sense of frustration amongst most workers. . . . The practical problem of preventing infantile paralysis has not been solved. It is even doubtful whether it ever will be solved."[3]

This lack of progress had compelled plain folk to prod the experts with their own hunches and ideas. Albert Sabin got a flood of letters suggesting that polio came from rotten fruit, horse manure, a "lusty sneeze," and the smoking habits of pregnant women. Concerned parents warned Peter Olitsky that "ripe corn," "bird droppings," and "mold on cream-filled layer cake" were causing the latest epidemics. One woman told him of her "polio revelation" the night before: "In the midst of my troubled thoughts—as plain as day—a voice said to me: 'IT COMES FROM BEETLES.' I was actually startled and sat up in bed. Somewhere in that interrupted thought came the words, 'ground hog.'" Others sent along possible cures. A loyal dog owner from Ohio recommended canine feces. A doctor in Berlin sent a sure-fire remedy—injecting polio patients with their own urine—which had worked wonders, he said, in treating jaundice, herpes, and mumps. The doctor did list a few pesky side effects, including infection, joint pain, mental depression, sore throat, and a fever.

Albert Sabin dutifully responded to these missives. Compulsive and prickly, he'd fire back a few lines declaring the suggestion to be an offense against science, the work of a moron, or sometimes both. Yet Sabin himself was no stranger to the bizarre guesswork surrounding this mysterious disease. He once believed that polio was linked to diet (a lack of Vitamins B and E) and might be cured by "special chemicals" found in mother's milk.[4]

With so much still unknown about the disease, no line of thought seemed completely out of bounds. Francis took a special interest in the role played by houseflies and contaminated milk. A young Jonas Salk, working in Spartan isolation, thought that food and pollen allergies likely weakened the body's resistance to polio. Articles in respected scientific journals linked the disease to penicillin, pollution, house pets, and DDT. In England, an elaborate study of "temperature, rainfall, and vapour pressure" concluded, anticlimactically, that "meteorological readings" were of no value "in predicting the incidence of poliomyelitis."[5]

Most revealing, perhaps, were the "progress reports" of foundation grantees. A research team at the University of California tried unsuccessfully to find poliovirus in domestic animals. Another at Wisconsin could not explain why boys got polio more often than girls. (They suspected hormones.) A third at Minnesota studied "whether patients with acute poliomyelitis had nutritional deficiencies related to their susceptibility to the disease." (The answer seemed to be no.) The foundation also sponsored research on "various forms of chemotherapy," including "urea compounds and organic dies." ("All proved of no value. . . . Grant discontinued.") It even funded a number of secret studies, such as the use of cobra venom and curare to block the path of poliovirus into the nervous system. "Too dangerous," the grant committee reported. "Findings, objectively, are not encouraging."[6]

Such was the state of affairs when Basil O'Connor created a new post at the National Foundation—director of research—and filled it with a hard-nosed administrator named Harry Weaver. O'Connor had recently returned to the job full-time after spending much of World War II as head of the American Red Cross. Alarmed by the lack of progress on the polio front, he was determined to streamline the foundation's research agenda, a process guaranteed to inflame the grantees, who viewed the slightest erosion of their independence as an affront to the scientific tradition.[7]

Weaver faced an uphill fight. Some of the grantees opposed his appointment on principle; they didn't need anyone's "direction." Others warned him to tread lightly—to treat them as individuals pursuing different lines of inquiry and not "like a troupe of trained seals." Publicly, Weaver called for "group planning" and "a pooling of ideas." Privately, he spoke of individual selfishness and a woeful lack of coordination. After talking to a number of grantees, he told O'Connor what both men already suspected: "only an appallingly few [are] really trying to solve the problem of poliomyelitis in man."[8]

There was truth to this. The grand outline set forth by Thomas Rivers in 1938 for the conquest of polio had failed to light a fire. No one seemed to be in a hurry to move things along. Indeed, as the brilliant David Bodian later admitted: "The fact is that most of us [then] doing research on poliomyelitis were motivated mainly by curiosity, and by the challenges of the many unsolved problems concerning the interaction of virus and host, rather than by the hope of a practical solution in our lifetime."[9]

Weaver had a plan. He was banking on a vaccine to tame polio, the fiasco of the 1930s (Kolmer and Park-Brodie) notwithstanding. To his mind, there was no other choice. It was clear that polio could not be purged from the environment, nor its victims effectively quarantined. No one had found a way to block poliovirus from entering the body or to neutralize it with drugs or chemicals once it got inside.[10]

The emerging new class of antibiotics, which worked so well against bacterial infections, seemed to have no effect on viruses. The only reasonable solution, Weaver thought, was a vaccine that would stimulate the immune system to produce the antibodies needed to ward off this crippling invader before it attacked. There was an added benefit as well. Weaver saw his vaccine effort as an opportunity to recruit new talent— young researchers, with no prejudices or preconceived ideas, who shared his sense of *urgency* about the disease.[11]

In Jonas Edward Salk, he found exactly what he was looking for.

JONAS SALK GREW UP in the Jewish immigrant culture of New York City. Born on October 28, 1914, the oldest of three brothers, he lived in East Harlem, then the Bronx, and finally Rockaway Beach in the far reaches of Queens. Each stop reflected a modest gain in the working life of his father, Daniel, a grade-school dropout from Russia who toiled in Manhattan's garment district as a designer of women's neckwear and blouses. "He was something of a Willy Loman character from *Death of a Salesman*," wrote Lee Salk, the youngest child, "beaten down in business but still believing that success would soon be his."[12]

It never came, though he kept his disappointments to himself. Described as a warm but distant man, Daniel left the child-rearing duties to his wife, Dora, who ran a very tight ship. She, too, was an unschooled Russian immigrant, best remembered for pushing her three sons relentlessly to excel. "She wanted to be sure that we all were going to advance in the world," Jonas recalled. "Therefore we were encouraged in our studies, and overly protected." The boys dubbed her "The Duchess— ruler of the house."[13]

All three would become doctors of a sort: Jonas the researcher, Herman the veterinarian, and Lee the psychologist. But it was clear that Dora viewed her first-born as the special child—the *Wunderkind*—a perception Jonas rather immodestly embraced. "There was a photograph of me when I was a year old," he said, "and there was that look of curiosity on that infant's face that is inescapable. I have the suspicion that this curiosity was very much part of my early life. . . . I tended to observe and reflect and wonder."[14]

At the age of 12, Salk entered Townsend Harris, a public high school for intellectually gifted students. Named for the nineteenth-century merchant and diplomat who founded the City College of New York, it had long been a launching pad for the talented sons of immigrant parents who lacked the money—and pedigree—to attend a top private school. Some viewed Townsend Harris as a perfect meritocracy: thousands applied each year, with admission limited to the top 200 competitors in a written exam stressing vocabulary and math. By the 1920s, Townsend Harris was overwhelmingly Jewish, filled with students every bit as ambitious as Jonas Salk. "It was as if somebody had finally invented a sport," a journalist noted, "in which Jews could be world champion."[15]

Students at Townsend Harris crammed a four-year liberal arts curriculum into three. More than half of them dropped out or flunked out along the way—the motto was "study, study, study"—but those who remained were all but guaranteed admission to the City College of New York (CCNY). For working-class immigrant families, City College represented the apex of public higher education. Getting in was tough, but tuition was free. Competition was intense, but the rules were fairly applied. No one got an advantage based on the accident of birth. By 1930 Jews comprised more than 80 percent of its student body. Indeed, the last prominent national fraternity on campus had closed its doors in 1913, complaining that "the Hebrew element is greatly in excess."[16]

The facilities at City College were barely second rate. There were no research laboratories. The library was inadequate. The faculty contained few noted scholars. What made the place special was the student body that had fought so hard to get there—"a den of precocious boys," wrote James Traub in his history of City College, "at once coddled and driven by their parents, pale and frail, fierce and argumentative, pushy, awkward, sensitive, naïve, and fearful." From these ranks, of the 1930s and 1940s, emerged a wealth of intellectual talent, including more Nobel

Prize winners—eight—and PhD recipients than any other public college except the University of California at Berkeley.[17]

Salk entered City College a month before his sixteenth birthday, a common age for a freshman who had skipped multiple grades along the way. He hoped to study law, he recalled, but his mother disapproved. She "was always able to put me in a state in which, when I had anything to say that was contrary to what seemed to be her wishes, I would stutter and stammer. And she didn't think I'd make a very good lawyer." This, perhaps, is true, although Salk's rather mediocre first-term grades as a pre-law student may have played a role as well. His transcript shows a D in French, a C in English, and a B in history.

Test scores were calculated precisely at CCNY, where the very hint of grade inflation was tantamount to heresy. A student could make "honors" by maintaining a B average in all courses and a B+ in the major subject. Though Salk reached neither plateau, his record did improve when he switched to the pre-med program in his sophomore year, earning consistent Bs in biology. His transcript contains seven grades of A—about one per term. His worst marks came in hygiene (gym), where regularly got a D.[18]

Salk's college years coincided with the height of the Great Depression. Student activism was especially intense at CCNY, reflecting the political currents swirling through New York's Jewish community. The student newspaper, *Campus*, hummed with stories about left-wing petitions and rallies, one leading to a scuffle in which the hidebound college president, Frederick Robinson, rushed from his office to spear some protestors with an umbrella: "ROBINSON RUNS AMOK ON CAMPUS," screamed one headline. "MADDENED PRESIDENT ATTACKS STUDENTS."

The City College cafeteria was an ideological war zone, with Stalinists, Trotskyites, and Socialists passionately defending their turf. In 1934, Salk's senior year, a number of athletes created the Varsity Club to defend the campus against political disruption. "Some called the formation a step towards student Fascism," said the student yearbook. "The term ended on a note of sadness."[19]

In later life, Salk would speak glowingly of the impact that City College had upon his career. Yet, his attachment to the college during his four years as a student was superficial at best. There is little to suggest that he experienced much of anything at CCNY beyond the grind of class work, preparation, and exams. His name did not appear in the numerous articles about the political protests that dominated campus life. He joined no clubs, held no offices, won no honors, played no sports, made no lifelong friends. Below each yearbook photo is a space reserved for the graduate's achievements. Salk's is completely blank. At City College, he left no visible footprints.[20]

Salk began medical school at an age—nineteen—when most students were starting their second year of college. At five feet nine and 130 pounds, with thick glasses and thinning brown hair, he was five inches taller and twenty pounds heavier than the day he had entered City College. Though his parents had scraped together $1,000 for tuition and other expenses, Salk would soon be paying his own way with scholarships and odd jobs. For the first time in his life, he was largely on his own.[21]

His college grades were just good enough to earn him admission to New York University (NYU) College of Medicine. Located in three cramped buildings along lower First Avenue, NYU based its modest reputation on a handful of famous alumni such as Walter Reed, who helped conquer yellow fever, and a small but growing cadre of researchers, including William H. Park, the public health specialist, and Thomas Francis Jr., an expert on viruses. Tuition at NYU was comparatively low; better still, it did not discriminate against Jews.[22]

That alone made it special. Most of the surrounding medical schools—Cornell, Columbia, Pennsylvania, and Yale—had rigid quotas in place. In 1935 Yale accepted 76 applicants from a pool of 501. About 200 of these applicants were Jewish, and only five got in. The dean's instructions were remarkably precise: "Never admit more than five Jews, take only two Italian Catholics, and take no blacks at all." For Salk and hundreds like him, NYU was the only game in town.[23]

Salk loved the challenges of medical school, in contrast to the drudgery of his undergraduate days. He excelled at almost everything, earning top grades in anatomy, bacteriology, chemistry, physiology, pathology, and pharmacology. Like most medical schools, NYU had recently upgraded its curriculum to emphasize laboratory work and clinical application. Salk's first trimester, for example, contained three hours per week of anatomy lecture followed by ten hours of microscopic anatomy laboratory and another ten hours of gross anatomy laboratory. With the dean's permission, Salk attended faculty seminars and exhibited, in the dean's words, "an extraordinary fund of information for an undergraduate medical student." But it was the laboratory work, in particular, that gave new direction to his life. At the urging of Keith Canaan, a distinguished biochemist, Salk took a leave of absence following his first year to study in Canaan's lab. Returning to medical school in 1936, he did clinical work in surgery, obstetrics and gynecology, pediatrics, and preventive medicine, while spending his elective period under the wing of Thomas Francis, who had begun to experiment with a killed-virus influenza vaccine. The association, Salk recalled, stirred a deep interest in the concept of human immunity to disease.[24]

At NYU, there was no blank space beneath Salk's graduation photo. Indeed, the yearbook blurb spoke volumes about his personal growth and academic progress.

> Took advantage of our naivete in that eerie first year to teach us some chemistry . . . liked us so much that he's been with us ever since. . . . seems to have researched in every laboratory on First Avenue without exception. . . . Can probably call more faculty members by their first name than anyone in school. . . . Surprised nobody in particular by obtaining a Mt. Sinai appointment. . . . at present rate will be professor of medicine in about 2 years.[25]

The day after his graduation, Salk married Donna Lindsay, a master's candidate at the New York College of Social Work. The two had met in Woods Hole, Massachusetts, where the Lindsays vacationed and Salk had spent summers in a lab. Their wedding plans pleased neither family. Dora Salk refused to believe that the cultured Lindsay, a Smith College graduate, Phi Beta Kappa, could possibly be Jewish. And Elmer Lindsay, a wealthy Manhattan dentist, viewed Salk as a social inferior, several cuts below Donna's former suitors.

In the end, Elmer agreed to the marriage on two conditions. First, the ceremony must wait until Salk could properly be listed as "Dr." on the wedding invitation. Second, the groom must elevate his rather pedestrian status by adding, of all things, a middle name. Following a tense, if somewhat hilarious negotiation, the couple chose "Edward," a favorite of British royalty. On June 9, 1939, Donna Lindsay became the wife of Dr. Jonas Edward Salk.[26]

Few hospitals in Manhattan had the status of Mount Sinai, particularly among the city's Jews. To intern there, a friend of Salk's recalled, "was like playing ball for the New York Yankees. . . . Only the top men from the nation's medical schools dared apply. Out of 250 who sought the opportunity, only a dozen were chosen. . . . Most went on to some sort of distinction. It was no place for a shrinking violet."[27]

Salk quickly made his mark. Though determined to pursue a career in research, he showed tremendous skills as a clinician and a surgeon. Yet it was his leadership as president of the house staff of interns and residents at Mount Sinai that best defined him to his peers. The key issue for many of them in 1939 was not the fate of the hospital, but rather the future of Europe. Hitler's invasion of Poland had plunged the continent into war. When several interns responded by wearing badges to signify support for the Allies, the hospital director warned them to stop. Caregivers, he said, must not upset their patients.

The interns went to Salk. He recommended that everyone wear the badge as an act of solidarity. The gesture worked; there was no further interference from the administration. "Jonas was a very staunch guy," an intern recalled. "He never took a backward step on that issue or, for that matter, any other issue of principle between us and the hospital."[28]

What exactly had triggered his political interest? A number of factors were at work: the Great Depression, the rise of Fascism in Europe, the daily suffering he encountered on his hospital rounds. But the most important one, it appeared, was the influence of Donna Lindsay Salk.

A fervent supporter of social and political causes at Smith, she had continued on that path after graduation, attending a school of social work widely known for its left-wing outlook. "My mother was an activist," said Darrell Salk. "Part of it was based on her passion for the underdog, and part of that, I suspect, was a rebellion against the life of privilege she had led. What she offered my father was a political outlet for his growing humanitarian concerns"[29]

When the couple first met in 1938, Salk's perspective barely reached beyond the lab. A few months later, he was attending political rallies, signing petitions, joining "Communist-front" groups, and leading protests at Mount Sinai. None of this seemed especially daring or dangerous in the Depression era, when Stalin's Russia was seen as a bulwark against Hitler's Germany, and left-wing radicalism was in vogue. But the political mood would change dramatically in the coming years, bringing new fears, different enemies, and bitter recriminations. What Salk could not have known—and may never have learned—was how close he would come, a decade later, to having his career destroyed on grounds that he posed a "security risk" to his country.[30]

Late in 1941, with his internship at Mount Sinai coming to an end, Salk wrote to Thomas Francis, his old mentor, inquiring about a job. Francis had recently left NYU to become chairman of the Epidemiology Department at the University of Michigan's School of Public Health. He was running experiments on a new influenza vaccine, and Salk wanted in. "I am hard put to articulate the satisfaction I derived from my [previous] work [with you]," he told Francis. "Its degree is measured by the depth of my hope that there may be a place for me in your new laboratory."[31]

Michigan, however, was not his first choice. Salk had tried—and failed—to find research positions at Mount Sinai, which frowned upon hiring its former interns, and at the Rockefeller Institute, where anti-Semitism probably played a role. His wife, Donna, had just settled into her job as a social worker, and his parents were pressing him to start a private practice close to home.[32]

With his options dwindling, Salk applied for a National Research Council fellowship, which could be used to fund a one-year appointment at Michigan. Francis took it from there. "Dr. Salk is very intelligent," he wrote his friends on the fellowship board. "I esteem his abilities highly and would welcome the opportunity to have him work with me." This said, Francis offered the requisite assurance: "Dr. Salk is a member of the Jewish race but has, I believe, a very great capacity to get on with people."[33]

The fellowship solved one problem, but another quickly arose. With the nation now at war, the military needed doctors. Following Pearl Harbor, Salk's New York draft board "advised" him to apply for a medical commission in the Army. Otherwise, it warned, he would be classified I-A—meaning immediate induction.

Salk wrote back, insisting that his fellowship to study influenza had a "direct bearing on the war effort." His draft board strongly disagreed. "I am not saying anything in disparagement of the fine work you have been doing," replied the colonel handling Salk's case. But physicians, he thought, had "more important things to do . . . in the present emergency than devoting themselves to research problems."[34]

Once again, the ubiquitous Dr. Francis intervened. Having just been chosen to head the Army's Commission on Influenza, he pressed hard for Salk's deferment, calling him "an essential investigator" in a field "of great importance to National Defense." A few weeks later, Salk penned Francis the good news from New York: "Just to let you know that I've been put in Class II-A [occupational deferment] by the Local Draft Board. Will be out—bag and baggage by early Saturday afternoon."[35]

THOMAS FRANCIS—T.F. or Tommy to his friends—was a pioneer in the rapidly expanding field of virology. The son of a steelworker and part-time minister, he grew up in Western Pennsylvania, attended Allegheny College on scholarship, and received his medical degree from Yale in 1925. Moving to the Rockefeller Institute, Francis joined an elite research team preparing vaccines against bacterial pneumonia. But he soon switched diseases, the story goes, on the advice of Tom Rivers, a towering figure at Rockefeller, who told him: "Look, Francis, there are a hell of a lot of guys in this country who are working on pneumonia, but nobody. . . knows anything about human influenza. Why don't you jump on the virus bandwagon fast and get to work?"[36]

Francis became the first American to isolate human flu virus, and the first scientist to pass the disease to mice, providing researchers with a cheap and plentiful source for experimentation. Among his discoveries was an entirely new strain of influenza—called type B—that speeded the production of more effective vaccines. "I think you can see from this," said Rivers, "why I was excited about Tommy Francis."[37]

Rivers was not alone. The coming of World War II thrust Francis, now at Michigan, into public view. As the nation built the largest fighting force in its history, the health of the troops became a primary concern. Recruits from all parts of the country were living and training together in close quarters, raising the threat of infectious disease. Influenza was a particular dread, given the awful memories of World War I.

Until that time, Americans knew very little about influenza; the pandemics of the past had barely touched the United States. Then in 1918 came the Spanish flu, named for the place where it was rumored to have begun. The sickness spread through Europe, striking (but rarely killing) soldiers at the front. For reasons still not clear, it faded in late spring, then reappeared in a deadly form, decimating the battlefield before reaching the port of Boston in late summer. By conservative estimates, one American in four took sick and at least a half million died. No part of the globe was spared. The Spanish flu devastated Western Samoa and wiped out Eskimo villages in Alaska. By year's end, it had infected half the world's population and killed one person in twenty, taking a greater toll, say medical detectives, "than any other disease in a period of similar duration in . . . history."[38]

This flu was not only lethal, it also picked on those who normally showed the greatest resistance to disease: young adults. The war, no doubt, played a central role in the choice of victims. "Troops lived in overcrowded, extremely unhygienic conditions," wrote one analyst, "and large groups of them moved rapidly from place to place. These are exactly the conditions which encouraged spread of airborne viruses." Furthermore, "many were stressed, exhausted, and poorly nourished— just the people who succumb most easily to infections." The U.S. Navy claimed influenza rates of 40 percent in 1918, the Army, 36 percent. A doctor visiting Fort Devens, northwest of Boston, saw the victims being carted into the base hospital. "They are placed on cots," he observed, "until every bed is full. . . . Their faces soon wear a bluish cast; a distressing cough brings up the blood-stained sputum. In the morning the bodies are stacked about the morgue like cord wood." Among American military personnel, the death toll from influenza (44,000) almost matched the number killed in battle (50,000).[39]

The flu was gone by late winter, leaving as quickly and mysteriously as it had come. Though America would experience no serious outbreaks in the next twenty years, military leaders still worried about a recurrence as the nation entered another world war. Needing a safe, effective vaccine against this potential threat, they quite naturally turned to one of the nation's leading expert on influenza: Thomas Francis.

Most virologists at this time favored the live-virus theory of vaccination. In the tradition of Jenner and Pasteur, they believed that the best way to stimulate high antibody levels in the blood, and thus produce a strong, lasting immunity to a given disease, was through a vaccine containing attenuated (or carefully weakened) live virus. The key, they thought, was to create a low-grade natural infection in the body, something that a killed virus vaccine could not do.

Francis disagreed. Immunity, he argued, did not require a natural infection. If properly prepared, a killed-virus vaccine could trick the immune system into believing that the body was under attack by enemy invaders. The trick was to fully inactivate (or kill) the virus without destroying its ability to stimulate protective antibodies—a delicate balancing act. At NYU Francis had experimented with ultraviolet light to kill viruses; at Michigan he tried a formaldehyde solution commonly used in embalming fluid. The results, thus far, were inconclusive.[40]

Francis was a natural choice for the Army commission. For one thing, his lab was up and running; his experiments were well under way. For another, his killed-virus vaccine provided a margin of safety that live virus advocates could not so easily claim. There was no chance that a properly killed virus could ever revert to virulence, triggering an epidemic among the troops. If Francis failed, so be it; he would not bring disaster in his wake.

The Salks arrived in Ann Arbor in the spring of 1942. Facing a tight wartime market and appalled by the university's substandard housing units, they rented an old farmhouse outside of town. "[It] reminded me of one of those back-to-the-land movements you used to hear about during the depression," said a friend who visited them, with Donna canning her own vegetables and Jonas chopping wood for the stove. According to "reliable" FBI sources, the couple remained active in politics, pushing radical causes and spouting rhetoric described by one informant as "far left of center."[41]

Donna quickly found a job as a social worker, while Jonas discovered a research environment tailor-made to his interests. In addition to generous funding from the Army, Francis had just won a large grant from the National Foundation for Infantile Paralysis "to train virologists and study virus diseases." This placed Michigan in a very select group of research institutions—able to recruit new faculty, attract top graduate students, hire the best technicians, and upgrade its laboratories.[42]

For Salk, a remarkable apprenticeship began. He would spend six years at Michigan, moving up the academic ladder—too slowly, he felt—from a research fellow to a research associate to an assistant professor of epidemiology. Each year, Francis would write Salk's draft board for an extension of the II-A occupational deferment, describing his assistant, quite correctly, as "impossible to replace." And each year, Salk would take on new responsibilities from Francis, who spent weeks on the road as director of the Army's Commission on Influenza. "This was as active a period as any in my life," Salk recalled. "At the age of twenty-nine, I took over [the laboratory] in Tom's absence. . . . It was quite a responsibility."[43]

Like Francis, Salk was intrigued by the potential of a killed-virus vaccine. He saw no reason why an approach that had proved successful against the bacterial toxins of cholera, typhoid, and diphtheria should fail to work against a viral disease. In the laboratory, Salk and his colleagues ran experiments on both the formalin used to kill influenza virus—a numbing game of trial and error—and the adjuvants designed to enhance a vaccine's power. Knowing that influenza had many different strains, and that immunity to one did not confer immunity to the others, they scoured the country for every available strain, hoping to give their vaccine the widest protective value.[44]

The Army, of course, offered researchers something truly unique: a chance to run large-scale human trials under carefully controlled conditions. In the fall of 1943, several thousand soldiers took part in an influenza experiment. Half were given a vaccine packed with "killed" strains of type A virus; the other half got a harmless placebo. The results were encouraging. Those injected with the real vaccine experienced significantly lower rates of influenza that season. The killed viruses had produced a strong antibody response.[45]

But follow-up experiments proved far less successful. The problem was not with the concept of a killed-virus vaccine, but rather with the virus itself. Influenza is tricky. The type A virus is known for its ability to undergo significant antigenic variation: the individual strains keep shifting—occasionally, as in 1918, with catastrophic results. Thus, a flu vaccine will only work when it contains the proper strain for the current season, and that involves a good bit of guesswork and luck. No one knew this better than the cautious Thomas Francis, who was loath to oversell either his product—or himself. Asked privately about the effectiveness of his flu vaccine, Francis said: "I believe that if a strain of virus is encountered similar to the one which is included in the vaccine, there should be protection." At worst, he added, "I do not believe it will do harm."[46]

Over time, the student-mentor relationship between Salk and Francis began to wear thin. As the junior partner, Salk increasingly sought public recognition for his work, lobbying to have his name appear first, as senior investigator, on research papers sent out from the lab. As Francis recalled, "He used to tell me, 'Everyone knows who *you* are. It doesn't matter whether your name is first or last.' You can't really dislike this in the man, you know. You've got to admire ambition, especially when it's combined with the kind of ability this fellow had."[47]

Most times, Francis acquiesced. But occasionally, he noted, Salk's ambition got the better of him and problems arose. "I remember one paper he wrote," said Francis, "that didn't seem to me to substantiate some of the conclusions he drew. I told him so, but he said he thought the inferences were warranted by reason if not by hard data. . . . I told him we didn't do things that way in our place. Then he said he thought he'd send the paper in anyhow. I told him if he did he had better go with it. That was that."[48]

Salk didn't dispute this version of events. "My striving was strong and unconcealed," he admitted. "I wanted to do independent work and I wanted to do it *my way.*" Francis had a well-earned reputation as a worrier—finicky, skeptical of grand theories, fearful of mistakes. "Tommy is a fella," groused one senior colleague, "who just hates to make up his mind." His instincts were those of an epidemiologist—"oriented toward the control of disease, rather than its academic contemplation."[49]

Salk, at this stage, took a more freewheeling approach. "There may have been times when I made more of my data than might have been expected," he said, "but I was not functioning in the expected way. . . . I was attempting to elucidate the *interaction* of man and virus in a field which was accustomed to viewing the two separately. I engaged in extrapolation because I had always felt that it was a legitimate means of provoking scientific thought and discussion. I engaged in prediction because I felt it was the *essence* of scientific thought. The fact that neither extrapolation nor prediction was popular in virological circles seemed to me to be a shame."[50]

This was as far as Salk would ever go in criticizing his mentor. He owed him far too much. But there were others in the younger generation who viewed Francis as something of a fossil, a fussy administrator with declining scientific skills. "Have you seen Tommy's paper in the recent *Bacteriological Reviews*?" a friend wrote to Salk. "A more garbled discussion I have never read. . . . And amazing it is that Francis is president of that organization."[51]

By war's end, Salk could see his time at Michigan coming to an end. He was still a research associate earning $4,700 a year. He had no tenure, no job security, no promise of future employment. And Donna Salk had recently stopped working to care for their first child, Peter, born in 1944.

Strapped for money, Salk took a dangerous step. Without seeking permission, he talked to officials at Parke-Davis, a major drug company interested in producing a flu vaccine, about a part-time consulting job. When Francis found out, all hell broke loose. He accused Salk of undermining the entire research team, and then lectured him, rather sanctimoniously, about the virtues and sacrifices of academic life. "To undertake such a [position]," he wrote in a biting memorandum, "would immediately weaken the entire outlook of the department and give advantages to one individual which are not justified. . . . If this is a matter of Dr. Salk's feeling . . . then he must leave."[52]

Salk backed off, with good reason. He had nowhere else to go. And Francis, keenly aware of Salk's expertise, was reluctant to push him out the door. A month later, in an obvious peace offering, Salk received a choice assignment to investigate the spread of influenza among American soldiers in occupied postwar Germany. It was the first time he had been outside the United States. Writing from Frankfurt on captured Nazi-SS stationery—"Heil Hitler," he joked—Salk told Francis that their hard work had paid off. "I feel confident that vaccinated troops did quite well," he said, adding that there was "not the remotest suggestion of an outbreak of any kind anywhere in the American zone."[53]

In 1946 Salk was promoted to assistant professor and given a moderate raise, to $6,000 per year. It was the best he could do, said Francis, who knew it wasn't good enough. After six years of apprenticeship, Salk needed to break free. He already had applied for vacancies at the University of California and Case Western Reserve, but both had turned him down. He had talked with Mount Sinai about a teaching position, but the funding proved too small. Then, in 1947, came word of a job at the University of Pittsburgh, which had just established a virus research program and was looking for a director.

The position lacked status. Pittsburgh was off the map as a research institution. Although the search committee told Salk that "several other people" were being considered for the position, the job was his to turn down. When Salk accepted it—seeing potential where others saw only oblivion—his colleagues were stunned. "Tommy Francis thought I was making a mistake," Salk recalled. "So did everyone else. I can remember someone asking me, 'What's in Pittsburgh, for heaven's sake?' and I answered, 'I guess I fell in love.'"[54]

Before departing, Salk sent Francis a heartfelt note of thanks. He had learned well from his mentor; the training he received would lay the foundation for his later work on polio. The faith in a killed-virus vaccine, the experiments with formaldehyde, the use of adjuvants, the mass-testing techniques—all had come from his association with Tommy Francis. "I have referred in the past to the 'baptism of fire' to which you subject your associates," Salk wrote, "and I feel that the rigorous standards and trials, which you apply to yourself as well, provide the temper and strength that can be achieved in no other way. I know the trademark 'made by Francis' has and will continue to provide opportunities and I shall endeavor, in my future activities, to deserve this label."[55]

The professional paths of Jonas Salk and Thomas Francis would cross again, eight years later. This time the world would be their stage.

IN 1883, A POPULAR GUIDEBOOK of cities described Pittsburgh as "the Great Furnace of America," the engine driving its industrial revolution. "In truth, she is a smoky dismal [place], at her best," the book added. "At her worst, nothing darker, dingier or more dispiriting can be imagined."[56]

Six decades later, this portrait still rang true. Home to much of the nation's steel industry, ringed by mining towns like Coal Bluff, Coal Brook, and Coal Valley, Pittsburgh remained one of America's bleakest cities, known for its choking pollution and working-class swagger. In the winter months, when temperature inversions kept the smoke and soot from reaching the atmosphere, the city rarely saw the sun. The sky grew so dark that streetlights blazed in the daytime. A study done in the 1940s had Pittsburgh leading the country in the rate of pneumonia and most other respiratory ailments. When describing their city, local newspapers were fond of quoting the writer James Parton, who had passed through quickly almost eighty years before. "Pittsburgh," he wrote, "is hell with the lid taken off!"[57]

The region's history spoke of big fortunes and bloody labor battles—Carnegie, Westinghouse, and Frick; Homestead, the United Steel Workers, and the Molly Maguires. In 1947, the year that Jonas Salk arrived, Pittsburgh suffered two coal strikes, a three-month electrical workers' strike, and a 27-day power strike—the nation's first ever—that shut down the city. For its part, Pittsburgh's upper crust—Andrew Carnegie excepted—was notorious for ignoring civic problems and social concerns. "The provincialism of Pittsburgh," Salk wrote a friend, "is very striking."[58]

There were breaks in the darkness, however. Following World War II, a new generation of power brokers led by Richard Mellon, heir to the Mellon family banking empire, and Mayor David Lawrence proposed an ambitious master plan for redeveloping the city, known as the Pittsburgh Renaissance. The plan emphasized generous spending to upgrade parks and libraries, control pollution, and create a world-class medical complex at the University of Pittsburgh.[59]

The medical school was an obvious priority. No one doubted its potential—or dismal current standing. As the only such facility between Philadelphia and Cleveland, it served a region with more than six million people. Yet the buildings were in disrepair, it had no major hospital on site, and there were few serious researchers or clinicians to be found. The biggest shock at Pittsburgh's medical school, Salk recalled, was discovering that most of his colleagues "were part-time instructors who earned their living in the private practice of medicine and had neither the time nor inclination for basic research."[60]

There was discrimination as well. The medical school had no Jews on its permanent faculty. "The student body was remarkably homogeneous," wrote one observer, "with only the small Jewish contingent and two or three women in each class to disturb its otherwise all-male, Anglo-Saxon character." Interestingly, the job of screening Jewish applicants was done by a group of prominent local Jews, mostly doctors and businessmen, whose private recommendations for admission were then rubber-stamped by the administration. These men not only accepted the quota system, they appeared to control it.[61]

It fell to William McEllroy, newly appointed dean of the medical school, to turn things around. "It would be hard to understand the total lack of interest in the medical school if you didn't live through it," he recalled. "Somebody would give $500 and think he'd done a generous thing." McEllroy was smooth and persistent. Cultivating the city's moneyed elite—the Mellon and Chalfant families, the Carnegie Foundation and Westinghouse Electric—he got them to do what they'd never even thought of doing before: to open their wallets to the medical school. McEllroy used their gifts to support research, create new faculty positions, and attract first-rate talent, including Arthur Mirsky, the acclaimed psychiatrist, and Benjamin Spock, the world's most celebrated pediatrician. His vision, said an associate, was "to turn Pitt into a school of national stature, a school comparable to Harvard."[62]

McEllroy had a good sense of the future. Seeing virology as a coming field, young enough for newcomers to find a niche and popular enough to attract outside funding, he endorsed a virus research program at the university to be supported mostly by private grants. In 1946, the medical school received $30,000 in seed money from the National Foundation for Infantile Paralysis to get the project up and running. Needing an ambitious researcher to head the program, and seeing no likely candidates on the Pittsburgh campus, McEllroy guided the search that hired Jonas Salk.

Exactly what was promised, other than a joint appointment in the virus research program and the medical school, would soon become a sore point between the two men. "I didn't have much to offer him," McEllroy recalled. "A lab that wasn't even finished. A moderate salary. A promise to give him a free hand and to help get any financial assistance he might need. Really, I think Jonas came here on faith."[63]

In part, that was true. Salk clearly bought into McEllroy's vision of Pittsburgh's shining future. There was great work to be done, and big money to be tapped. "Here was a metropolitan area east of the Mississippi River," Salk noted, "a wealthy community which was talking about environmental and cultural rehabilitation." What he expected was McEllroy's hand in reaching out to local donors. Salk wanted his fair share.[64]

It didn't come quickly. At Michigan, Salk had worked in spacious, fully equipped quarters, surrounded by a small army of colleagues and staff. At Pittsburgh, he was given two bare rooms in the basement of Municipal Hospital, adjacent to the medical school. His new staff consisted of a single "secretary-technician." There were no graduate students to train. His research colleagues, three in number, worked on plant viruses, a subject of little interest to Salk.

He could have pulled out. Tommy Francis had left the door open for his return to Ann Arbor, but Salk knew there was no turning back. Pittsburgh offered him exactly what Michigan could not: the chance to be independent, to build his own shop. So he pushed forward, waging "a kind of guerilla war," as one colleague put it, for space, funding, and respect. He won a small grant from the Sarah Mellon Scaife Foundation for new equipment, and slowly expanded within the hospital basement— "a closet this week, an extra office [the] next." These were small victories, to be sure, but his confidence grew. "All goes well," he wrote in November 1947, "and I feel that the unlimited potentialities of this place will be realized."[65]

A few weeks later, Salk prepared an elaborate memo for McEllroy about his research plans "for the next several years." At seven single-spaced pages, it outlined both the diseases that Salk intended to study and the funds he hoped to raise. The list included polio, influenza, measles, and the common cold in that order, with the first two getting the lion's share of ink.[66]

Influenza made perfect sense. It was Salk's primary area of expertise. The Army had allowed him to take his influenza grant to Pittsburgh, and he expected to continue his research there. His goal, he told McEllroy, was "to evolve a vaccine . . . to be effective against future epidemic strains."[67]

But polio? Salk was a novice in the field. He claimed, years later, that "everybody else was fooling around with the polio thing, so I thought I'd play around with it, too." A better explanation—the one he admitted to privately—is that the phrase "polio research" was likely to be heard, and rewarded, at the nation's most generous private funding agency. "It is hoped," he wrote, "that the National Foundation for Infantile Paralysis will be interested in supporting the projects outlined."[68]

The most revealing part of this memo is not what it said about polio, but rather what was missing. Salk spent several pages on ways to diagnose and measure the disease, yet he never mentioned the word "vaccine." The omission seems odd in light of his future success. In truth, it spoke volumes about the painfully slow progress of polio research since the early days of Simon Flexner at the Rockefeller Institute. In 1910 the production of a safe, effective polio vaccine seemed a few short months away. It hadn't happened, of course, and the roadblocks encountered since that time had soured many researchers on the prospect of *ever* finding a workable vaccine. Was it really possible to vaccinate against polio? In 1947, the answer still was very much in doubt.

7

Pathway to a Vaccine

A T THE INSTITUTE FOR REHABILITATION IN WARMS SPRINGS, Georgia, there is a Polio Hall of Fame. Seventeen bronze busts line the gallery walls. Fifteen are of scientists, the most celebrated being Albert Sabin and Jonas Salk. Two are of esteemed laymen, Basil O'Connor and Franklin Delano Roosevelt. Together, these four men represent the public face of polio—the courageous victim, the devoted foundation leader, the brilliant researchers with their lifesaving vaccines.

There is no bust of Harry Weaver in this museum, and precious little praise for him. Like everyone else who ever worked for the National Foundation, he lived in the giant shadow of the man who ran the show. But Harry Weaver was special. As director of research from 1946 through 1953, he successfully harnessed the diffuse, free-floating energy of these fifteen polio specialists, among others, and focused it—too narrowly, some complained—toward a single goal. It was the charismatic O'Connor who led the national crusade against polio. It was the coldly efficient Weaver who provided the scientific blueprint for success.

Weaver did not have imposing academic credentials. Most of his career had been spent teaching anatomy at Wayne State University in Detroit. He had worked for a time on the relationship between polio and nutrition, a once-promising subject that had come up dry. What distinguished him, most agreed, was his "wonderful quality of being bold." He saw no problem in asking of others what he, as a scientist, had failed to accomplish himself. "In research," said Tom Rivers, "you often need a person like [Harry] around, you know, someone . . . to encourage people to see what the grass is like on the other side. In other words, a catalyst. Harry Weaver performed that function beautifully."[1]

Weaver saw polio research as applied science—seeking a specific solution to a particular problem. For him, the solution to polio lay in a successful vaccine, and the problem in developing one lay in the foundation's obvious failure to lead. For years, its grantees had been inching along on disparate, often esoteric projects, ignorant of each other's findings, and painfully slow to challenge the accepted truths about the disease. Not everyone fit this mold, but there were too many who did, Weaver thought. It was time for a change.

Vaccines already had proved successful against other viruses—smallpox and rabies being notable examples. And a vaccine that effectively immunized humans against poliovirus stood a good chance of ending the disease, since humans appeared to be the only natural hosts. To Weaver, the simmering feud between live-virus and killed-virus advocates didn't much matter at this point. Indeed, the foundation was willing to bankroll both sides at once. What did matter was removing the obstacles that had been stalling polio vaccine progress for years.

This would not be easy. Big changes would have to be made in the way that large grants were funded, administered, and reviewed. Weaver knew that the medical school had now supplanted the independent institute as the dominant force in biological research. "In fact," he wrote, the better schools "are today more nearly institutions for the conduct of research than they are schools for the training of physicians and teachers. In [some of them], extra-institutional funds in support of research may equal or even surpass the total of funds available for the support of all the remaining activities of the institution."[2]

The problem, Weaver noted, was that these "extra-institutional funds" were not as beneficial as they first appeared. Medical school administrators learned rather quickly that winning a large outside grant for scientific research, while no doubt prestigious, could be more of a drain than an asset. The sticking point involved indirect costs. "The acceptance of [outside funds]," said Weaver, "has forced the institution to expand its physical facilities, its administrative, technical, and secretarial staffs, and to spend more money for maintenance and for public utilities, to mention only a few examples."[3]

Weaver ran into this problem after only a few weeks on the job. The National Foundation had agreed to fund a grant proposal from the

Bacteriology Department at Harvard, but the university administration had resisted, complaining about the high overhead it would be forced to cover. Weaver responded with a promise to pay a portion of these indirect costs, based on a complicated formula he had worked out himself. Harvard then accepted the grant.[4]

Over time, Weaver simplified the process. With the approval of Tom Rivers and Basil O'Connor, he added "a specified percentage" to each foundation grant, ending "the need for [my] time-consuming formula." The new rules were:

If the grant is $10,000 or less, the amount of the grant will be increased by 46%.

If the grant is between $10,001 and $30,000, the amount of the grant will be increased by 46% for the first $10,000, and 38% of all remaining.

If the grant is more than $30,000, the amount of the grant will be increased by 46% of the first $10,000, 38% of the next $20,000, and 6% of all remaining.

These funds could be used to further "good research that may properly be expected in institutions for higher learning," a catchall for anything not already covered in the grantee's original budget. "We believe," said Weaver, "that this new policy provides a [good] mechanism . . . to defray a more equitable share of the total cost of conducting programs of research." Few disagreed.[5]

Weaver also moved to overhaul the foundation's novel policy of offering long-term grants, begun in 1942. These grants, lasting up to five years, had allowed researchers to think in terms of larger projects. The problem, Weaver discovered, was that the foundation had done a poor job of tracking the grantees. "The failure of our Medical Advisory Committee to review [their] annual progress and contemplated research," he complained, "is not conducive to [formulating] the best possible attack on the problems of polio."[6]

Weaver wanted more flexibility. He did not think it reasonable that a five-year grant totaling $100,000 must be doled out automatically at $20,000 per year; the decision, he said, should be made by the grantee and the foundation, depending on current circumstances. But Weaver demanded accountability as well. Those making strong progress would be encouraged to apply for supplemental funding. Those making little or no progress could have their grants terminated before the five years were up. The key was to put the money into the hands of the right people.[7]

The use of indirect costs and long-term grants would revolutionize the way medical research was conducted in the United States. Other foundations soon picked up these models, and the government did, too. Harry Weaver had turned funding into an art form.

To PRODUCE AN EFFECTIVE VACCINE, three basic problems would have to be solved. First, researchers would have to determine how many different types of poliovirus there were. Second, they would have to develop a safe and steady supply of each virus type for use in a vaccine. Third, they would have to discover the true pathogenesis of polio—its route to the central nervous system—in order to fix the exact time and place for the vaccine to do its work. All were elementary, if essential, parts of the puzzle.

These problems had been haunting scientists for years. What Weaver added was a sense of direction, the outlines of a plan. Step one seemed obvious to him. Within months of becoming research director, he launched the most ambitious program in foundation history to examine and type every strain of poliovirus known to scientists around the world. A successful vaccine would have to protect against each different type, and no one was certain how many there were. The logistics were daunting. Hundreds of strains would have to be located, transported to special laboratories, and studied in numbing detail.

Some viruses, such as smallpox, are extremely stable; others, like influenza, are always in flux, requiring almost yearly modifications of the vaccine. Where did polio fit in? Simon Flexner still claimed there was only one type of poliovirus; researchers in Australia thought there were at least two; others guessed there might be three. The answer was anybody's guess.

There was, of course, only one way to find out. Start typing. To oversee the process, Weaver established a committee that placed well-known researchers like David Bodian of Johns Hopkins, Tommy Francis of Michigan, and Albert Sabin of Cincinnati alongside novices such as Pittsburgh's Jonas Salk.

The senior members did none of the actual typing. Their job was to lay down the scientific ground rules and then legitimize the results. The work itself was farmed out to the lesser lights for good reason: they were the only ones who could be found to do it. Typing viruses was a very dull task, the sort of thing that a Francis or a Sabin would normally give to a technician or a graduate student. This was not the fast track to a Nobel Prize. Indeed, as Weaver himself admitted: "I know of no problem in all the medical sciences that was more uninteresting to solve. The solution necessitated the monotonous repetition of exactly the same technical procedures on virus after virus, seven days a week, 52 weeks a year, for three solid years."[8]

Why, then, would anyone take part? When Weaver visited Salk in Pittsburgh, he laid out the reasons in lavish detail. Salk would receive a generous multiyear grant from the foundation. His medical school would be reimbursed for all the indirect costs it incurred, such as maintenance, utilities, and insurance. Polio may not have been Salk's chosen virus—influenza was—but the timing was right. "Weaver represented a liberating force," Salk recalled. "The original attractiveness of Pittsburgh had been the apparent openness of the situation there, but then the openness had proved illusory. And now Weaver came along, willing to provide me with funds and work and people and facilities to be administered and organized by me."[9]

Salk now had a foot in the door. The foundation's first check—for $41,000—arrived in 1948, and money poured in from other sources as well. The Army renewed Salk's grant for influenza research, a project of abiding interest to him, while the Sarah Mellon Scaife Foundation agreed to fund the parts of his laboratory "that will not be used for polio investigations."[10]

Salk's quarters were located in Pittsburgh's Municipal Hospital, a regional center for the treatment of infectious disease. In the years following World War II, the widespread use of "wonder drugs" such as penicillin had dramatically thinned the hospital's population, creating lots of unused space. Salk moved quickly into the vacuum. By 1949, he had claimed two full floors, one containing his laboratories, offices, and a glassware sterilization room; the other housing the monkey quarters, complete with "ventilating facilities, cages, cage cleaning equipment, and an incinerator." Ironically, the largest remaining ward in the hospital was for polio patients—a constant reminder of the job that lay ahead. A nurse recalled that "ambulances literally lined up outside the place. There were sixteen or seventeen new admissions every day. One of our resident physicians never went to bed for nights on end, except for stretching out on a cot in his clothes. We nurses never got home, either. To leave the place you had to pass a certain number of rooms, and you'd hear a child crying for someone to read his mail to him or for a drink of water or why can't she move, and you couldn't be cruel enough just to pass by. It was an atmosphere of grief, terror and helpless rage."[11]

Salk's operation kept expanding. Between 1949 and 1953, he would garner almost a million dollars in grants from the National Foundation, with $255,000 more going for indirect costs. He would also receive $140,000 from the Army for his influenza research and a host of smaller donations. His laboratory alone would account for almost 90 percent of his medical school's entire outside funding in these years.[12]

Salk's first grant provided for both "key personnel," with "minor participants." Salk hired well, finding people who shared both his vision and his workaholic ways—people who could see their current plodding tasks as the start of something special, the creation of a lifesaving new vaccine. The original group included Jim Lewis, a bacteriologist; Byron Bennett, the chief technician; Tony Penko, the lead animal handler; and Lorraine Friedman, the office manager. Lewis did the monkey work: inoculations, bleedings, autopsies, and tissue harvesting. He also performed the surgery that separated these primates from their organs in which the poliovirus would be grown. Bennett supervised the equipment and processed the tissue and blood samples provided by Lewis. A problem drinker, nicknamed "the Major" for his service in the Army Medical Corps, Bennett was "a pillar of strength," according to fellow workers, "most comfortable when working alone." Lorraine Friedman, a Pittsburgh native, took what she thought was a temporary job as Salk's personal secretary—and stayed on for the next forty years.[13]

BY THE TIME THIS MAMMOTH PROJECT was up and running, a key question had been partially answered. How many types of poliovirus existed? At least three, said David Bodian, who released his finding in 1949. Bodian's study demolished the fiction that all poliovirus was the same. Yet, because he had used a small sample of strains in his experiment, it seemed likely that a larger sample might bring a larger result. If so—if the foundation's typing project discovered four distinct types of poliovirus, or five, or fifteen—it would mean big trouble for the production of a vaccine.

Salk's laboratory did the bulk of the testing. Dozens of strains were examined, using the stools, the throat cultures, and, in fatal cases, the nerve tissue of polio victims and their families. Many of the samples Salk received were collected by other foundation grantees—

From the laboratory of Dr. Francis: Texas, Mahoney, Hjluberg, and Minnesota.

From the laboratory of Dr. Sabin: Obe, Ten, Wal, Ric, Fin, Fro, Hopk, Hof, and Per.

From the laboratory of Dr. Paul: Rosenthal, Bunnell, Greach, and Searle.

From the laboratory of Dr. Bodian: Coady, Elkins, Smith, Greenleaf, Weekly, and Vetter.[14]

Each sample came with a short description. Thus, "The Minnesota virus was originally isolated by us from the nervous tissue removed at autopsy from Mrs. Ethleen Chase on 7-24-46, who was living in Minneapolis at the time of the epidemic and who succumbed three days after onset of bulbar type of poliomyelitis. . . . [It] has been stored under dry-ice refrigeration in a sealed glass ampule."[15]

Or, "The Mahoney virus . . . was originally isolated in a rhesus monkey which received a pooled stool suspension representing Patricia, Mary, and Fred Mahoney. The stools had been collected on 9-10-41. These individuals, residing in Akron, Ohio, had been contacts of cases of poliomyelitis but were not ill themselves. [The virus] has been through six monkey passages and [was] stored in sealed glass ampules in the dry-ice box."[16]

The Mahoney strain turned out to be the most virulent one of all. Its use in a polio vaccine—even a killed-virus vaccine—would spark enormous controversy in the coming years.

The typing program lasted from 1949 to 1951. All told, it cost the foundation more than $1,200,000, with a large chunk going to the care and purchase of monkeys. This outlay solved a nightmarish problem. Monkeys were essential to polio research. They remained the basic experimental animal for studying the disease. But monkeys were expensive and hard to get. Many died in transit. Others arrived in awful shape, sick with pneumonia and dysentery, and nearly always undernourished. As Thomas Francis complained in a letter to the National Foundation: "Of the 100 monkeys you shipped us, two were dead on arrival and three died in the next few days. The condition of the group in general was very disappointing." It was not uncommon for researchers to scour the local zoo in search of castoff animals. Some even requested pregnant monkeys, hoping to breed the animals themselves. They were "going nuts," a foundation official recalled. "They'd get ready to do a piece of research. No Monkeys."[17]

Most researchers favored the cynomolgous monkey from the Philippines because it appeared to closely mimic the polio experience of humans, with the virus entering through the mouth and replicating in the gastrointestinal tract. But these animals were scarce and delicate, so American labs looked to the Indian rhesus monkey, a more resilient and plentiful source.

The Indian government was happy to oblige. Exporting rhesus monkeys was good for the economy, providing both foreign currency and local employment. Workers were needed to capture the animals and carry them "on shoulder poles to the nearest railway station and from there to New Delhi," where they were put on airplanes for the four-thousand-mile trip to London, and then on to New York. Furthermore, a thinning of the monkey population appealed to government officials, because monkeys were responsible for destroying ten percent of India's crops.[18]

There was a problem, however. Because monkeys are sacred in the Hindu religion, concerns were raised about their mistreatment by non-Hindus during their capture, their travel, and their time in the laboratories. One such mishap, in which 390 monkeys died of suffocation at a London airport, almost caused Indian officials to ban future exports. In response, the National Foundation agreed to monitor this process, and to promise that the monkeys would be well cared for and used only for polio research.[19]

The bargain made sense. In 1949, the foundation established a special facility known as Okatie Farms in rural South Carolina to process the monkeys arriving from abroad. Veterinarians screened them for disease, and nutritionists supervised their diet. Once in shape, they were trucked to foundation grantees throughout North America. ("We should like to have 50 conditioned cynomolgous monkeys, three to five pounds, delivered monthly," said Tommy Francis in a typical request.) The cost was about $26 per animal, including transportation. "Okatie," said an observer, "was in its way a little Warm Springs for monkeys."[20]

More than 17,000 of them would be sacrificed in the typing project alone. The procedure went like this: fecal samples from human polio victims were injected into the brains of monkeys, who were exercised daily to look for telltale signs of polio. When paralysis appeared, the animals were destroyed so their brains and spinal cords could be harvested for poliovirus. Tissue-serum mixtures of the virus were then injected into the brains of healthy monkeys. Those that received a known Type I strain and recovered were considered to have immunity to all other Type I strains. "They now would be inoculated with virus of an unknown type. If they proved susceptible to infection, it would mean that the unknown strain belonged to Type II or Type III. . . . The tests then would have to be conducted all over again, using the same unknown virus to challenge monkeys immune to Type II or Type III."[21]

While the typing program certainly expanded Salk's reach within the foundation, it also marked his lowly position in the calcified pecking order of polio research. Salk got an early whiff of this at a meeting of the typing committee, when he posed what he thought was a modest query about procedure. "Albert Sabin . . . turned to me and said, 'Now Dr. Salk, you should know better than to ask a question like that.'" It was, Salk recalled, "like being kicked in the teeth. I could *feel* the resistance and the hostility and the disapproval. I never attended a single one of those meetings afterward without that same feeling."[22]

Salk bit his lip and played the role of junior partner. He visited Sabin's lab in Cincinnati, offered the appropriate compliments, and even spent the night at Sabin's home. He thanked Sabin profusely for sending him reprints of articles and new strains of virus to be typed. It counted for little. Sabin didn't think much of Salk, and never would. He viewed him as an errand boy for the National Foundation, ambitious but mediocre, who would do whatever Harry Weaver wanted in order to advance. In an early letter to Salk, reviewing a draft paper on the typing project, Sabin dropped a heavy hint of the trouble that lay ahead. "You have made a number of references of extraordinary praise, etc., to the National Foundation," he wrote. "My own reaction is that this is perhaps in bad taste. . . . It is quite obvious that this entire project was sponsored by the National Foundation, and I can see no need for expressions regarding the help that was given by [them]."[23]

The final results of the typing project were reassuring. David Bodian's prediction had held up well. The 196 tested strains of poliovirus all fit neatly into three distinct types. The poliovirus "family" was remarkably, *conveniently*, small.

Type I contained 82 percent of the strains, followed by Type II with ten percent, and Type III with eight percent. Researchers gave each one a nickname. Type I was called "Brunhilde," after a chimpanzee from Bodian's lab; Type II was dubbed was "Lansing," in memory of a deceased polio victim from that Michigan city; Type III was named "Leon," for a young Los Angeles boy who had also died from the disease.[24]

Though some researchers suspected there might be other types of poliovirus, time would prove them wrong. Among the skeptics was Albert Sabin, who wondered whether Salk had overlooked the possibility of subtypes common to other diseases. This time, Salk put deference aside. Sabin's second-guessing clearly hurt. He might not be Sabin's equal in terms of reputation, but he felt sure he had no peer in terms of thoroughness and detail. "After working with influenza viruses, in which the existence of subtypes is quite clear," he fired back, "I am quite unimpressed by the differences among the poliomyelitis viruses." The evidence, in fact, showed a "remarkable homogeneity in antigenic structure." This case was closed.[25]

ONE POINT NOW WAS CERTAIN. A polio vaccine would have to protect against all three virus types to be successful. This was a huge step forward, though key problems still remained. After four decades of trial and error, nobody had been able to grow poliovirus that was safe enough, or plentiful enough, for use in a vaccine. All previous attempts had failed.

It wasn't for lack of effort. In 1907 an obscure Yale biologist named Ross Harrison made what some have hailed as "one of the ten most important discoveries in Western medicine." It was the concept of tissue culture: the ability to grow and nurture living cells in vitro, outside the hosts—plant, animal, and human—from which they came. "Harrison's discovery," wrote two distinguished researchers, "has made possible the study of living organisms at the cellular and even the molecular level, and the development of modern vaccines, including those for poliomyelitis, measles, mumps and rabies. . . . Indeed, because of tissue culture more has been learned about the basic mechanism of disease in the past fifty years than in the previous five thousand."[26]

Tissue culture seemed perfectly suited for the study of polio, which, like other viruses, can exist only in living cells. Yet success did not come quickly. In 1936 Sabin and Peter Olitsky of the Rockefeller Institute had shown that poliovirus could, indeed, be grown in test tube cultures. That was the good news. The bad news was that it would only grow in nervous tissue.[27]

There was a logical explanation for this, though no one knew it at the time. The poliovirus in vogue at the institute was Simon Flexner's "MV," a highly neurotropic strain, unable to grow in anything *except* nervous tissue. And by using it in their experiments, Sabin and Olitsky had confirmed the mistaken belief that poliovirus could not survive anywhere else.

This presented a dilemma for researchers, since the nervous tissue of monkeys was known to cause encephalomyelitis, an inflammation of the brain and spinal cord, when injected into human beings. If Sabin and Olitsky were correct—if poliovirus would only grow in dangerous nerve tissue—then how did one go about harvesting it for use in a vaccine? In the matter of polio, at least, the promise of growing a *safe* virus in tissue culture had reached a dead end.

And there the matter stood. It was not easy to challenge the wisdom of Simon Flexner and two leading lights from the nation's most respected research institute. "That work was so meticulously done that I believed it was absolutely correct," Tom Rivers recalled. "Hell . . . every working virologist that I know believed it, with the possible exception of John Enders at Harvard."[28]

Today John Enders is one of the most revered figures in the history of medicine. In the 1940s, however, his reputation was scant, to say the least. Born in Connecticut in 1897, the son of a prominent banker, Enders had served in World War I, worked briefly in real estate, and tried a graduate program in British literature before earning a doctorate in microbiology in 1930. Joining the Harvard faculty, he began his lifelong study of viral diseases, especially measles and mumps. Unlike many of his colleagues, he was not an MD. "Very few people in those early years were particularly burnt up about Enders, because he was a quiet person and published modestly," said Rivers, "but those who followed his work [knew him] to be a careful and ingenious investigator."[29]

Enders left his teaching position in 1947 to head the infectious disease laboratory at the Children's Hospital of Boston. The move caused some surprise. "Most ambitious scientists would have considered this as a comedown or at least a step in the wrong direction," a colleague recalled. But Enders thought otherwise. To this rumpled, self-confident Brahmin of independent means, the reduced status and lower salary were of little concern. At the age of fifty, he sought the best environment to get on with his work.[30]

Enders set up shop in four rooms of a vacant building next to Children's Hospital. A small part of his funding came from a $200,000 research grant given to Harvard by the National Foundation, which barely knew he was alive. Among the first recruits to his laboratory were two pediatric residents interested in studying viral disease, Fred Robbins and Tom Weller. The men had roomed together at Harvard Medical School before serving in World War II. Neither showed much interest in polio. At Children's Hospital, Robbins began to work on digestive diseases, while Weller tried to grow chickenpox and mumps viruses in tissue culture.[31]

By 1948, the art of in vitro cultivation was rapidly advancing. The introduction of antibiotics such as penicillin and streptomycin made it simpler to maintain sterile cultures by cutting down on bacterial contamination. New techniques were being employed to gently roll the test tubes, exposing the tissue inside to the proper amounts of fluid and air. And Tom Weller discovered that the tissue would survive longer if the nutrient medium was changed at regular intervals, about every four days.[32]

The great breakthrough in Enders's lab that year came largely through scientific intuition. "One day, when Tom and I were preparing a new set of cultures," said Fred Robbins. "Dr. Enders suggested that since we had some poliovirus stored in the freezer, we might inoculate some of the cultures with this material, which we did." The cultures contained both nerve and non-nerve embryonic tissue. Four were injected with chickenpox virus, four with Lansing Type II poliovirus, and four were left as controls.

Weller and Robbins were skeptical. Why should they succeed when the likes of Sabin and Olitsky had already failed? But Enders had a hunch. "It was in the back of my mind," he recalled, "that, if so much poliovirus could be found in the gastrointestinal tract, then it must grow somewhere besides nervous tissue." And, he added, "I'm a very stubborn man."[33]

His instincts were correct. The Lansing strain grew not only in the nervous tissue, but in bits of skin, muscle, and kidney tissue as well. In the following months, a series of experiments using Type I and Type III poliovirus proved equally successful. Simon Flexner had been wrong; so, too, had Sabin and Olitsky. It had taken forty years—and numerous dead ends—to solve one of polio's greatest riddles.

The implications were enormous. By cultivating these viruses in a test tube, rather than in the brain or spinal column of a monkey, researchers could get a much better look at the changes occurring inside polio-infected cells. Far more important, a safe reservoir of poliovirus had now been created, free from the contaminating effects of animal nerve tissue. And that, in turn, made possible the mass production of a vaccine. "I'll tell you one thing," Tom Rivers recalled, "that report sure as hell captured everyone's attention. . . . It was like hearing a cannon go off."[34]

Enders took it all in stride. In truth, polio had never been his main research interest. He was more intrigued by other viruses, especially measles, for which he would later develop a popular vaccine. Yet polio turned the modest Enders into an uneasy celebrity. His election to the National Academy of Sciences in 1953 was followed one year later by the Nobel Prize in Medicine and Physiology. (Other Nobel laureates in 1954 included Ernest Hemingway and Linus Pauling.) When the official word came from Stockholm, Enders made it clear that he would accept the honor only as part of a team that included his junior colleagues, Robbins and Weller. In doing so, he set a standard for generosity against which future researchers, Jonas Salk in particular, would be judged—and found wanting.

BY 1951 TWO OF THE MAIN OBSTACLES to developing a successful polio vaccine had been removed. Researchers had shown that three distinct types of poliovirus existed, and that each could be grown in safe non-nervous tissue. These discoveries, coming so close together, raised hopes that polio could be prevented, and perhaps even cured.

There was much to do, of course, before human testing could begin. Memories of the Kolmer and Park-Brodie fiasco were fresh enough to give anyone pause. Furthermore, the effectiveness of a polio vaccine was still a matter of some debate. A generation of research had shown that poliovirus entered through the nose and traveled directly to the central nervous system without first reaching the bloodstream. If this were true, it meant that a vaccine designed to stimulate antibodies in the blood, the natural defenses against infection, would do no good.

This interpretation reached back to the early days of Simon Flexner, whose various theories about polio had dominated the research agenda for as long as anyone could recall. His institute remained a key center for polio studies, and he ruled it like a personal fiefdom, jealously guarding his turf. As Peter Olitsky, chief of the Rockefeller Institute's virology lab, confided to a colleague: "Dr. Flexner affirmed that all work on polio research is his field, that my department (and myself) are to conduct work in this field only by invitation."[35]

By the 1930s, Flexner had soured on the notion of producing a successful polio vaccine. Still insisting that poliovirus entered the central nervous system through the nose, he encouraged Olitsky to begin working on a "chemical blockade." The idea, quite simply, was to stuff the nasal pathway with chemicals in order to keep poliovirus from entering the body. "Protect the Nose and Prevent Polio" became the rallying cry.

In 1936, Sabin and Olitsky dutifully ran "blockade" experiments on monkeys. Meanwhile, public health officials in Alabama used a solution of picric acid (a poisonous acid) and alum on human volunteers. When the results proved disappointing, stronger chemicals were urged. The following year, children were sprayed with zinc sulfate during a polio outbreak in Toronto. The chemical proved useless in stopping the epidemic, and several children suffered "a complete and evidently permanent loss of the sense of smell."[36]

The message seemed obvious. "We have no evidence whatsoever," Sabin admitted, "that spraying chemicals can prevent poliomyelitis in human beings." There was an unintended benefit, however. The dismal failure of "chemical blockade" forced researchers to look again at how poliovirus entered the body.[37]

Sabin took the lead. In a breakthrough experiment in 1941, he gathered material from human autopsies to show that poliovirus, while plentiful in the alimentary tract of polio victims, was rarely found in the nasal passages. He "traveled around to different sites," recalled Dorothy Horstmann, who first met Sabin in the morgue of a Tennessee hospital. "He came with all his paraphernalia and did the autopsy in an extremely complicated procedure. . . . An instrument was never used twice so that one specimen was not contaminated by another. The results proved beyond any doubt the olfactory pathway was not involved in the human disease. . . . This was not an infection that traveled by the nasal route."[38]

At Johns Hopkins, Howard Howe and David Bodian tried a different approach. After first severing the olfactory nerves of a chimpanzee, they fed it large doses of poliovirus by mouth. The animal quickly succumbed to the disease, as the researchers had expected, despite the elimination of the nasal pathway.[39]

Flexner's theory lay in shreds. Researchers now viewed the alimentary canal, not the nose, as the obvious portal of entry. And this discovery, in turn, stirred new hope for a vaccine. If poliovirus entered through the mouth and worked its way down the digestive tract, then it must travel through the blood before entering the central nervous system. If so, a vaccine designed to raise antibody levels in the bloodstream would be able to neutralize the virus *before* serious damage was done.

Among the first investigators to look in this direction was Dorothy Horstmann, a member of Yale's crack polio unit. "I started working on this problem very early," she recalled. "I collected blood from every patient that came into the hospital during the 1943 polio epidemic [in New Haven]. I remember very well, 111 blood specimens were tested . . . and [poliovirus] was recovered from only one. . . . It wasn't a very good batting average, so we thought it was something that perhaps didn't happen very often."[40]

Horstmann was intrigued by that one case, however—a nine-year-old girl who "would never have been admitted to the hospital if there had not been an epidemic." Except for some slight neck pain, the little girl showed no outward signs of polio. Was it possible, Horstmann wondered, that poliovirus was only present in the bloodstream during the brief period before a victim took sick and the physical symptoms became apparent?

To test this theory, Horstmann began a series of experiments on chimpanzees. She fed them poliovirus by mouth—"the natural route of infection"—to determine if, and when, it turned up in their blood. The results were dramatic. Poliovirus was detected within days of the feedings. In a personal letter to Horstmann in 1953, John F. Fulton, Yale's distinguished historian of medicine, raved: "This disclosure is as exciting as anything that has happened in the Yale Medical School since I first came here in 1930 and is a tremendous credit to your industry and scientific imagination. . . . It is also medical history!"[41]

Working independently at Hopkins, David Bodian reported almost identical results. What was going on? Why had previous researchers been unable to detect poliovirus in the blood? The answer was deceptively simple: they had waited too long to begin looking.

When poliovirus enters the blood, it creates the very antibodies that will soon destroy it. Thus, poliovirus can be found there only during a brief period of incubation *before* these antibodies have formed to do their work. In a few cases, the virus will reach the central nervous system, causing paralysis and sometimes death. But even then, its presence can no longer be detected in the blood, since the antibodies it has produced have fully neutralized the virus.

In theory, at least, the puzzle had been solved. Research had found the time (early in the infection) and the place (the bloodstream) for the battle to be waged. "It meant," said John Paul, "that small amounts of virus which invaded the blood could probably be overcome by relatively small amounts of circulating antibody, and by this means could be blocked from gaining access to the central nervous system. . . . At one fell swoop, the problem of immunizing man had been rendered easier than was expected."[42]

Polio would be conquered through a vaccine.

SIMON FLEXNER, THE FATHER OF MODERN POLIO RESEARCH, did not live to see most of his long-held theories discarded, one by one. Nobody had done more to raise scientific interest in this disease or in the field of virology as a whole. And nobody had done more to shape the parameters of the polio debate in ways that walled off new approaches, diverse opinions, and fresh ideas. In an article published in 1946, Flexner still insisted that there was but one type of poliovirus—a position he had held, and defended, for his entire career. His words, fittingly, were the last ones he would ever write about the disease. He died later that year.

8

The Starting Line

Nineteen forty-nine had been a mixed year on the polio front. Dramatic breakthroughs in the laboratories had raised public hopes sky high for the development of a lifesaving vaccine. But a record surge in polio numbers had raised public fears as well. Only twice in the current century—1916 and 1946—had more than 25,000 cases been reported. In 1949, the total reached 42,000, making it the worst year on record by far. *Life* magazine described polio as the nation's leading public health threat—"sudden" "capricious," "uncontrollable." The *Saturday Evening Post* called it "the most dreaded of youthful afflictions."[1]

In fact, it was no longer just a disease of the young. Researchers noted that people in their twenties and thirties were at much greater risk than before, and that the chances of serious paralysis and death seemed to rise dramatically with age. In addition, epidemics were being tracked in definite cycles—hitting an area hard, infecting large parts of the population, creating widespread natural immunity, and then returning in force when a fresh pool of unprotected victims emerged. In places such as New York City, a serious outbreak could now be *expected* every five years.

Public fear of polio had long been linked to public optimism about a cure. They were two parts of the same message, skillfully honed over the years by Basil O'Connor and the National Foundation for Infantile Paralysis. "Give us your time and your money," it said, "and together we will smite this awful plague."

In 1949, the message grew bolder. As the number of polio victims increased, so, too, did the need for donations to fund laboratory research and patient care. For the first time, the foundation claimed that victory over the disease was not simply inevitable, it was *imminent*. "The conquest of polio," it declared, "is now in sight."[2]

These words—so prophetic today—sparked rebellion in the ranks. A number of the foundation's own grantees accused it of deceiving the public in a shameless attempt to raise more money. In a blistering letter to O'Connor, Albert Sabin came close to calling him a liar. There were "no assurances" of preventing polio in the near future, or *ever*, he sniffed, and to say otherwise was "irresponsible," "unwarranted," and "unkind."

Sabin had another concern as well. He did not like the scientific direction in which the foundation was headed. By promising a quick solution to the polio problem, it had given a distinct advantage to those who supported the simpler killed-virus approach. Though Sabin had barely begun his own quest for a vaccine, he worried that live-virus advocates like himself would be shunted aside, with dire consequences, he warned, for the future of polio research.[3]

Sabin was a master at fusing his own needs and ambitions to larger humanitarian concerns. Within days, he had recruited other prominent grantees to join his revolt. As the pressure mounted, O'Connor took a small step backward by withdrawing the comments that had started the fuss. "Maybe we over-dramatized," he admitted. "But we are losing no time in attacking the mystery in our medical laboratories. These things are possible because the people of the country have supported the movement to the hilt. Those are the *facts*."[4]

Still, O'Connor didn't waver in his belief that faster was better in the search for a vaccine, that speed truly mattered when lives were at risk. What he wanted to know, and quickly, was: Who would get there first?

IN THE FALL OF 1949, Jonas Salk wrote to John Enders requesting a sample of "foreskin tissue culture material" for study in his Pittsburgh lab. There was an ulterior motive at work here, which Enders fully understood. Salk had ambitious plans. He was looking for the best way to produce safe poliovirus for use in a vaccine, and he needed to know whether Enders was moving in that direction, too. "I do not want to intrude on any things that you might be doing or want to do," he said, with appropriate delicacy. "I hope you will feel perfectly free to be very frank with me, particularly if you have already made plans to do any studies of this sort on your own."[5]

At first Enders politely turned him down. "We are, at the moment, engaged in some pilot experiments on the immunizing effect of the material," he explained, "and I would prefer to have the results . . . in hand before . . . wishing anyone else to undertake any large scale investigation."[6]

What Enders didn't say was that he and his colleagues, Fred Robbins and Tom Weller, were at odds over what to do next. The two younger men were anxious to begin work on a polio vaccine; Enders was not. He viewed the project as routine, even boring, the sort of thing best done in "a commercial establishment." Furthermore, he didn't believe that a killed-virus vaccine would ever provide adequate protection against polio, or that a live-virus vaccine could be safely developed without years of painful trial and error. Nothing about this endeavor seemed quite right to Enders. "Our laboratory is not set up for vaccine production," he said, noting that future breakthroughs on the polio front might well come from "chemotherapeutic approaches" to the disease. Deciding to pass, Enders generously shared his tissue culture techniques with Salk and others. But his perceptions of the young scientist from Pittsburgh were not especially favorable. Enders did not view Jonas Salk, then or later, as a serious force in the field of virus research.[7]

THE TEAM BEST POSITIONED to move forward quickly on a vaccine was working at Johns Hopkins. The top researchers there—David Bodian, Howard Howe, and Isabel Morgan—had done more to unravel the mysteries of polio than any other group. In 1941 Bodian and Howe had determined the route of entry for poliovirus to be the alimentary canal, not the nasal passages, as scientists had long believed. Bodian had also been the first to predict that at least three types of the virus existed, and to show, along with Dorothy Horstmann, that polio had a brief but significant "viremic phase" in which the virus traveled through the bloodstream into the central nervous system.[8]

The Johns Hopkins team had also introduced a vital new player into polio research: the chimpanzee. It spent great sums of March of Dimes grant money to buy several dozen of these primates, with extraordinary results. "Chimpanzees were to prove nearest to man with respect to [polio]," wrote one authority. "It was a conspicuous step forward." Howe and Bodian grew fond of their chimps, giving each a nickname as it entered the lab. "We inoculated Zombie," Howe would tell Bodian. Or, "Bozo's brain is so beautiful that I am thinking of writing a little more on it alone." At a scientific conference in 1952, Tom Rivers actually scolded Bodian for using the word "he" to describe one his chimps, claiming it made animals the "equal of men." "Well," said a perplexed Bodian, "he *wasn't* a she." "Well," Rivers replied, "*it* is an it!"[9]

Isabel Morgan joined the Johns Hopkins group in 1944. "By good fortune, I met her at Woods Hole," Bodian recalled, "and induced her to come to Baltimore." The daughter of two prominent biologists—her father, Thomas Hunt Morgan, received the Nobel Prize in 1933 for his work on chromosomes and heredity—Isabel Morgan graduated from Stanford and earned her doctorate in bacteriology at the University of Pennsylvania before joining the Rockefeller Institute in 1938. She worked in Peter Olitsky's lab, studying immunity to viral diseases such as polio and encephalomyelitis. In a confidential memo, Olitsky described her as "a woman of great originality [who] refuses to accept so-called established statements of fact unless they are proved valid beyond any doubt in her own mind."[10]

Morgan's obvious talents, however, did not lessen the discrimination she faced. Her salary at the Rockefeller Institute was well below what her male colleagues were earning, and the research awards invariably went to men. As Tom Rivers recalled, "few Ph.D. ladies ever had much of a chance for advancement at the institute during the early days." It was a key reason Dr. Morgan looked elsewhere.[11]

At Johns Hopkins, she began a series of experiments to immunize monkeys against polio with a killed-virus vaccine. She grew the poliovirus in nervous tissue—monkey brains and spinal cords—before inactivating it with formaldehyde. The results were promising. Her vaccinated monkeys were able to withstand a series of intracerebral injections containing high concentrations of live poliovirus. None showed symptoms of the disease. "I need hardly repeat," said Rivers, "that until the time she did her work, most virologists believed that you couldn't immunize against poliomyelitis with a formalin-inactivated vaccine. She converted us and that was quite a feat."[12]

But the progress ended there. In 1949, at the very height of her career, Dr. Morgan left Johns Hopkins to marry Joseph Mountain, a former Air Force colonel who worked as a data processor in New York. The couple moved to Westchester, where she took a job with the county's Department of Laboratory Research. She was 38 years old. The yawning chasm between the laboratory at Johns Hopkins and the one in Westchester can be gleaned from the correspondence of Peter Olitsky. In 1953, the director of the Westchester lab sent Olitsky a copy of a scientific paper he was hoping to publish. Olitsky, a man noted for his kind and patient demeanor, tore the paper to shreds. Sensing he had gone too far, Olitsky wrote a second letter apologizing for the harshness of his criticism. He also advised the director that it would be wise for him to clear all future publication attempts with Dr. Morgan. "I have the fullest confidence in her scientific judgment," said Olitsky. "She can be of greatest aid."[13]

Morgan spent much of her time as a homemaker and a stepmother to her husband's young son, Jimmy, who had a learning disability. "Ibby loved science, but she loved her new family even more. I'm certain of that," said David Bodian's wife, Eleanor. "Dave, of course, saw it as a tremendous blow for his lab and for polio research, but everyone understood. It was a different time. A woman like Ibby had a hard choice to make, and she made it."[14]

After Morgan left Johns Hopkins, no one there emerged to aggressively pursue her work. Bodian was more interested in the pathology of polio than in the development of a vaccine. And Howard Howe, the one most likely to build on Morgan's early successes, had neither the ambition nor the energy to match the relentless progress of future competitors such as Jonas Salk. "It wasn't our field," said Bodian, "and it wasn't our taste."

Would Morgan have beaten Salk to the polio vaccine had she remained at Johns Hopkins? It's certainly possible since Salk had barely entered the starting gate by 1949. The Hopkins lab was first rate in every way. Morgan had the knowledge, the technique, and the funding to move forward quickly on her killed-virus vaccine.

She was held back, however, by her reluctance to do human testing. This certainly made sense. Morgan, after all, began experimenting at a time when poliovirus was grown exclusively in nervous tissue, with the potential for a deadly allergic reaction. Though the breakthrough by John Enders would forever solve this problem, it still took a special kind of daring in the early 1950s to move from testing in animals to testing in children. Indeed, Isabel Morgan later told friends that she had shuddered at the thought of taking that fateful next step under *any* circumstances. Unlike Salk, she didn't feel completely confident about her vaccine. In truth, she never got the chance.[15]

Her story is etched in tragedy. In 1960 her beloved stepson Jimmy was killed in a midair plane collision over New York City while returning home from college for his Christmas break. Morgan quit her job, got a master's degree in biostatistics from Columbia, and went on to work as a consultant at the Sloan-Kettering Cancer Institute in Manhattan. She died in 1996, without ever returning to the field of polio research.

At a memorial service the following year, a former colleague spoke movingly of the qualities that had set her apart. "Looking at Isabel Morgan Mountain's career," he said, "and the ways in which she shaped it in response to blissful or sad events affecting her personal life, one can only be impressed by her adaptability, her courage, and, in science, her profound and lasting influence."[16]

At the very least, she had blazed the trail that Jonas Salk would follow to completion.

IN PEARL RIVER, NEW YORK, no more than twenty miles from Isabel Morgan's Westchester laboratory, a young Polish immigrant was working secretly on his own polio vaccine. His name was Hilary Koprowski, and his experiments would soon ignite a firestorm within the scientific world.

A graduate of the Warsaw University Medical School, Koprowski, had fled to Brazil with his wife, Irena, a biologist, after the Nazis invaded their homeland in 1939. Taking a job with the Rockefeller Foundation in Rio de Janeiro, he had worked for several years on a live-virus vaccine to combat yellow fever. From there, the Koprowskis came to the United States, settling in Pearl River, home of Lederle Laboratories, the pharmaceutical division of American Cyanamid, which hired him as a researcher in 1945.[17]

Koprowski had many talents. An accomplished pianist, fluent in a half-dozen languages, a connoisseur of fine food and wine, he both inspired and intimidated people with his worldly charm, volcanic temper, and willingness to take risks. His boss at Lederle was Herald Cox, a brilliant virologist who had trained at the Rockefeller Institute. Cox assigned Koprowski to a new polio project, designed to produce a live-virus vaccine. "It was apparent from an early stage," said a student of their relationship, "that Koprowski was not the kind of man to submit to control on matters of detail; if one was going to employ such a personality, the only thing to do was to hand him a broad assignment and leave him alone." Cox left him alone.

At Lederle, opinions of Koprowski varied widely. At one end were coworkers who described him as a ruthless man "of extreme ambition" and "very limited conscience." At the other were those who saw him as a medical pioneer. "One of [his] great scientific gifts," a colleague noted, "is being able to smell what's going to be important," and to pursue it relentlessly. "He's not always right. . . . But by and large, his gambles usually pay off."[18]

Lederle was a company on the move. Its scientists had recently synthesized vitamin B and developed aureomycin, a powerful antibiotic. The grounds at Pearl River resembled an Ivy League campus, with stately buildings, duck ponds, and manicured lawns. And the facilities rivaled the Rockefeller Institute in terms of laboratory space, equipment, and technical support.

Even better, the polio experiments it conducted did not have to pass muster with the National Foundation's research committees or conform to often finicky rules. Lederle Labs had no interest in mimicking the academic culture that prevailed at Michigan or Johns Hopkins or Yale. Its aim was simple: to develop a safe and profitable vaccine.

Like Isabel Morgan, Koprowski began his polio experiments before the tissue culture discoveries of John Enders. In 1947 he injected a strain of Type II (Lansing) poliovirus directly into the skulls of mice. Next he removed the brain matter, mixed it into a saline solution, and passed the souplike substance through groups of cotton rats until the poliovirus had been properly "attenuated" (weakened) for use in a vaccine.[19]

Koprowski fed the vaccine orally to nine chimpanzees. Then he gave them doses of virulent Type II poliovirus to see whether his vaccine offered any protection. All nine remained polio-free, suggesting that it did.

What worked for animals, of course, did not necessarily work for people. Though research suggested that the oral feeding of chimpanzees mimicked the human condition, this was hardly proof enough. The next step for Koprowski involved a powerful but unwritten rule of scientific research. Before testing his oral vaccine on other humans, he must try it on himself.

This tradition, going back centuries, was still very much alive. In 1903, Jessie Lazear, a member of Walter Reed's medical team on yellow fever, had died after allowing himself to be bitten by an infected mosquito. A decade later, Joseph Goldberger had demonstrated that pellagra was noninfectious by injecting himself with the blood of its victims, eating pieces of their scaled-off skin, and even swallowing a vial containing bits of their feces. In the 1930s, polio researchers John Kolmer, William Park, and Maurice Brodie had all vaccinated themselves before experimenting on children.[20]

Koprowski's moment came in 1948. Late one winter afternoon, he and his assistant, Thomas Norton, whipped up a "polio cocktail," using a Waring blender to turn the pieces of rat spinal cord and brain tissue into a gray "oily glop." The two men drank from small glass beakers, tilting their heads to fully drain the liquid. It tasted a lot like cod-liver oil, they agreed. "Have another?" asked Norton. "Better not," Koprowski replied. "I'm driving."[21]

TWO YEARS LATER, in 1950, Koprowski tested his live-virus vaccine on children. The site was Letchworth Village, a nearby state institution opened in 1912 as a haven for "the feeble-minded and epileptic." Located in the pastoral farm country of New York's Hudson Valley, Letchworth had earned a good reputation among health professionals, despite occasional press reports of overcrowding and patient abuse.[22]

Koprowski's contact there was George Jervis, the laboratory director, who had done important work in the field of mental retardation. The two had collaborated on a research paper and become personal friends. According to Koprowski, Dr. Jervis had begged him to test his polio vaccine at Letchworth in the name of public safety. It seemed that the children were playing in their filth and throwing feces around the dorm. "To a virologist, that is like playing with live hand grenades," wrote Koprowski's biographer. "Jervis was terrified that Letchworth would soon be wiped out by polio if something wasn't done."[23]

Koprowski first fed his attenuated virus to a "nonimmune human volunteer." When the child showed no symptoms of illness, the test was widened to include nineteen others, each getting "a tablespoon of infectious material" in half a glass of chocolate milk. Koprowski did not tell Herald Cox about the test, nor did Jervis bother to notify New York state officials. The reason, Koprowski later admitted, was the certainty of being turned down.[24]

It is not clear whether Jervis got consent from the children's parents or simply took on that responsibility himself. When Koprowski published the results in 1952, his use of the word "volunteer," which included two children so helpless they had to be fed the vaccine though stomach tubes, prompted the British medical journal *The Lancet* to note:

One of the reasons for the richness of the English language is that the meaning of some words is continually changing. Such a word is "volunteer." We may yet read in a scientific journal that an experiment was carried out with twenty volunteer mice, and that twenty other mice volunteered as controls.[25]

Koprowski viewed these experiments as a positive first step. All the "nonimmune children had developed" Type II polio antibodies, and none showed signs of the disease. In 1951, Koprowski discussed his results at a scientific roundtable on polio sponsored by the National Foundation—enemy territory, to be sure. All the big grantees were on hand: Bodian, Francis, Rivers, Paul, Sabin, and the newcomer Jonas Salk. Few of them had even heard of Koprowski, the "commercial scientist" from Lederle Laboratories.

These roundtables often resembled free-for-alls. There were no points awarded for good manners or tact, Thomas Rivers recalled. "You had to be prepared to be ripped apart. It didn't matter who you were: if you got up to talk you were a fair target. That was the function—to examine results and test ideas. Why should anybody be scared?"[26]

Certainly not Koprowski, who could more than hold his own. As he began speaking that day, the group was restive and his words did not immediately sink in. He could hear Thomas Francis turn to Salk and ask, "What's this—monkeys?" Salk replied, "No, children," and all hell broke loose.

The idea of testing live virus in humans was controversial enough. But the notion of experimenting on children, in secret, with a virus grown in animal nerve tissue, seemed like a whopping mistake. "How dare you," said Albert Sabin. "Why did you do it? Why? Why?" Koprowski replied that *someone* had to take the next step, so it might as well be him. "You are not sure about this, you are not sure about that," Sabin shot back. "You may have caused an epidemic."[27]

Koprowski held his ground. He believed that the Letchworth tests, secret or not, fit well within the margins of accepted scientific practice. Indeed, while heroic stories abounded about Louis Pasteur saving the life of a nine-year-old boy with rabies, and Edward Jenner testing his smallpox vaccine on his infant son, it was *institutionalized* children—those in orphanages, alms houses, and asylums—who had borne the brunt of medical testing in Europe and the United States. They were ideal subjects—isolated, captive, easily studied and controlled. They were oblivious to the good or harm that an experiment could do, and in no position to resist.

Some of this testing had been beneficial, such as the experiments carried out in French orphanages which had helped develop a diphtheria antitoxin. But much of it was barbaric, with children being denied proper nourishment, injected with dangerous substances, and subjected to intense levels of pain.[28]

When Koprowski went to Letchworth, he was not working in a vacuum. The so-called Nuremberg Code of 1947, adopted in response to Nazi medical atrocities, had set down a series of ethical guidelines for researchers to follow. Among these was the need for informed consent—an elastic goal when dealing with children. Most ethicists agreed that such experiments could be undertaken with the blessing of a parent or a guardian, when children were "peculiarly suitable" as test subjects, when there was "no discernable hazard" to their health, and when they might "directly benefit" from the results.[29]

Whether the Letchworth experiments met all, or any, of these criteria would become a matter of angry debate. What is clear is that Koprowski had crossed a divide that others soon would be crossing as well. Years later David Bodian would praise the human testing done at Letchworth as a "turning point" in the development of a successful vaccine. It was, he said, the natural—and courageous—next step in the battle against polio.[30]

Koprowski recalled Letchworth with typical bravado. "If we did such a thing now," he said recently, "[we'd] be put in jail and the company would be sued." Of course, he added, "If Jenner or Pasteur or Theiler or myself had to repeat and test our discoveries [today], there would be no smallpox vaccine, no rabies vaccine, no yellow fever vaccine, and no live oral polio vaccine."[31]

As with so much else in the life and career of Albert Sabin, the true motives for his assault on Koprowski that day are hard to untangle. No one denied that Sabin could be obnoxious. His best friends described him as arrogant, egotistical, and occasionally cruel. Yes, Albert was a know-it-all and something a bully, they would say, but he did it for a cause. He was an ethical man, a defender of scientific principles, unfailingly generous to those who shared his lofty goals. "With his white shock of hair," a colleague recalled, he "evoked images of the Old Testament prophets. . . . He often told us what we needed to know but were not all always willing to hear."[32]

Others, though, saw a different Albert Sabin—a sharp-elbowed careerist, jealous, hypercompetitive and determined to punish those who invaded his turf. "Sabin was a mean goddamn bastard," said Maurice Hilleman, a pioneer in vaccine research. "Smart. But a brainsucker. He went from one field to another, always sneaking in." Asked years later to explain Sabin's glowing obituaries, Hilleman snapped: "Hell, everyone would have enjoyed writing that one."[33]

The real Sabin, it appears, lay somewhere in between. Sprinkled through the correspondence of polio researchers are letters praising him for his generosity and others damning him for his duplicity. In one, a colleague at the Rockefeller Institute, Walter Schlesinger, accuses Sabin of taking too much credit for a collective discovery—a charge Sabin denied. "But then, that's our boy," Schlesinger confided, "and all of us who know Albert admire him and detest him at the same time for the same reasons. He deserves a comeuppance."[34]

Albert Bruce Sabin was born in Bialystok, Poland, near the Russian border, in 1906. When he was fifteen, his family came to the United States to escape the murderous pogroms that erupted there following World War I. The Sabins settled in Paterson, New Jersey, an immigrant textile center, where his father took a job as a weaver. Fluent in Polish and German, but knowing no English, Sabin was tutored by a cousin who encouraged him to avoid the dead-end life of the silk mills by getting an education.

According to Sabin, he went to the principal at Paterson High School and handed him his records, written in Polish. The principal asked for a translation. "He said, 'Where would you be now?' I said I was the equivalent of a sophomore in high school, and he replied, 'I'll put you in as a sophomore; if you flunk, you start over. If you pass, you continue.'" It was, Sabin added, "a very nice arrangement."[35]

Sabin passed. He powered through high school, working long hours on the side. Then, in a remarkable stroke of luck, an uncle by marriage—a dentist living in Manhattan—offered him a deal. "He said that if I would come to live with them, he'd pay my tuition if I became a dentist too," Sabin recalled. "So in 1923, I went to pre-dental school at New York University and then two years of dental school."[36]

Sabin hated the dentistry but loved the science. The courses in pharmacology and biochemistry turned his interest toward medical research; so, too, did the publication of two best-selling books. "*Microbe Hunters* by Paul de Kruif was a great stimulus," Sabin noted. "And then *Arrowsmith*, and all that. I said, 'That's me. That's the life I want to lead.'"[37]

When Sabin quit dentistry in 1926, his uncle cut him off. With no money for medical school, and no hope of being admitted, he called upon the one person he knew with the power to help—William Hallock Park. Sabin had taken Park's graduate course in bacteriology as a dental student. "I gave him a hard-luck story," Sabin said. "I must have broken his heart." Park offered Sabin a menial job in his laboratory. He also opened the door to medical school. Park had that sort of influence. As a bacteriologist, he had prepared the first diphtheria antitoxin used in the United States. And as director of New York City's Bureau of Laboratories, he had become a towering figure in the field of public health. Park had been at New York University since 1900, serving as department chairman and medical school dean. He was "my champion," Sabin recalled: "the illustrious, gentle and warm-hearted Dr. Park."[38]

When Sabin couldn't pay his tuition, Park got him a scholarship. When Sabin needed money for food and rent, Park found him a part-time job at Harlem Hospital, taking sputum samples from pneumonia patients. "I didn't have much time to be very good student," Sabin recalled, "because I had to rush from the medical school to the hospital, work till late at night, then study a couple of hours, get up in the morning, and take the subway back."[39]

Still, the job paid other dividends. To Park's amazement, Sabin developed a method for the rapid typing of pneumococci, turning what had been an overnight process into one that now took two or three hours. Park proudly called it "the Sabin method" and claimed that it saved lives. He also submitted the results to a scientific journal, which earned his student a kind of celebrity status at NYU. When Sabin graduated in 1931, his yearbook blurb caught the future all too well:

Walls reverberate a beautiful voice,
It's mello, basso, it's strong and it's choice,
Is't Stentor? Still—not the drop of a pin,
No; 't is none other than the great Sabin.
He taught the pneumococcus how to type,
And thereby did save the white mouse's life.
Altho he's apart and sometimes aloof.
Soon we'll be proud to say, "I knew that goof."[40]

The summer following Sabin's graduation saw a major polio outbreak in New York City. As a house physician at Bellevue, NYU's teaching hospital, Sabin got to see the disease at close range. In 1933, he published his first article on the subject, beginning a career in polio research that would span six decades. No one, wrote John Paul, "ever contributed so much effective information—and so continuously over so many years—to so many aspects of poliomyelitis, as Sabin."[41]

One of his tasks at Bellevue was to perform autopsies on polio victims, a skill that would serve him well in the future. The job took on a personal edge when a researcher in Park's laboratory, William Brebner, died from a monkey bite. Sabin assisted in the autopsy and wrote up the case: "Dr. W.B., 29 years old, engaged in experimental work on poliomyelitis . . . was bitten on the dorsum of the left ring and little fingers. The wounds . . . were superficial . . . and Dr. B. continued his work. . . . " Within days, however, Brebner's body cramped up, his temperature rose to 104.8, and he complained of "pain in the upper extremities." His breathing slowed as paralysis reached his chest. "Despite partial aspiration . . . and other supportive measures, he lived only 5 more hours."[42]

Some suspected polio. Others blamed a herpes virus common to monkeys. But Sabin claimed to have discovered an entirely new agent, which he called virus B in Brebner's honor. "Well, Sabin was never bashful," said Tom Rivers, "and he came up to the [Rockefeller] institute . . . to show me his work." Rivers was impressed. The case was strong, he recalled, and it got even stronger when "several other workers were bitten by monkeys and died, and this same virus was recovered."[43]

Sabin's reputation soared. In 1934 he won a fellowship from the National Research Council to study viruses at the elite Lister Institute in London. As elsewhere, his personality and work habits evoked a powerful response. When he applied for a position at the Rockefeller Institute, J.C.G. Ledingham, director of the Lister Institute, sent this message to New York: "I hear you are [thinking of] taking on Dr. Sabin. I should warn you that for Heaven's sake don't! While he has a brilliant mind, he has used up every monkey in the place!"[44]

Sabin got the job. "God, he was a sight," said Tom Rivers, describing the "British" Sabin who returned from his twelve-month fellowship abroad. "He wore tweed jackets and fancy vests and smoked a pipe. He was the most elegant dresser in the entire Institute, but more important, he quickly showed that he was also capable of doing elegant work in the laboratory."[45]

That, at least, was what Rivers said in public. Privately, he spun a rather different tale, recalling how he blistered the young man's pretensions: "God damn you, Sabin! You can't turn a cheap East Side Jew into an Englishman in one year! Don't you ever come to see me with spats on again. Don't you ever speak to me in that broad accent again." Rivers noted, with great relish, that his words had done some good. "You know, by God, he went back to being an East Side Jew, and he's been all right ever since."[46]

In truth, Rivers did speak highly of Sabin's work to Simon Flexner. But he also made it clear that he had no room for Sabin in his own division at Rockefeller Institute and would like him assigned to someone else. He recommended Peter Olitsky, a Jew, who quickly agreed. "Having worked successfully with geniuses before," Olitsky recalled, "I was anxious to have him as an associate."[47]

Sabin entered a workplace loaded with young talent. The list of those who apprenticed under Peter Olitsky in these years reads like a who's who of the later polio crusade—Herald Cox, Walter Schlesinger, Jerome Syverton, and Isabel Morgan, to name a few. But even here, Albert Sabin stood apart from the rest. His nonstop schedule was duly noted by colleagues with a mixture of awe and contempt. He didn't go on vacations or take Sundays off. He worked. Forced by Olitsky to go on a short honeymoon in 1934, Sabin wired his boss: "MARRIED . . . HAPPY . . . BACK NEXT WEEK."[48]

His experiments drew widespread attention. Using monkeys, for example, he demonstrated that bulbar polio—the most serious form— occurred more frequently after tonsillectomies, when the nerves of the mouth and the throat were directly exposed. His finding, confirmed by others, led many doctors and dentists to postpone tonsil, adenoid, and major oral surgery during the summer polio season.[49]

One of the great benefits of the Rockefeller Institute was the interplay among researchers. Early on Sabin met Max Theiler, a South African émigré who took a fatherly interest in his career. Theiler was then experimenting with a live-virus vaccine for yellow fever. (Its success would earn him the Nobel Prize for medicine in 1951.) As Tom Rivers recalled, no one "ever had to draw Albert a picture of the implications of any virus research. He always had a mind and imagination of his own." But Theiler's work had a profound impact on Sabin by strengthening his belief that lasting immunity to disease depended upon a natural infection with a living agent—in short, a live-virus vaccine.[50]

Working life at the institute was not without its drawbacks. Like others there, Sabin felt hamstrung by the influence of Simon Flexner, whose firmly held theories about polio still dominated the field. Though Flexner could be very generous to junior colleagues, one rule was absolutely clear: polio was the director's primary domain. Nobody worked on the disease without Flexner's express permission—an arrangement that tied the hands of those seeking new approaches to the disease. As a junior member and a man with great survival instincts, Sabin was extremely deferential in his dealings with Flexner.[51]

In 1939 Sabin got an offer from the University of Cincinnati to become an associate professor of pediatrics in the medical school and a research fellow in virology at the Children's Hospital. The $6,000 annual salary—about double his current pay—was certainly appealing. And, the joint appointment allowed him to mix clinical work and laboratory research in an independent setting, where he alone would determine the agenda. Sabin's letter of resignation was brief but sincere. "After a great deal of deliberation, I have decided to leave 'home,'" he said, "and have a try at the opportunities offered by the Children's Hospital Foundation."[52]

Though hardly among the nation's top medical schools, Cincinnati had a number of strong departments, with pediatrics heading the list. "Albert has been a very happy member of our group," the department chair wrote Olitsky. "He has been a great stimulant . . . and it is a fine thing that we are able to have him with us." The Sabins bought a house in one of Cincinnati's finer neighborhoods, with a garden, fruit trees, and a large expanse of lawn. "I've become a country squire," he told a friend. "I shall have to watch out that my work does not decrease as my comforts increase."[53]

He needn't have worried. In 1939 Sabin won the Theobold Smith Medal, awarded by the American Association for the Advancement of Science to "men under thirty-five" for his work on "infantile paralysis and the properties of viruses." A year later, the *New York Times* profiled a discovery of his regarding a possible cause of arthritis, and the popular magazine *Science* credited him with identifying a type of encephalitis never before seen in North America. For Cincinnati, Sabin was a godsend—a rising star with a gift for the spotlight.[54]

But problems soon emerged. Conditions at Cincinnati could not hope to match those at the Rockefeller Institute, where the laboratories were supremely well-stocked. "It is going to be almost impossible to do any polio research for some time," Sabin complained. "There are only 25 monkeys in the Cincinnati zoo. I bought only 4 and had to spend $12 a piece. While they do breed here, they haven't gone in for it in a big way, i.e. the zoo people, not the monkeys."[55]

For this problem, at least, there was a solution. In 1939 Sabin won his first grant from the National Foundation—$7,000. "Together with my regular budget," he told Olitsky, "it gives us quite a sizeable sum to work with." The foundation liked its money spent quickly, as a visible sign of progress, and the prolific Sabin was happy to oblige. "I have just received another $11,300 grant," he wrote John Paul in 1941, "and I expect to use it all in the next six months."[56]

To most people he knew, Sabin described life in Cincinnati in glowing terms. To Peter Olitsky, his mentor and confidant, he told a different story. He had made a mistake in leaving the institute and hoped to come back "home."

Part of the problem was intellectual. Sabin missed the high-powered atmosphere of the institute, the fluid give-and-take of ideas, the contact with "scientifically more congenial people." And part of the problem was personal. Sabin did not much like doctoring to children. "I am not a pediatrician," he wrote Olitsky, "and after two years' experience, I know I don't want to be one." The plain truth, he said, is that "I am not happy here and it does not seem to be the place where I hope to spend the next ten, perhaps most fruitful, years of my life."[57]

Olitsky was sympathetic. He agreed to "feel out Tom Rivers on the matter," but his approach didn't go well. "Though Tom admires your wonderful work, your capacity, your drive to do everything yourself," Olitsky reported, "I cannot say that [his] reaction to my overtures was what you would consider pleasant." Rivers preferred to "admire" Sabin from a safe distance—in this case, about 600 miles.[58]

Like Jonas Salk, Sabin spent World War II studying viral diseases for the military. Unlike Salk, Sabin joined the armed forces and rose to the rank of lieutenant colonel in the Army Medical Corps. Where Salk's specialty had been influenza, Sabin worked on sandfly fever, a nasty but nonfatal illness common to soldiers in the Mediterranean, and Japanese B encephalitis, a sometimes deadly disease affecting the central nervous system. Much of his duty was spent in the Middle East, where, he told a friend, "I have been working in the only way I know—without pause or rest."[59]

Sabin had to put polio on the back burner. "It's definitely not a military *problem*," he agreed, although it did seem to strike more American and British soldiers—men between the ages of 20 and 40—than anyone had anticipated. "The only mystery as I see it," he wrote Olitsky, "is why the incidence is so much higher among [our] troops than among the natives." Sabin suspected that the natives, widely exposed to poliovirus as infants, had experienced the mild, natural infection that produces lifelong immunity. Many soldiers, by contrast, were encountering the virus for the first time.[60]

With the war over, Sabin returned to Cincinnati. His dreams of moving elsewhere had largely vanished. The medical school rewarded him with a professorship in research pediatrics, meaning he could see patients when he wished or not at all. Sabin would now work full-time in the laboratory, his only real home. He envisioned a stepped-up research effort against polio run by scientists, not bureaucrats, and led by experienced people like himself. As many would come to learn, his was not a voice to be taken lightly.

9

Seeing Beyond the Microscope

AMERICA NEAR THE MIDPOINT OF THE TWENTIETH CENTURY was quite different from the country we know today. The population of around 150 million included a small and declining number of foreign-born residents, the result of strict immigration quotas imposed in the 1920s. Most African Americans still lived in the South, where racial segregation was the law. Blue-collar workers outnumbered white-collar workers, and labor unions were at their peak. Major league baseball had only sixteen teams, none west of St. Louis. There were no shopping malls or motel chains or felt-tip pens. Commercial television was just beginning, rock music a few years away. Tobacco companies placed cigarette ads in medical journals. It cost three cents to mail a letter and a nickel to buy a Coke.

Marriage rates were at an all-time high, while divorce rates were declining. Cities were losing population. A huge middle class had developed, accompanied by suburban living, a baby boom, and an explosion of consumer goods. According to public opinion polls, most Americans were bullish about their future, having survived the Great Depression and emerged victorious from World War II. All things seemed possible; an almost palpable optimism prevailed.

In Pittsburgh Jonas Salk was living this postwar American dream. He and Donna had bought a house in the suburbs large enough to accommodate their three children—Peter, 8; Darrell, 6; and Jonathan, 2. Now a full professor at the medical school, Salk was earning $12,000 a year, more than twice the national average. He ran one of the best-equipped virus laboratories in the world. Grant money was pouring in.

His name had begun to appear in news stories about a possible break-through on the polio front. He was only thirty-six years old.

His schedule was grueling, with conferences, publications, and grant proposals piled on top of his research projects and administrative duties in the lab. He could barely find time for his family, much less the politics and activism of his earlier years. He assumed that the book had been closed on his political past. It turned out he was mistaken.

THE FEELINGS OF NATIONAL CONFIDENCE and optimism that flowed from World War II told one part of a complicated story. There were deep anxieties as well. In the fall of 1945, a prominent journalist observed: "There is no use dodging what is now plain: a serious cleavage has developed between Russia and the Western democracies." Before long, that cleavage had become a rupture, popularly known as the cold war. The Soviet advances in Eastern Europe, the Berlin Blockade, the "fall of China" to communism—all added fuel to the fire. At home, meanwhile, a series of spectacular spy trials led many to conclude that Russian agents and their sympathizers had penetrated deep into the fabric of American society. J. Edgar Hoover, the powerful FBI director, claimed that the United States now had one communist for every 1,814 people—a truly menacing ratio considering that Russia had only one communist for every 2,771 people in 1917, when the Bolshevik revolution occurred.[1]

President Harry Truman viewed such charges as wildly overblown. In private, he portrayed Hoover's FBI as a potential Gestapo. Yet Truman was a political realist, who understood the danger of appearing "soft" on communism as the cold war heated up. In 1947 he established the nation's first Federal Loyalty-Security Program, requiring the FBI to run background checks on all civilian workers in the executive branch. Those suspected of disloyalty—a term that ranged from outright espionage to "sympathetic association" with groups deemed "subversive" by the U.S. attorney general—faced the prospect of dismissal. Among the early targets was Jonas Edward Salk.[2]

Shortly after moving to Pittsburgh in 1947, Salk had been selected by the U.S. surgeon general to be a consultant in the field of epidemic disease. The appointment, though rather routine, meant a lot to a young scientist on the move. Salk viewed it as a key marker in his professional life, a sign of his growing stature and success. He noted it proudly on his early resumes and kept listing it over the years as larger honors poured in. As a consultant to the federal government, Salk was subject to a background check. Trouble came quickly. FBI agents regularly swapped information with staffers from the House Un-American Activities Committee (HUAC), which kept extensive files on "subversive groups," complete with their publications and membership lists. As luck would have it, a HUAC report had once cited an obscure journal called *Social Work Today* as "pro-Communist." And *Social Work Today* had once lauded the good deeds of Jonas E. Salk, then an intern at Mount Sinai Hospital in Manhattan.[3]

Between 1948 and 1952, the FBI carried out more than four million of these federal background checks. In cases where "derogatory information" was found, the Civil Service Commission could order a full field investigation of the employee, an exhaustive procedure involving FBI offices throughout the country. In all, the bureau handled about 20,000 such probes, involving less than one percent of the federal work force. Salk got caught in this dragnet.[4]

Four FBI field offices took part in his investigation. Agents fanned out to interview friends, colleagues, and neighbors. Others combed suspect publications and membership lists in search of his name. The first probes, conducted in 1950, linked Salk to several "pro-Communist" groups during his years at Mount Sinai and at the University of Michigan. In 1941 he supposedly joined the "Communist-controlled" American Labor Party. In 1946 he allegedly served as secretary-treasurer of the Independent Committee of the Arts and Sciences and Professions of Michigan, a group cited by HUAC, among others, as pro-Communist. In between, it was said, he had joined, contributed to, or appeared on the mailing lists of the National Council of American-Soviet Friendship, the American Association of Scientific Workers, the New York Conference for Inalienable Rights, and Russian War Relief—all "reliably reported" to be Communist fronts.[5]

The FBI compiled a mountain of raw information. Salk's confidential file runs to more than three hundred pages. Agents found his American Labor Party registration card by sifting through voter records at the New York City Board of Elections. They linked him to Communist fronts through verbal tips and mailing lists provided by "informants of known reliability." They even produced the affidavit showing that Salk had added the middle name "Edward" in 1938.

The most damaging information came from interviews at the University of Michigan. Two of Salk's former colleagues described him as "far left of center," "outspoken in praise of Russia during World War II," and a "guiding spirit" behind numerous Communist fronts on the campus. The bureau's Detroit office reported that Salk's younger brother Lee, a student at the university in these years, had belonged to a "Marxist Study Group," as well as the local Communist Party, while living with Jonas and Donna. In addition, the Salk brothers had supported a campaign by the Campus Inter-Racial Association "to compel Ann Arbor barbers to cut the hair of students regardless of race."[6]

Salk's full field investigation reached the surgeon general's office in the summer of 1950, an ominous season marked by the arrests of Julius and Ethel Rosenberg for conspiracy to commit atomic espionage and by the start of the Korean War. The contents set off predictable alarm bells; army security officers, concerned mostly with Salk's activities in Ann Arbor, asked the FBI to re-interview his primary accusers. This was done with some reluctance, given the bureau's hefty cold war workload. "Case reopened for additional information upon request of the Department of the Army," reads a 1951 memo in Salk's file.[7]

The second round of interviews went better for him. Questioned more pointedly this time, Salk's accusers were unsure of themselves, unable to recall specific details, and unwilling to give sworn depositions. One of them even put a sympathetic face on Salk's political outlook, which, he said, "seemed to support the ideas of the Soviet regime."

> [Source] stated that during this period of time [Salk] was dissatisfied, extremely bitter, and fearful of the future. He stated that [Salk] appeared to be frustrated as a result of repressive influences in his appointment at the University . . . and remarked that it was quite possible that [Salk's] ideas . . . are simply a release from that frustration.

What emerges from these various FBI reports is Salk's powerful commitment to left-wing activism at an early stage in his life, a commitment encouraged by his wife, Donna, and ignited by the twin crises of the 1930s, the Great Depression and the rise of Nazi Germany. There was nothing clandestine about his behavior. At Mount Sinai and again at Michigan, Salk immersed himself in radical politics and in medical research, seeing a clear humanitarian connection between the two. Phrases like "an extremely honest man, outspoken in his views" and "so honest that he could not help express the way he felt" appear throughout the FBI interviews. Colleagues—critical and friendly— noted Salk's devotion to equal rights, fair employment, and better health care. They recalled him picketing businesses that refused to serve minorities, protesting loyalty oaths for faculty members, and advocating socialized medicine. Few, however, regarded his behavior as in any way threatening to the United States. "With the exception of two professional associates," the FBI report concluded, "all other individuals interviewed during the course of this investigation recommend subject highly."[8]

The Civil Service Commission agreed, ruling Salk "eligible on loyalty." It did not summon him to a hearing. Had it done so, he might have been dropped as a consultant and denied a security clearance. And that, in turn, could have ended his scientific career. Universities in early cold war era were notorious for terminating faculty members with "political problems." So, too, were the private granting agencies that depended so heavily on public donations. It is hard to imagine a scenario in which the image-conscious National Foundation would have chosen a "loyalty risk" to lead its meticulously scripted battle against polio.[9]

Salk probably knew of these probes. Would he have not received some signal from one or more of the dozens of people interviewed by the FBI? Surprisingly, however, he made no mention of his "loyalty problems" in his extensive correspondence with friends and colleagues and officials at the medical school and beyond. And he never mentioned these problems to his children, two of whom worked closely with him in their later professional lives. "Had he been aware of all this, I think he would have told us," said Darrell Salk. "On the other hand, he never talked about his radical politics, either. He seemed to slam the door on that part of his life."[10]

Apparently so. The FBI reports filed from Pittsburgh portray a dramatically different Jonas Salk, a man with no political identity. "Neither the appointee nor his wife has taken an active part in community affairs since their arrival [in 1947]," said one. "Appointee unknown to Pittsburgh confidential informants," said another. "Fellow employees believe him loyal." Salk's life was different now. He had a lab to run and a career moving forward at breakneck speed. Every ounce of his energy was directed toward a single goal: a vaccine against polio.[11]

There is an interesting footnote to this episode, however. Several years later, a number of University of Pittsburgh faculty members, horrified by the lynching of a black teenager named Emmett Till in Mississippi, invited a minister to campus to speak about racial terror in the

South. Salk attended the event, at which money was raised and a local civil rights newsletter begun. "I asked Jonas about his reaction," a colleague recalled, "hoping to discuss the matter with him and get his thoughts. He informed me that he had not read the newsletter. In fact he was no longer receiving it; he had asked the minister to remove his name from the mailing list. 'Why?' I asked. The answer shocked me. . . . Jonas [said] that now that he was becoming a public figure it was not good for his name to be associated with partisan causes. He did not want any attachment . . . to a potential 'left-wing' group. One must realize that this was the McCarthy era, an important context in which to judge his actions."[12]

Donna Salk, meanwhile, was busy raising three young boys. In later years, when the children were older, she would lend her name to a host of thoroughly mainstream groups and causes, such as the League of Women Voters and the Pittsburgh Commission on Human Rights. Though the local press would sometimes describe her as "an advocate for the underdog," she took great pains to portray herself as a traditional housewife and mother, "carrying out my beliefs and principles in a voluntary capacity." In 1950s America, it was the safe and natural thing to say.[13]

THE RULING OF THE CIVIL SERVICE COMMISSION came at a pivotal time. Truth be told, the typing program that had triggered Jonas Salk's career in polio research soon bored him to tears. Salk learned quickly that David Bodian had been right: there were three distinct types of poliovirus, and the chances of finding another one were slim. It was clear, he wrote Harry Weaver in 1949, "that the Leon virus represents a third immunologic type . . . unrelated to Brunhilde or Lansing." And equally clear, he added, that the full picture would emerge "before this year is up."[14]

Salk had bigger plans. In the spring of 1950, he revealed them to Weaver in meticulous detail. Besides typing virus strains, Salk admitted, his lab had begun to experiment on "the prevention of poliomyelitis by immunologic means." Monkeys had already been tested with vaccine solutions containing live and killed poliovirus—a hint, it appears, that Salk was keeping both options open. Work was also proceeding on the use of adjuvants—vaccine additives designed to jolt the immune system—as well as on different techniques for inactivating poliovirus, such as formaldehyde and ultraviolet light.

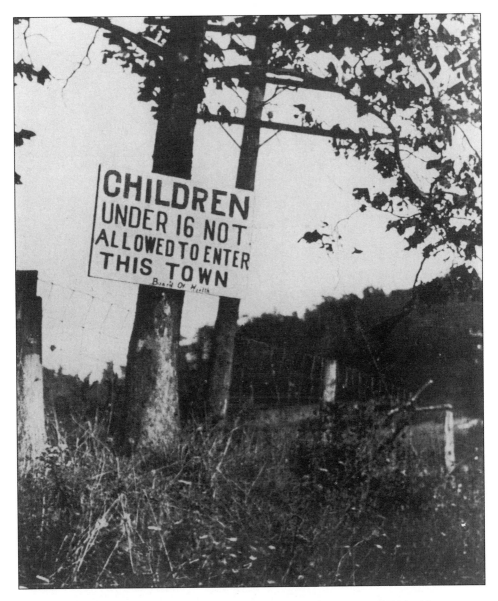

The United States experienced its first major polio outbreak in the summer of 1916, with the epidemic centered in New York City. Many surrounding communities closed their doors to outsiders, using heavily armed policemen to patrol the roads and rail stations in search of fleeing New Yorkers and their children. The epidemic lasted through October, claiming 27,000 American lives. New York City reported 8,900 cases and 2,400 deaths, 80 percent being children under five. *March of Dimes.*

Polio was still a "new" disease to most Americans when it victimized Franklin D. Roosevelt in 1921. Thirty-nine years old, robust and athletic, with a cherished family name, he seemed an unlikely candidate for a disease that appeared to target children from the slums. Paralyzed from the waist down, Roosevelt would go to great lengths to disguise his disability from the public. Photographers were discouraged from taking pictures of him in a wheelchair; reporters and columnists rarely mentioned his paralysis. For his part, Roosevelt spent his life in search of a cure. These rare photos, taken in the 1930s, show him fishing in his leg braces and exercising in the pool at Warm Springs, Georgia. Right, *March of Dimes;* below, *AP/Wide World Photos.*

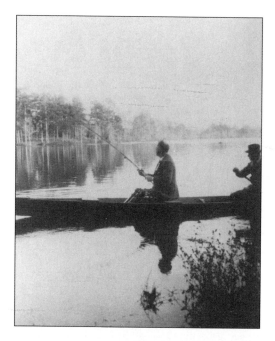

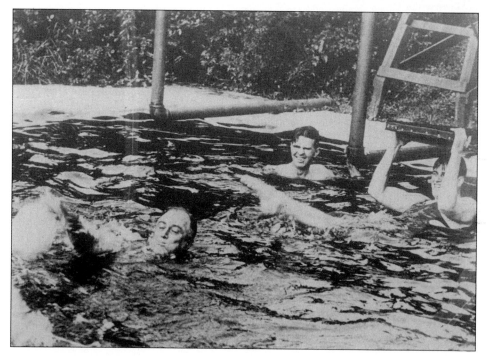

When FDR decided to return to politics in 1928, he chose his Wall Street law partner, Basil ("Doc") O'Connor, to run the Warm Springs Foundation. A decade later, Roosevelt selected O'Connor to head up the newly created National Foundation for Infantile Paralysis. Raised in the Catholic working-class town of Taunton, Massachusetts, a graduate of Dartmouth College and Harvard Law School, O'Connor turned the National Foundation into the largest voluntary health organization of all time. Its success in raising

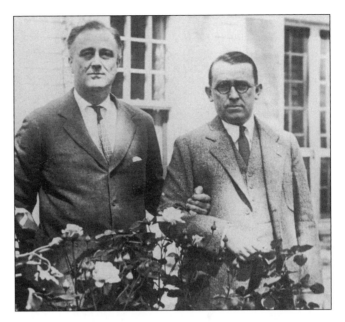

money, generating publicity, caring for polio patients, and sponsoring medical research would serve to redefine the role—and methods—of private philanthropies in the United States. *March of Dimes.*

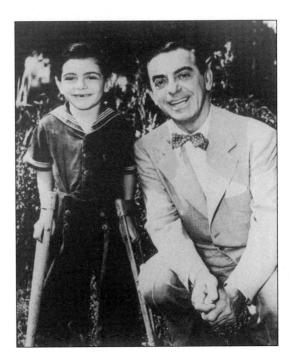

From the start, the National Foundation relied on the star power of celebrities such as Eddie Cantor to raise funds. A veteran of vaudeville, silent movies, and the *Ziegfeld Follies*, Cantor had emerged in the 1930s as the nation's highest-paid performer, starring in big-budget Hollywood musicals while hosting a popular weekly radio program. In 1938, Cantor suggested the fund-raising approach that would become a staple of future polio campaigns: the "March of Dimes." *March of Dimes.*

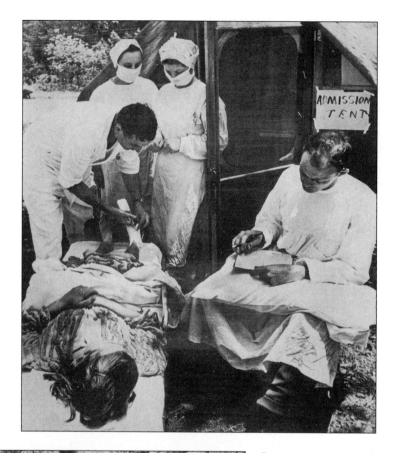

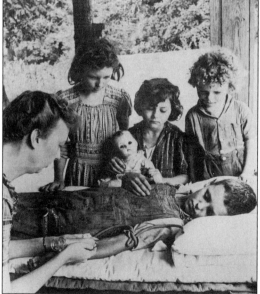

In summer 1944, a polio epidemic tore through the Catawba River Valley of rural North Carolina, its epicenter being the furniture-making town of Hickory. Public events were cancelled, and swimming pools, movie theaters, and libraries were closed. People drove through town with their car windows rolled up, and trains sped through without stopping. Viewing the crisis in Hickory as both a humanitarian challenge and a public relations bonanza, the National Foundation worked with local officials to build and staff a makeshift polio hospital in 54 hours. Iron lungs and medical supplies were flown in; orthopedic nurses arrived from the University of Minnesota and physical therapists from Johns Hopkins. The Yale Polio Unit sent in a team of physicians, including Dorothy Horstmann, pictured here drawing blood from a patient. Before closing its doors, the hospital treated 454 patients. Two-thirds were said to have "recovered completely." *March of Dimes.*

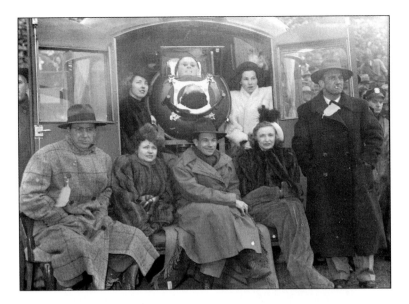

The iron lung became the most terrifying symbol of polio's destructive power. Invented in 1928 by a Harvard University engineer named Philip Drinker, this airtight chamber was designed to assist patients with damaged breathing muscles by exerting a push-pull motion on the chest through alternating pressure that forced the diaphragm to expand and contract.

Above: Though not intended for long-term use, the iron lung became a home of sorts for severely paralyzed patients such as Fred Snite, Jr. (pictured here watching a Notre Dame football game). Stricken with polio in 1936, Snite would spend the rest of his life in an iron lung, becoming a well-publicized voice for polio survivors. "If it's God's will that I be cured I will be; if not I won't," he said. "I figure I have a right to ask only one thing: the strength to face up to it." *Notre Dame Archive.*

Below: An iron lung ward in a Boston hospital during an epidemic in the 1950s. *March of Dimes.*

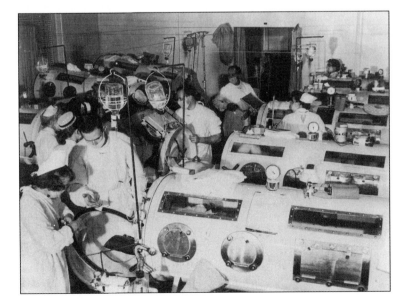

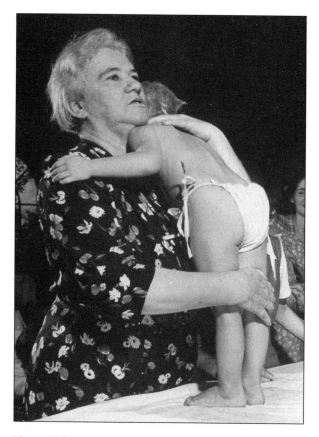

No one did more to modernize the ways in which polio
patients were rehabilitated than Sister Elizabeth Kenny,
shown here demonstrating her methods before an appreciative
audience in Arkansas in 1942. Seeing polio as a spasm of the
muscles rather than a disease of the nerves, the Australian-
born Kenny rejected the traditional philosophy of polio
aftercare, which called for immobilizing the damaged limbs
with splints and body casts, in favor of a more active therapy
that relied on hot packs and exercise to loosen and reeducate
the "alienated" muscles. By the 1940s, Kenny had become an
international celebrity, scorned by the medical establishment
but adored by millions of faithful supporters. *Ed Clark/Getty
Images.*

Facing Page

In 1946, the March of Dimes introduced its first official polio poster child, Oregon's Donald
Anderson. The poster contained two photographs, the first showing Donald at age three in
his hospital crib, bandaged and braced. The second one showed him at age six, striding
confidently into the future. Donald also posed with numerous celebrities, such as Yankee
slugger Joe DiMaggio. The message was simple: a beautiful child, once perilously close to
death, had been restored to health through the contributions of ordinary Americans to the
March of Dimes. In truth, Donald Anderson's road to recovery was far more difficult than
the public ever knew. *March of Dimes.*

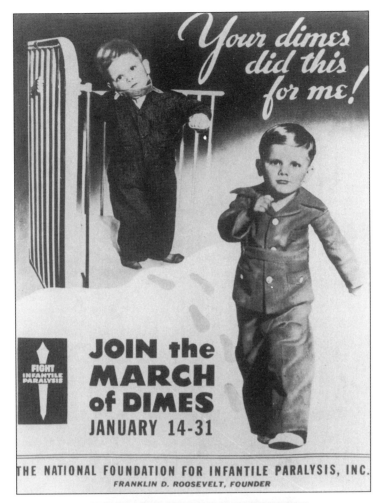

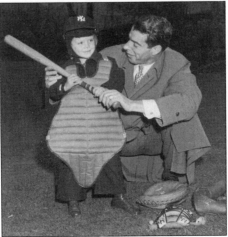

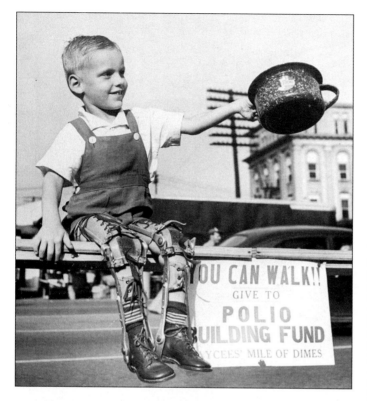

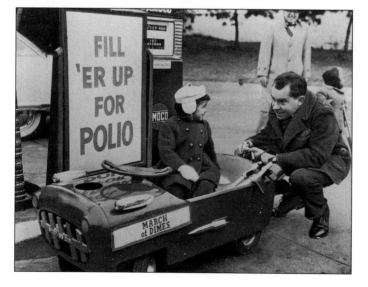

The March of Dimes relied heavily on polio patients and public figures to raise money for the cause. The top photo shows a child in leg braces soliciting funds for a new polio hospital in High Point, North Carolina, in 1946. *Martha Holland/ Getty Images.* The bottom photo is of Vice President Richard Nixon pumping gas for polio in 1954. *March of Dimes.*

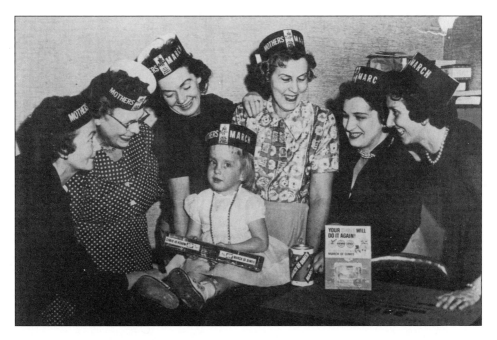

In 1950, the local March of Dimes chapter in Phoenix, Arizona, organized a "Mothers' March on Polio" to raise funds through a door-to-door canvass of every neighborhood in the city. People were urged to show their support for the march by leaving a porch light burning to welcome the volunteers. The Mothers' March spread quickly to other towns and cities, involving tens of thousands of women and becoming, for one night each year, the largest charitable army in the nation. *March of Dimes.*

Monkeys and chimpanzees proved invaluable in the war against polio. Not only did they become the basic experimental animals for studying the disease, but their kidneys were used to grow and harvest the poliovirus that went into the polio vaccine. In 1949, the National Foundation established a special facility known as Okatie Farms in rural South Carolina to process the thousands upon thousands of monkeys arriving from India, the Philippines, and elsewhere around the world. *Getty Images.*

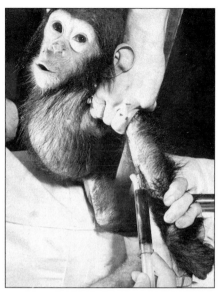

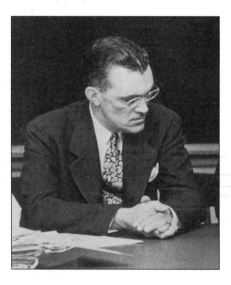

Harry Weaver is one of the unsung heroes of the polio crusade. As the National Foundation's director of research from 1946 to 1953, he led the effort to develop a successful vaccine. By changing the way in which grants were funded, administered, and renewed, Weaver sped the pace of medical research in the United States. *March of Dimes.*

To produce an effective polio vaccine, several problems had to be overcome. As late as the 1940s, researchers still were not certain how poliovirus entered the body, how many types of the virus existed, or whether it circulated in the blood. Perhaps the biggest hurdle, however, involved the growing of poliovirus safe enough for use in a vaccine. In 1948, John Enders (left), Thomas Weller (right), and Frederick Robbins discovered that poliovirus could be grown in test tube cultures of non-nerve animal tissue, providing a safe and plentiful reservoir of the virus. For their efforts, the three were awarded the Nobel Prize in 1954—the only polio researchers to be so honored. *March of Dimes.*

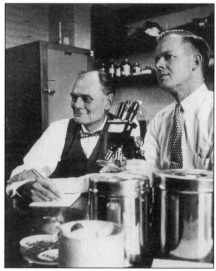

Working at Johns Hopkins, Isabel Morgan was the first researcher to successfully test a killed-virus polio vaccine on monkeys. In 1949, at the very height of her career, Dr. Morgan left Johns Hopkins to marry and raise a family. Had she continued her pioneering polio research, some believe she might have been the one who developed the vaccine that was mass-tested by the National Foundation in 1954. At the very least, Morgan blazed the trail that Jonas Salk followed to completion. *Courtesy Barbara Morgan Roberts.*

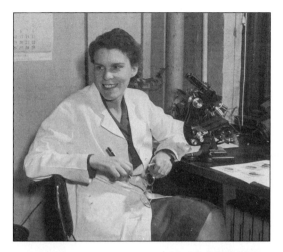

Working at Lederle Laboratories in Pearl River, New York, Polish-born researcher Hilary Koprowski developed a live-virus oral polio vaccine in the late 1940s, years before Jonas Salk and Albert Sabin produced polio vaccines of their own. Brilliant, outspoken, and controversial, the pioneering Koprowski would be plagued by concerns regarding the safety of his vaccine. *Yael Joel/Getty Images.*

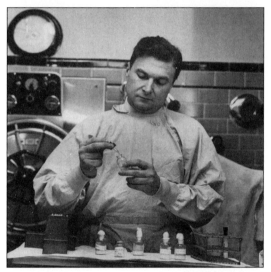

With generous funding from the National Foundation, Jonas Salk set up his laboratory in a hospital building on the University of Pittsburgh campus. Salk hired well, finding staffers and researchers who shared both his scientific vision and his workaholic ways (pictured here is Ethel Bailey). Over time, however, the extraordinary achievements of this group would be partly shadowed by claims that Salk did not fully acknowledge the crucial role played by his associates in the development of the polio vaccine. *March of Dimes.*

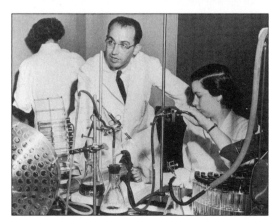

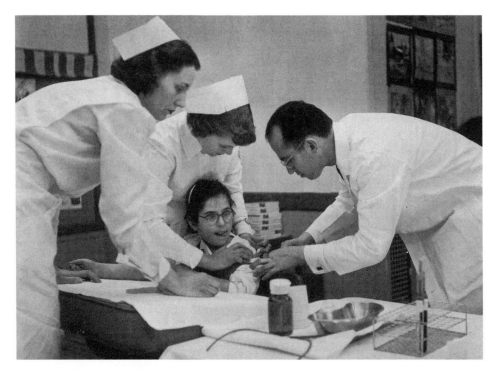

As a prelude to the mass vaccine trials of 1954, Jonas Salk tested his polio vaccine on children and adolescent "volunteers" in two institutions near Pittsburgh—the D. T. Watson Home for Crippled Children and the Polk School for the Retarded and Feeble-Minded. In this era, such human testing was a common practice. Salk had already inoculated his family with the vaccine. He received the enthusiastic support of the administrators running both local institutions and got parental permission for these vaccinations wherever possible. Some researchers, however, were uncomfortable about using institutionalized children for medical experiments. "An adult can do what he wants," complained Tom Rivers, the National Foundation's top medical advisor, "but the same does not hold true for a mentally defective child. Many of these children did not have mommas and papas, or if they did their mommas and papas didn't give a damn about them." *March of Dimes.*

Facing Page

The year 1952 would be the worst on record, with more than 57,000 cases nationwide. The 1952 polio season started before Memorial Day, gained ferocious momentum in the summer months, and pushed well into October.

Top: At a time when there was no way of preventing the disease, the National Foundation circulated a list of "polio precautions" for parents to follow. Towns and cities across the United States tried to prevent the spread of polio by closing swimming pools, libraries, and movie theaters, spraying DDT from trucks and airplanes, and encouraging children to play indoors. *March of Dimes.*

Bottom: A polio ward in Greensboro, North Carolina. *Getty Images.*

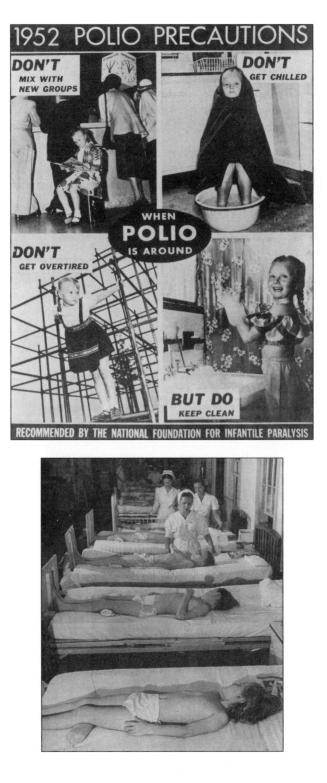

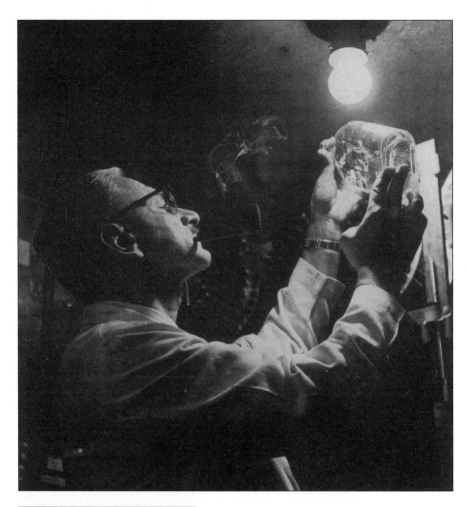

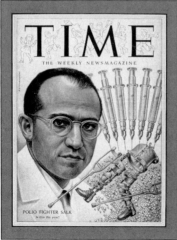

The bitter rivalry between Albert Sabin and Jonas Salk would dominate the polio vaccine crusade for half a century, beginning in the late 1940s and lasting until their deaths in the 1990s. Salk was the favorite of National Foundation administrators, especially Basil O'Connor, who understood that Salk's killed-virus vaccine could be developed more quickly than Sabin's live-virus vaccine. Sabin had the support of most polio researchers, who believed that the natural infection produced by a live-virus vaccine was essential in creating a powerful and permanent immunity to the disease. Sabin consistently belittled Salk, calling him "a kitchen chemist." Many scientists, unused to seeing one of their own grace the cover of *Time* magazine, viewed Salk as someone more interested in generating publicity for himself than in toiling anonymously in the laboratory, where a true researcher belonged. Sabin photo, *March of Dimes; Time* cover, *Time/Life Photos*.

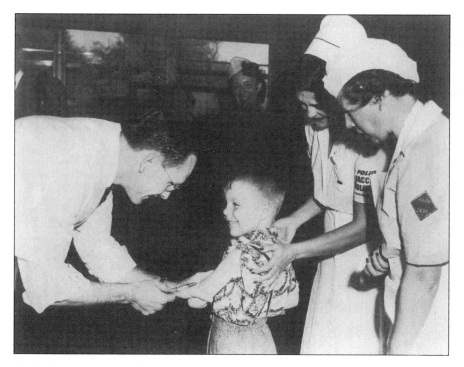

On April 12, 1954, Dr. Richard Mulvaney injected Salk polio vaccine into the left arm of six-year-old Randy Kerr at the Franklin Sherman elementary school in McLean, Virginia, beginning the largest public health experiment in American history. "I could hardly feel it," boasted the nation's first polio pioneer. "It hurt less than a penicillin shot." *March of Dimes.*

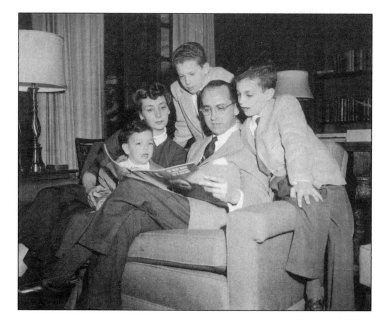

Jonas and Donna Salk and their three children, (left to right) Jonathan, age five; Peter, eleven; and Darrell, eight, relaxing in Ann Arbor, Michigan, on April 11, 1955, the day before the Francis Report was made public. *AP/ Wide World Photos.*

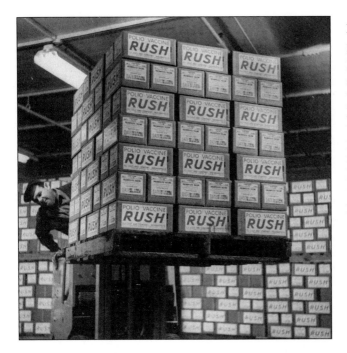

Anticipating that the Salk vaccine trials of 1954 would prove successful, National Foundation President Basil O'Connor contracted with several major drug companies to manufacture nine million doses of polio vaccine for the coming year. Under enormous pressure, the federal government licensed these doses in great haste, without proper supervision or testing. The consequences were severe. More than 200 polio cases were traced to contaminated lots of vaccine produced by Cutter Laboratories of Berkeley, California. Most of the victims were severely paralyzed; eleven people died. This photo shows the Salk vaccine being rushed to market early in 1955. *Al Fern/Getty Images.*

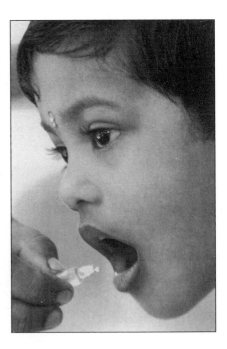

Polio still haunts isolated parts of the world despite persistent efforts to make it extinct. Three countries presently account for more than 95 percent of the remaining cases— Nigeria, India, and Pakistan. Here a child is being given drops of the Sabin oral polio vaccine in Madras, India, as part of the ongoing global polio eradication campaign. *M. Lakshman/AP/Wide World Photos.*

The next step was the big one: human testing. Salk was unaware of Hilary Koprowski's recent vaccine experiments with children; almost no one had been told of these tests, yet Salk didn't dare move without Weaver's approval. What he stressed, therefore, was his *willingness* to begin such testing the moment foundation officials gave him the green light. It was exactly the sort of message—eager, confident, aggressive— that seemed to separate him from the pack. "I think that the time has come," he told Weaver, for "these experiments to be carried out in man."[15]

Salk dealt frankly with the subjects he had in mind. He recommended both "institutionalized children" and "inmates of prisons" who might be coaxed to volunteer. "I have investigated the local possibilities for such an experiment," he said, "and find . . . there are institutions for hydro-cephalics and other similar unfortunates. I think we may be able to obtain permission for a study."[16]

Weaver's response was revealing. He appeared to seek a middle ground—a way of reminding Salk of his current responsibilities without thwarting his ambitious future plans. "I will have to insist," he be-gan, "that all funds expended from the appropriation set up to support the program of typing be expended exclusively for typing experiments." Of course, Weaver added, there was nothing to stop Salk from filing a new grant application aimed at "studies of the character you have out-lined." The words "human testing" were never mentioned, though Salk could hardly have missed the point. "I am very grateful to you," said Weaver, "for setting down your thoughts in such great detail."[17]

In the summer of 1951, Salk attended the Second International Po-liomyelitis Congress in Copenhagen, Denmark, to deliver the report of the virus typing committee. Though the results had been widely reported beforehand, it was symbolism that mattered most. The invi-tation, carefully scripted by Harry Weaver, marked Salk's emergence as a top polio researcher, elevating him to a level many thought he didn't deserve.[18]

The trip to Europe aboard the liner *Stockholm* made these feelings rather clear. To Salk, a week at sea with Albert Sabin was an experi-ence to be endured—and never repeated. "He really is a remarkable fellow," Salk recalled. "During the voyage . . . it became obvious to anyone who had not heard of it before that I was a nice young whip-persnapper from Pittsburgh, going to Denmark to report on some drudgery I had performed. I might have failed abysmally, it seemed clear, if Albert had not been up in the flies, pulling the strings and setting the standards. I was not quite Charlie McCarthy and Albert was not quite Edgar Bergen, but you can't have everything. It was an amusing trip."[19]

But also a lonely one. In truth, Sabin's perception was widely shared by others in the field. There was not a lot about the public Jonas Salk to cause the gods of science to stand up and take notice. His vita didn't contain the words "Rockefeller Institute" or include a prestigious fellowship year abroad. There were no links to Harvard, Johns Hopkins, or Yale. He lacked the breadth and brashness of a Sabin, the commanding presence of a Tom Rivers, the stunning originality of a David Bodian, the blueblood pedigree of a John Enders or a John Paul. His mentor, Thomas Francis, was widely respected but conservative to a fault. And Salk was marooned out there in Pittsburgh, fiddling with an old-fashioned killed-virus vaccine and doing the dog's work that his betters refused to do. In the tight, clubby world of virus research, he remained an outsider. A good technician, perhaps, but a lightweight as a thinker. He didn't fit in. He never would.

Salk's speech in Copenhagen was overshadowed by the presentations made by Enders, who reported the details of his 1948 tissue culture breakthrough, and then by Sabin, who did his best to explain why he and Olitsky had failed to achieve this breakthrough themselves. For the trip home, Harry Weaver reserved Salk a cabin on the *Queen Mary*, flagship of the Cunard Lines and the finest vessel afloat. He wanted Salk to meet Basil O'Connor, a fellow passenger on the ship. Weaver sensed they would get along well.

In some ways, it seemed a rather odd match. O'Connor was something of a dandy, brusque and bombastic, with his big cigars, hand-tailored suits, a suite at the Waldorf, and a corner table on hold at Manhattan's swank "21." His persona was almost guaranteed to offend a research scientist, and often did. Yet O'Connor had a lot in common with Salk, Weaver thought—in substance, if not in style. Each man came from a poor immigrant background and had been the first in his family to attend college. Each saw his work as his religion and had a perfectionist's eye for detail. Each looked upon the conquest of polio as a goal to be achieved quickly—not as a distant, elusive dream.

The two men met over dinner on the *Queen Mary*, joined by O'Connor's daughter Bettyann. The year before, in a remarkably cruel twist of fate, Bettyann Culver had phoned her father to say, "I think I've got some of your disease." At the age of 30, this mother of three was almost completely paralyzed on her left side. Her husband and one son suffered milder cases of polio at the same time. Following months of rehabilitation at Warm Springs, Bettyann Culver had regained movement everywhere except in her abdomen, where a set of muscles was permanently destroyed. "I never dreamed," said Basil O'Connor, "of polio hitting us."[20]

That ocean journey home began a friendship that would span the next twenty years. Where Thomas Francis had introduced Salk to the cloistered world of medical research, Basil O'Connor would launch him into the dizzying world of celebrity science. From their very first meeting, when he carefully gauged Salk's compassion for the plight of Bettyann Culver, O'Connor believed he had found someone special—a scientist who connected his laboratory work to the lives of ordinary people. O'Connor put it simply: "He sees beyond the microscope."[21]

By 1951, with the typing program now behind him, Salk moved seamlessly to the next plateau. Funding was no longer a problem. A huge grant from the National Foundation had just been approved. And Salk used much of it for physical expansion and new personnel, the object being to produce large quantities of safe poliovirus, a process made possible by the tissue culture breakthrough of John Enders and his colleagues a few years before. Salk acquired more lab space by taking over much of the basement of the largely vacant Municipal Hospital. He then hired Percival Bazeley, a veterinarian from Australia, to run the virus production process.

Bazeley is among the many faceless heroes of the polio crusade. A pioneer in the field of antibiotics, he had worked as a researcher at the prestigious Commonwealth Serum Laboratories in Melbourne before joining the army during World War II and commanding a tank battalion in New Guinea. In 1943, Bazeley was sent to the United States to study the methods for mass-producing penicillin. "He did it under the pressure of wartime," an Australian biographer noted, "incredibly fast, and with the amazing achievement that we were the first country in the world to provide penicillin to the civilian population." Bazeley had contacted Harry Weaver about returning to America to work on polio, and Weaver had passed his name on to Salk. Bazeley's vision was to produce poliovirus in the massive quantities required for the development of a successful vaccine.[22]

He wasn't alone. Working beside him were two recent additions to the Pittsburgh laboratory, Julius Youngner and Elsie Ward. Youngner, a World War II veteran associated with the Manhattan Project, had earned his PhD in microbiology from the University of Michigan. Specializing in cell culture techniques, he had worked at the National Cancer Institute before coming to Pittsburgh. Ward, a zoologist, specialized in growing viruses and keeping them alive. She served as Youngner's technician.[23]

Their job was to reproduce the Enders model in Salk's laboratory, growing poliovirus in non-nervous tissue. But their first attempt, using monkey testes, brought meager results. The good news was that cell cultures could be obtained without sacrificing expensive monkeys. The bad news, Youngner noted, was that "using monkey testicular tissue did not lend [itself] to large scale production of virus. [So] I began to look for more practical techniques."[24]

"After some intense work," Youngner added, "I realized that monkey kidney was the answer." A single such organ, properly handled, could produce enough raw material for 6,000 shots of polio vaccine. The process was exacting, to say the least. Though all the monkeys came from the foundation's Okatie Farms in South Carolina, Salk demanded that each one be given a "physical" by Jim Lewis and his staff. This done, the animal was anesthetized and its kidneys removed. The cortex (outer layer) was then separated, chopped into tiny fragments, and "rinsed several times with salt solution to remove blood and debris."[25]

The next step was the most ingenious. On his own, Youngner revived a largely forgotten process, developed at the Rockefeller Institute in 1916, that used trypsin, a powerful pancreatic enzyme, to separate tissue fragments into individual cells. The process was known as trypsinization, and without it the whole project might have failed. More cells meant more particles on which to grow poliovirus, the key to mass-producing a vaccine.[26]

There was good news from beyond Pittsburgh as well. In 1951 researchers at the University of Toronto's Connaught Laboratories developed the first synthetic nutrient for sustaining tissue culture, naming it "Medium 199" to denote the number of tries it took to get the product just right. Composed of more than sixty ingredients, from complex vitamins to simple table salt, Medium 199 provided an ideal diet for the monkey kidney cells, dramatically increasing their yield. Ever better, it did not contain the animal serums used in previous nutrient solutions, making it much safer for human use.[27]

The kidney cells were then seeded with live poliovirus. Kept in a gently rocking incubator, with the nutrient medium replaced every few days, the mixture was harvested, placed in large glass bottles, and passed through a series of sensitive filters to screen out impurities. What emerged, in the end, were impressive quantities of pure, undiluted virus.

Now came the matter of choosing the proper strains. This was a tricky business, a balance of risk and reward. Some strains were potent but dangerous, others tired but safe. "Essentially what is being searched for," wrote one observer, "is a [strain] powerful enough to cause immunity and yet docile enough to do no harm."[28]

It was a game of trial and error, testing and tinkering, and few knew it better than Jonas Salk. "We just put them in a race to see which performed most satisfactorily in tissue culture," he recalled. "Three of them gave brilliant, startling results, destroying monkey and human tissue right before our eyes. It was thrilling." To Salk, the logic was simple: a thorough process of inactivation could kill one virus strain as safely and easily as it could kill another. Confident of his methods, he chose the most virulent strains.[29]

Salk was making a public statement, showing supreme confidence in his laboratory and in himself. For Type I, responsible for more than 80 percent of all paralytic polio cases, Salk selected the controversial Mahoney strain, isolated in the lab of Thomas Francis in 1941. For Type II, he picked MEF (Middle East Forces), isolated at the Rockefeller Institute from the spinal tissue of a British soldier who had died during a polio outbreak in Egypt in 1943. For Type III, he chose the Saukett strain, isolated by Salk himself from the feces of a young polio victim at Municipal Hospital. "Others have spent years trying to find better ones," he noted. "So have I. But nobody has found one."[30]

The crew then inactivated these strains, one by one, employing the methods that Salk had learned at Michigan and refined in Pittsburgh. Repeated testing had shown that the best way to kill poliovirus was to use formaldehyde at a ratio of 250:1, keeping the mixture "immersed in an ice water bath" at one degree Celsius. Too much formaldehyde would reduce the vaccine's power to immunize against disease; too little might leave dangerous virus particles undisturbed. There was an art to it. The formaldehyde could not simply be poured into a vat and sloshed around. It needed to touch, envelop, and inactivate every drop of the mixture, a process known as "cooking" that demanded precision at each stage.

Numerous safety checks were run along the way. Julius Youngner invented a remarkable color test to note the presence of live virus in the vaccine. Monkeys were injected and watched for signs of polio. If even one took sick, the entire batch was destroyed. If all went well, the monkeys were sacrificed a month later and microscopically examined for any invasion of poliovirus. "I was overwhelmed by the complexity of this whole procedure," wrote a journalist with access to the laboratory, "[but] Salk insisted that the polio vaccine was 'one of the simplest medical preparations to manufacture.'"[31]

FOLLOWING THE COPENHAGEN CONFERENCE, Harry Weaver created an Immunization Committee to advise him on the development and testing of a polio vaccine. The twelve members—including Bodian, Enders, Francis, Paul, Rivers, Sabin, and Salk—ran the gamut of scientific thinking. There were live-virus advocates and killed-virus advocates (notably Francis and Salk). There were those who wanted human testing to begin sooner rather than later, and those who cautioned about the dangers of undue haste. There were even a few who questioned the scientific basis for a vaccine. As one member said: "A disease caused by a virus [usually] so benign that it safely immunizes well over 99% of the population without recognizable illness is obviously not a suitable subject for mass immunization if attended by *any* measurable risk. . . . Thousands [will be] injected who do not need it for every one who does."[32]

There were so many disparate voices on this committee—so many self-interested parties—that gridlock was inevitable. The first meeting, in December 1951, was devoted to Salk's recent killed-virus experiments on monkeys. Most members were skeptical. Their training had taught them that true immunity depended upon a natural infection, something that only a *living* agent could create. They didn't believe that a killed virus could produce antibody levels that were high enough or durable enough to protect against polio. And they worried that Salk, in confronting this dilemma, might be tempted to juice up his vaccine with the most potent strains of poliovirus known to science, a recipe for disaster if anything went wrong.

Salk spoke with quiet confidence that day. His experiments on monkeys had produced a powerful antibody response, he said, strong enough to neutralize a shot of live poliovirus to the brain. None of the monkeys had contracted polio or experienced an adverse reaction to his vaccine. Though Salk could make no claims about long-term effectiveness—it was still too early for that—his message was clear. The time for limited human testing had arrived.

The committee made no such recommendation. And Harry Weaver didn't request one, knowing full well it would have been turned down. Salk's presentation had been solid; it just hadn't changed any minds. To most of those present, the use of the virulent Mahoney strain, supplemented by a potentially dangerous adjuvant, seemed to argue *against* the effectiveness of a killed-virus vaccine. As Albert Sabin noted: "I am one of those people who believes that, if it is at all possible—this is theoretical—to infect an individual with an attenuated live virus, you have got your best immunizing agent."[33]

The majority agreed.

THE PROJECT WOULD HAVE TO BE DONE in secret. Only Tom Rivers, Harry Weaver, and Basil O'Connor were aware it. Unknown to the Immunization Committee, Salk had already convinced authorities at two local institutions—the D. T. Watson Home for Crippled Children and the Polk School for the Retarded and Feeble-Minded—to supply him with "volunteers."

Since minors were involved, the National Foundation for Infantile Paralysis wanted personal consent to protect itself against law suits and bad publicity. At the Watson Home this wasn't a big problem. Salk spoke to many of the parents himself, assuring them that the tests were safe and vital to "posterity." He proved to be a perfect ambassador for the project—a devoted scientist with three young boys of his own. Few turned him down.[34]

The Polk School was a harder sell. It contained patients with IQ scores "under 50," many of whom were long-term wards of the state. Until the 1940s, authorities in Pennsylvania had allowed public institutions to host all sorts of medical experiments. But times had changed; in 1944 the attorney general had intervened to stop a major vaccine trial at a state facility, claiming the government could not allow patients to be used as "guinea pigs" in a project where "many might suffer serious side effects" and "some might even die."[35]

There was a loophole, however. The 1944 ruling had involved a drug company that hoped to market a measles vaccine for profit. "Research for the benefit of the public may be one thing," the attorney general had written, "but participation . . . of mental patients for the benefit of a commercial laboratory engaged in a private enterprise, however laudable, may be quite a different one." Salk's vaccine project had an obvious humanitarian bent. It wasn't designed to make anyone rich.

Furthermore, the Polk School had experienced a minor polio outbreak the previous year, so an experimental vaccine could be viewed as a safety measure, offering future protection against the disease. In a letter to state authorities, Polk Superintendent Gale Walker made this point and others in pleading Salk's case. A mental institution offered an ideal setting, he said. The patients lived in a "controlled environment," rarely leaving the grounds. They could be counted on to show up for blood tests and inoculations. Their medical records were complete and up-to-date. And they now had the chance to help others in their own special way. "My personal reaction is intensely favorable," Walker concluded. "I believe that in no manner could the charge of using [our] patients for guinea pigs be leveled at us and I feel the association of my Institution in this project would do much to assist us in our attempts to gain a little professional dignity and acceptance [in the outside world]."[36]

The state of Pennsylvania agreed. Salk could run his experiments, it said, obtaining the permission of parents and guardians wherever possible. At the National Foundation, the ruling was greeted with a mixture of excitement and unease. Tom Rivers had never liked the idea of using institutionalized children. He had gone along, reluctantly, because he believed in Jonas Salk and the promise of his vaccine. But his conscience told him that something was wrong. "An adult can do what he wants," Rivers said, recalling the experiments of that era, "but the same does not hold true for a mentally defective child. Many of these children did not have any mommas and papas, or if they did their mommas and papas didn't give a damn about them."[37]

The Watson Home and the Polk School had little in common. The former was a rather elegant facility, located on the former estate of David T. Watson, a turn-of-the-century Pittsburgh lawyer who had made his fortune representing such notables as Andrew Carnegie and Henry Clay Frick. Originally intended as a refuge for "crippled, indigent white females," the Watson Home had become a leader in the field of polio rehabilitation. In the 1940s, its medical director, Jesse Wright, had invented the "rocking bed," an ingenious contraption that freed numerous polios from the claustrophobic terror of an iron lung.

As a grantee of the National Foundation, Dr. Wright knew Salk personally and admired his work.[38]

The testing began in June of 1952. Since all the volunteers at the Watson Home were polio patients, there was little risk involved. Salk's strategy was simple. After taking blood samples, he injected his subjects with the type of killed virus that corresponded to the polio antibodies in their system. Those with high levels of Type I antibody were given Type I polio vaccine on the assumption that immunity already existed and no further damage could be done. Salk wanted to determine whether his killed virus vaccine could stimulate further immune activity in the volunteers, raising their antibody levels even higher. And if so, for how long?

The first to be vaccinated—Salk's "Subject No. 1"—was Bill Kirkpatrick, a sixteen-year-old high school sophomore who had been at D. T. Watson for almost a year. His story was familiar. Over Labor Day Weekend 1951, he had run laps at the local track to prepare for the coming football season. "I thought I had overdone it because I was physically very tired," he said. "My neck felt stiff. My skin felt chapped."

Kirkpatrick spent a feverish night at home. The pain was unbearable, he recalled. "It was just like someone taking a sledgehammer and beating it against your spine. I could feel my legs go soft like jelly and, all of a sudden, I couldn't move."[39]

A spinal tap confirmed the worst: Kirkpatrick had polio. He spent the next three weeks in quarantine at Municipal Hospital, seeing only "the masked and gowned medical staff" that included Salk. His weight dropped from 145 to ninety pounds, and his paralyzed legs looked like sticks. "My ambition was to be a doctor—a surgeon," Fitzpatrick recalled. "I knew a surgeon needed full use of his arms, and I prayed very deeply that they wouldn't be paralyzed."[40]

The isolation terrified him. Day and night he could hear the sounds of children sobbing and the hiss of the iron lungs. A girl he befriended there died. Moved to the Watson Home, Kirkpatrick began a vigorous program of rehabilitation that got him up and walking again with a back brace and two canes. (His arms were fine.) When word circulated that Salk was looking for volunteers, Kirkpatrick convinced his parents to let him take part. "The other kids were kind of frightened of this," he recalled, "so I stepped up to bat first."[41]

Salk gave most of the injections himself. Thirty volunteers received the Type I virus vaccine, two got the Type II, and eleven the Type III.

Salk returned frequently to check on their health. "When you inoculate children with a polio vaccine," he said later, "you don't sleep well for two or three months."[42]

The early signs were encouraging. No illness was reported among the volunteers, and their blood tests showed a significant rise in antibody levels. Meanwhile, Salk began his next round of vaccine tests at the Polk School, a grim institution, understaffed and overcrowded, 80 miles north of Pittsburgh. Polk was a troubling place to visit despite Superintendent Walker's enthusiasm for Salk's experiment. The patients were housed according to mental ability, with people of different ages crammed together. The wards had a stench that an outsider would not soon forget. More important, the experiments were riskier because the subjects didn't have polio. Blood tests showed that some of them possessed antibodies to one or more types of the virus, but that others had none. This placed a fair number of Polk volunteers in a high-risk category: young adults with no apparent immunity to the disease.

The experiments were designed to test the vaccine's safety and antigenic power. Salk tried his vaccine with and without a mineral oil adjuvant. He tinkered with the cooking process for killing the viruses. He injected some volunteers with a single type of poliovirus and others with all three types mixed together, a trivalent vaccine.

The Polk findings were even more impressive. The vaccine proved safe. It stimulated a high antibody response to all three types of poliovirus that persisted for months. Salk was ecstatic. "It was the thrill of my life," he recalled. "Compared to the feeling I got seeing those results under the microscope, everything that followed was anticlimactic."[43]

10

"Plague Season"

For Salk, there was reason to hurry. The year 1952 was the worst polio year on record, with more than 57,000 cases nationwide. The headlines screamed of "Plague Season" and "Polio Time." Twenty-one thousand victims suffered permanent paralysis and about 3,000 died. "The United States had never experienced a higher crest of the epidemiological wave," a journalist noted, "and never would again."[1]

Polio seasons were unpredictable. Some began in late May and burned out by mid-August. Others came in July and lasted through Labor Day. The 1952 season started before Memorial Day, gained ferocious momentum in the summer months, and pushed well into October. On July 4 a *Washington Post* headline warned: "Polio Cases Set Record So Far in '52." A week later, despite raising a record $41.4 million dollars in its annual March of Dimes campaign, the National Foundation for Infantile Paralysis admitted that 500 of its 3,000 local chapters were now bankrupt, having "expended all their funds" on medical bills and patient care. In response, foundation officials channeled several million dollars to epidemic areas, along with 332 respirators, 79 rocking beds, 240 nurses, 48 physical therapists, and tons of supplies. Never before had so much been needed so soon.[2]

What explained this swelling tide? Researchers pointed to the more careful reporting of polio cases by public health officials and to the better diagnostic techniques of doctors. Some believed that the increase was due, in large part, to the exploding birth rate in America: put simply, a larger pool of potential victims. Others noted the circulation of more virulent strains of Type I poliovirus—a phenomenon more easily documented than explained. A few blamed the dumping of new poisons into the environment, especially the pesticide DDT.[3]

Clearly, something dramatic had occurred. It was well known that the average age of the polio victim had been rising steadily over the years. In the great epidemic of 1916, the vast majority of reported cases had ranged from infants to four-year-olds. By 1940, however, the most vulnerable age group had become the five- to nine-year-olds, with a quarter of the new cases involving a victim between age ten and nineteen.[4]

On the other hand, the *incidence* of polio had remained relatively stable in the 1920s and 1930s at an annual rate of about four cases per 100,000. And here, quite clearly, is where the great change occurred. In the period 1940–1944, reported polio cases doubled to 8 per 100,000, doubled again to 16 cases per 100,000 for 1945–1949, and climbed further to 25 per 100,000 for 1950–1954, with the peak of 37 per 100,000 reached in 1952. In a remarkably prescient essay, published in 1947, Albert Sabin tried to link these rising numbers with the increased age of polio victims, posing questions that are still debated to this day. "Is it possible," he wrote, "that there is a time in infancy . . . when infection with poliovirus is predominantly inapparent and results in life-long immunity?" Probably, Sabin concluded. "Does it follow then, that epidemics begin to occur in a country when large numbers of children fail to acquire the polioviruses during that important phase of their life?" Probably. Is this why polio epidemics "seem to be affecting more and more the countries in which sanitation and hygiene, along with the general living standard, are presumably making the greatest advances?" Probably—though Sabin left the door wide open for further research. "If I have left the reader somewhat bewildered and with the impression that [we] do not know the answers," he concluded, "I must confess that it was precisely what I intended to do."[5]

In the plague year 1952, horror stories abounded. On Tuesday, July 22, 16-year-old Catherine Thiel came down with a fever. She had spent the day on her farm in Mapleton, Iowa, doing normal chores in the blazing sun. The family doctor arrived, gave her a shot of penicillin, and recommended ice packs for her throbbing head. Catherine seemed to rally; her fever went down, her appetite increased. But two days later, the telltale signs appeared: muscle ache, joint pain, a stiff neck. The doctor returned. His diagnosis: polio.

For parents Joe and Clara Thiel, the trouble was just beginning. On Wednesday, son Jerry, 13, felt too sick to work in the fields. On Thursday, daughter Jean, 4, had to be carried up to bed. On Friday, three more Thiel children, Francis, 10, Harry, 9, and Ronald, 3, complained of headaches and muscle pain. Over the weekend, 6-year-old Marcella "began to ache" and 12-year-old Ina Mae "went to bed crying." Before long, eleven of the 14 children had come down with polio. "It was kind of like a nightmare," said Clara Thiel.[6]

Polio hit the Iowa farmbelt hard in the summer of 1952. An epidemic in nearby Sioux City had swamped local hospitals. Hearing the news, Joe and Clara Thiel had warned their children to stay out of the Mapleton swimming hole and to wash up before eating. They had tested the well water—it was fine—and used extra DDT to drive away flies. Joe Thiel had even gone to town to buy the new "polio insurance" that paid up to $5,000 for each child under eighteen. The Thiels had done everything they'd been told to do, everything they could. Why had it happened to them?

There were no firm answers, only clues. The Thiels rarely left their farm. They had little contact with strangers. The widespread epidemic may have exposed the children to poliovirus for the first time in their lives. From the news stories, one learned that the two oldest Thiel children had recently left the farm but returned frequently for visits. Donald, an army private, was home on furlough from Fort Riley, Kansas, an enormous training center for new recruits. Joan worked as a delivery room nurse at St. Joseph's Hospital in Sioux City, site of the region's largest polio ward.

Nine of the eleven Thiel children recovered, two were left paralyzed, but no one died. It was even worse that September for a family living near Milwaukee. Four of the six children came down with bulbar polio, a dangerous, often fatal form of the disease that affects the cranial nerves responsible for breathing, swallowing, and speech. The oldest, a 17-year-old high school football player, complained one morning of a "severe headache and pain and weakness of his right arm and shoulder." Rushed to the hospital, he began to vomit and sweat profusely. Antibiotics were administered as well as plasma and intravenous fluids. By late afternoon, he could no longer cough or swallow. "He was placed on a respirator at 6:30 P.M., but continued to decline and died at 6:50 P.M."

The next morning, his four-year-old sister woke up with a headache and a stiff neck. She, too, was rushed to the hospital, where the prognosis looked good. Though complaining of a sore throat, she ate a good supper and "seemed to be sleeping and breathing normally." A few hours later, the resident on duty found her unconscious, with no pulse or respiration. "She was pronounced dead at 8:20 P.M."

The following day brought more tragedy. A second sister, age 8, was taken to the hospital after complaining of a "sore throat, headache, stiff neck, and a weak voice." She began to vomit and had trouble swallowing. The doctors responded with oxygen, penicillin, and plasma, put a suction tube down her throat, and placed her in an iron lung. "She continued to respond coherently to questions until 6:15 P.M., when she died."

It wasn't over. Two days later, a third sister, age 13, complained of "a severe headache with vertigo, nausea, and a mild fever." Given the same treatment, she, too, failed to recover. She vomited uncontrollably, her temperature shot up to 105, and her blood pressure fell. "She was markedly apprehensive," a doctor noted, "because she recognized her symptoms as similar to those of her brother and sisters." She died at 8 P.M.[7]

The message from Mapleton and Milwaukee was especially dire. Polio not only struck children individually, it devastated entire families as well. To polio researchers, this did not come as a surprise. The surest way to get the disease, they believed, was intimate contact with infected people. A glance at the 1916 New York City epidemic showed that about five percent of the 8,634 families attacked by polio had reported more than one case. During a 1943 outbreak in Los Angeles that figure had hit nine percent. Indeed, Salk's mentor, Thomas Francis had studied a case in which five children from one family had contracted bulbar polio and three had died.[8]

The speed with which the disease had ravaged these families made one point ominously clear: getting quick medical attention did not always help. Doctors and hospitals could do only so much. Wonder drugs and iron lungs and round-the-clock attention had failed to keep these children alive. In an era without a vaccine, it was a terrifying thought.

MORE THAN TWENTY YEARS had passed since Franklin D. Roosevelt, then governor of New York state, recruited his dutiful but disinterested law partner to join the flagging polio campaign. What began as a last-ditch attempt to save the troubled Warm Springs Foundation had matured into a medical crusade without precedent in American history. For this, Basil O'Connor deserved, and took, the lion's share of credit. He was a larger than life figure—the founding father of modern philanthropy, he liked to say—who worked for no salary but did everything first class. He lived on Manhattan's Park Avenue, dined at exclusive restaurants, stayed at the best hotels, and hosted meetings at the nation's most elegant resorts. His opulent quarters at the National Foundation for Infantile Paralysis were fit for a political czar. "I'll never forget his office," said researcher Dorothy Horstmann. "He sat at his desk directly opposite a large, full-length portrait of himself." Wearing handmade pin-striped suits with a white carnation in the lapel, O'Connor had come a long way from the working-class streets of Taunton, Massachusetts, which he frankly recalled as "one generation removed from servitude."[9]

Few worked harder. A founding partner at a New York City law firm, O'Connor spent virtually all of his time on "polio business," traveling hundreds of thousands of miles a year. "He sleeps only six hours a night," a friend wrote in the 1940s, "and except for eating, which one suspects is a health measure rather than a gustatory pleasure, sleeping and working are his whole existence." Notoriously demanding, intolerant of "buck-passing" and "indecision," he was forever prodding subordinates with testy notes:

> To heads of all Departments: I realize that there are occasions when matters have to be sent for my personal or confidential attention, but the practice has become so prevalent that what now attracts my attention is one that *isn't* marked "personal" and "confidential."

> [And]: Remind S.U.R. that as General Counsel I expect his *counsel!*

> [And]: So you both recommend *what*? Do not send memos such as this without a recommendation. I've said this *before*.[10]

O'Connor turned sixty in 1952. His wife, Elvira, was in very poor health; she would die three years later. His daughter Bettyann, a recent polio victim, was still struggling to recover. In June of 1952, O'Connor suffered a major heart attack; laid up for three months, he saw the fight against polio, increasingly, as a personal race against time. "I'm not foolhardy. I like living," he told a friend. "But it seems to me we place too much emphasis on how *long* we live, not how *well* we live." Jonas Salk noted the change in O'Connor's behavior following the heart attack, a time when most victims are thinking about slowing down their schedules, not speeding them up. "I think," said Salk, "he wants to make sure we lick this thing while he's still alive." For O'Connor, too, there was reason to hurry.[11]

Hershey, Pennsylvania, was among O'Connor's favorite spots. There was much that appealed to him there—the opulent expanse of the old Hershey estate, the grand nineteenth-century feel to its grounds and accommodations, the wafting aroma of chocolate from the local factory. Hershey was easily accessible to the major grantees, a comfortable train ride from Pittsburgh and Cincinnati, Baltimore and Philadelphia, Boston, New Haven, and New York. In January 1953 America's candy capital again played host to the National Foundation's contentious Committee on Immunization. O'Connor presided; Salk took center stage.

The committee, composed mostly of virologists, had no formal power. It played an advisory role in matters pertaining to immunization, which by this point meant the development of a vaccine. The problem was that a clear majority of the members could agree on almost nothing beyond the need to proceed slowly, a position at odds with the foundation's vow to the American people. O'Connor respected these grantees as scientists but reviled them as a deliberative group. The Hershey meeting would do little to change his mind.

Salk reported on his vaccine experiments at the Polk School and the Watson Home. "It was a tense meeting," he recalled, "and I was by no means the tensest person there." Shock, alarm, skepticism, jealousy—all spilled out at once. Some doubted the staying power of a killed-virus vaccine. Others raised safety concerns, especially acute with juvenile "volunteers." Was the inactivation process foolproof? Wasn't a mineral oil adjuvant potentially toxic? Couldn't monkey kidney tissue cause organ damage when injected into humans? Why use the Mahoney strain when less virulent options were available?[12]

The big question was what to do next. Did the limited success at the Polk School and Watson Home merit a larger field trial in the near future? Salk carefully avoided the issue, but others weighed in. Joseph Smadel, director of the virus laboratory at Walter Reed Army Hospital, spoke in favor of a big field trial, the sooner the better. Impressed by Salk's data, though by no means a fan of Salk's killed-virus approach, Smadel believed that the consequences of inaction clearly outweighed the risks. It didn't matter whether Salk had the final answer to polio. That would come later; people were dying now.[13]

But Smadel found few allies that day. One by one, the grantees begged to disagree. First Albert Sabin, then Howard Howe, then the great John Enders spoke of the long road that lay ahead. There was so much more to know, so much more to do. Scientists must set their own pace, oblivious to outside pressure. "I would suggest more experimentation along the lines that [Salk] is doing so admirably at the moment," said Enders, "and not enter into a large experiment which will inevitably be connected with a lot of publicity and may jeopardize the entire program"[14]

O'Connor said little. Harry Weaver remained mute. Salk had laid out his case; the other grantees had been informed. Their response was predictable, and there was no sense picking a fight. A few nights later, Weaver told the foundation's board of trustees about a promising breakthrough in the labs. While offering no specifics—no names or places—he spoke glowingly of a juiced-up, killed-virus vaccine, calling it "the kind of progress one is accustomed to see prior to the taking of an important forward step."[15]

To John Troan, a young reporter for the *Pittsburgh Press*, this code was not hard to decipher. Troan had good contacts inside Salk's lab. He had followed the University of Pittsburgh polio story from the start, educating himself about the science of vaccination and becoming a conduit for news that Salk himself wanted the public to know, often meeting with him at a Chinese restaurant near the medical school campus. Troan was well aware of the experiments being conducted at the Polk School and Watson Home; he even knew the results. What Harry Weaver had done, in making his remarks to the board of trustees, was to free Troan to publicly identify the man responsible for Weaver's optimistic words. "So far as anyone knows," Troan wrote the next day, "there's only one scientist in this country who is working on exactly this kind of vaccine. He is Dr. Jonas E. Salk."[16]

Word spread quickly. On February 9 *Time* announced some "solid good news on the polio front," quoting Weaver's upbeat prediction. More important, it gave the first whiff of serious celebrity to the man who would come to symbolize the miracles of laboratory science to an adoring public. Above the caption, "Ready for the big attack" was a photo of "Researcher Salk."[17]

Fellow grantees were appalled. Or so said Albert Sabin in a handwritten, advice-filled "Dear Jonas" note that arrived the next day. "Although it was nice to see your happy face in TIME," Sabin wrote, "the stuff that went with it was awful—I know you couldn't have had anything to do with it, for if you did they would have gotten the story straight." Sabin blamed the foundation—his old nemesis—for the trouble, claiming: "[They] have made unwarranted and premature promises before and there is nothing much we have been able to do about it. However, this is the first time they have made a public statement based on work which the investigator has not yet completed or had the opportunity to present . . . in a scientific journal." Sabin warned Salk to be careful, implying that his very career was at stake. "Please don't let them push you to do anything prematurely or to make liters of stuff for 'Harry Weaver's field tests,' until things have been carefully worked out, assayed, etc., so that you know what the score is before anything is done on a 'public scale.'" He ended with a flourish of "all good wishes and affectionate regards," adding his "very best to Donna and the boys."[18]

Actually, this was sage advice. There *was* a danger of moving too quickly. And the foundation had, indeed, violated tradition by commenting on work that had yet to appear in a scientific journal where the data could be carefully reviewed. The problem, of course, lay with the bearer of this advice. Albert Sabin was a rival with his own agenda, who had shown no interest in helping Salk in the past. He was widely viewed as believing polio research to be a zero-sum game, which meant that for him to win, others had to lose. There was no room in his world for two successful vaccines.

But Sabin wasn't alone. Salk got much the same advice from other grantees, including John Paul. After congratulating Salk on his excellent early results, Paul got down to business. "You must not," he wrote, "and no doubt will not be railroaded into doing anything that you yourself have not planned or desired." The implication was clear: Salk could side with his fellow researchers, who lived by the rules of science, or he could join forces with the National Foundation bureaucrats, who lived by the rules of fund-raising and public relations razzle-dazzle.[19]

Salk responded warmly to Paul. "Your wise words of caution," he said, "will be with me when we move into the future." Salk meant it. He had no immediate plans to begin large-scale human trials. His vaccine needed more work, more tinkering, and it had yet to be mass-produced. Salk saw no reason to choose sides at this point, though he clearly felt squeezed by both. "The talk by some about hurrying into

field trials" he recalled, "was as disheartening as the wearisome reviews by others of all the facts we had not yet established. Each school
of thought was unhelpful, really."[20]

What Salk wanted were the resources to move forward when he felt
comfortable with his vaccine. Unlike Paul, Enders, and Sabin, he was
thinking in terms of twelve to fifteen months, not five to fifteen years.
And this required a willingness to collaborate with the National Foundation. Where else could an ambitious polio researcher go in the United
States? The plain fact, in an era before massive federal involvement in
the public health field, was that the foundation ran the polio crusade.
It had financed Salk's laboratory, showered him with grants, supported
his controversial killed-virus theories, placed him on all the right committees, managed his growing celebrity, and brought him to the very
edge of scientific greatness. Like it or not—and both sides liked it more
than not—Salk and the foundation were bound together in ways that
no scientist and no philanthropy had ever been bound together before.

FOR YEARS, THE NATIONAL FOUNDATION HAD BEEN RAISING huge sums
of money by promising to vanquish polio. It was important, no doubt,
to showcase the generous aid being given to those already stricken, the
people in wheelchairs and iron lungs, but nothing mattered more to
the average donor than the ongoing research to prevent *new* cases of
the disease. That's what kept the money pouring in: the news of constant progress in the lab. "The Foundation's difficulty was that it could
not afford to be unpopular," a scientist observed. "It could not appear
sluggish or over-cautious. It was trapped within its own image of dynamic optimism."[21]

This image raised deep concerns among the foundation's own
grantees—not all, but most. Wary of public opinion, scornful of cheery
press releases, resentful of calls to speed up their research, they saw no
quick fix for polio and were unwilling to pretend otherwise. The threat
they posed was substantial. If given the chance, a majority of the Immunization Committee would surely refuse to endorse a large-scale
test of the Salk vaccine—this year, next year, and well into the future.
Though nonbinding, a vote of "no confidence" could prove devastating to the foundation's momentum.

When problems like these arose, O'Connor often looked to an old
ally for help. From his perch at the Rockefeller Institute, Tom Rivers

had popularized the field of modern virology, turning it from an appendage of bacteriological study into a fully independent discipline, "as much concerned with the fundamental problems posed by molecular biology," wrote his biographer, "as with the diseases caused by viral agents." In his time there, Rivers had hired or mentored a great many of the foundation's current grantees; as O'Connor's long-time unpaid advisor, he had formulated the guidelines for studying polio in the wake of the Kolmer and Park-Brodie fiasco. Rivers was no booster of Jonas Salk and his killed-virus vaccine. Except for recent conferences, their paths had rarely crossed. Rivers got involved in this controversy because Basil O'Connor asked him to. And because his conscience told him that a partial defense against polio was better than no defense at all. "I felt like Joe [Smadel]," Rivers recalled. "I was sure that Jonas had an inactivated vaccine that was safe [and] I can tell you that if I had a kid I wouldn't have hesitated for one minute to inoculate him . . . with Salk's vaccine."[22]

In February 1953 O'Connor invited an elite group of journalists, health officials, and medical researchers to his favorite haunt, the Waldorf-Astoria, to hear Salk speak about his progress. Sabin wasn't invited, nor Enders, nor Paul; there would be no dissenting voices. "Dr. Salk is over a barrel," said Tom Rivers in his opening remarks. "Terrific pressure is going to be put on him. Terrific pressure is going to be put on the Foundation and there is always a danger of going too fast. There is also the danger of going too slow, because if you have something that is good, the public should have it as soon as possible." Exactly how good? Like most virologists, Rivers favored a live-virus vaccine as the ultimate solution to polio. Yet he took issue with partisans like Albert Sabin, who saw little value in Salk's work, even as a stopgap until something better came along. The world couldn't wait "fifty years or ten years" for the "ideal vaccine" when there seemed to be an "effective [one] right now, when people are crying for it," Rivers declared. Innocent lives were at stake—children's lives![23]

It was a mixed endorsement, to be sure. Salk followed Rivers that day with a cautious account of his work, hoping to whet public interest without causing a stampede. "I don't even know that we have a vaccine yet," he told the group. "That term . . . should be understood . . . as a colloquial expression. We have preparations which have induced antibody formation in human subjects."[24]

Rivers was in no mood for semantics. The time for this sort of modesty had passed. "I think you have a vaccine, Jonas," he shot back. Salk chose not to argue the point.

The press had a field day. Some stories got it right: "Polio Conquest Nearer." Others went too far: "Hint Polio Vaccine Ready." The oddest item appeared in the syndicated column of Broadway gossip maven Earl Wilson ("It Happened Last Night"), who took time out from his normal round of celebrity spats and nightclub-hopping to report: "New Polio Vaccine: Big Hopes Seen." Shown the item, Salk was alarmed. His findings had yet to appear in a scientific journal. What was going on?

Salk went to see O'Connor in New York. Events were moving too quickly, he warned, and he no longer felt in control. His professional reputation was in jeopardy. He was embarrassed as a scientist. The only thing to do, Salk told O'Connor, was to level with the people: "I said I thought I might be able to exert a moderating effect if I went directly to the public myself and told them, perhaps by radio, exactly what the situation was and exactly why it was not yet time to count on polio vaccination."[25]

O'Connor loved the idea. He had friendly contacts at the networks. Getting Salk free airtime would not be a problem. Millions would tune in. The National Foundation would now have a lab-coated warrior to go along with its ubiquitous poster child. Americans could learn about the polio fight from a man who was actually fighting it. The publicity would be priceless.

Salk portrayed his appearance as a painful chore by a reluctant participant, an intrusion upon his precious time and privacy. But there were some—and the numbers would climb along with Salk's growing celebrity—who took a rather different view. "What adult would be naïve enough to think he could go on [national radio] to talk about a polio vaccine and expect to be allowed to retreat to his cloister afterward?" asked one critic. "Naïve, my foot. Whether he believes it or not, Jonas went on the air that night to take a bow and become a public hero. And that's what he became."[26]

His talk took place on March 26, 1953, at 10:45 P.M. The fifteen-minute show, broadcast nationally on CBS radio, was called "The Scientist Speaks for Himself." Introduced by Basil O'Connor, Salk provided a detailed summary of his own work and of polio research in general. He made two major points that night, one directed toward the public, the other toward his colleagues. To the former, he pleaded for time. "Although progress has been more rapid than we had any right to expect," he said, "there will be no vaccine available for widespread use for the next polio season." To the latter, he spoke with confidence, as an equal in the field. Noting that a "preliminary report" of his findings would soon appear in the *Journal of the American Medical Association*, Salk offered them a review. "In the studies that are being reported this week [in *JAMA*]," he said, "it has also been shown that the amount of antibody induced by vaccination compares favorably with that which develops after natural infection." In other words, his killed-virus vaccine had worked just fine.[27]

The scientist, indeed, had spoken for himself. And his message, mixing patience with optimism, struck a deeply responsive cord. "A polio-free world may be at the fingertips of a Pittsburgh scientist," read a typical news report, which described his vaccine as "still experimental but far beyond the mere test tube stage." Americans could wait on Jonas Salk, it appeared, because they finally had something worth waiting for, something concrete, something that they themselves had played a role in creating. "This is not only a triumph for American medical research," said an editorial carried by Hearst newspapers coast to coast. "It is also a triumph for every one of us who has given to the March of Dimes, which made the research possible. The dimes that we gave have produced a dividend of 1,000,000 percent or so in heart-warming experience in shared good."[28]

Basil O'Connor couldn't have said it better himself. A few weeks later, he announced the formation of a Vaccine Advisory Committee to begin planning the largest medical experiment ever attempted. The members included health experts from the federal government, the academic world, and the private sector. Conspicuously absent were the foundation's own grantees. "We formed [it] to break a logjam," Harry Weaver admitted. "The Immunization Committee was not able to function with the necessary dispatch. It could get entangled for months in technical debates. Furthermore, its members were virologists and the decisions on which we needed help were not exclusively virological."[29]

In reality, O'Connor didn't want their input. He knew all too well where they stood, and he feared that putting even one of them on the committee would open the door for the others. From the foundation's perspective, the issue was no longer *whether* the Salk vaccine was going to be mass tested, but rather how and when. If Albert Sabin wanted to refight old battles on the Immunization Committee, so be it. The Vaccine Advisory Committee would move forward with the business at hand. "The researcher's word is law in the laboratory," O'Connor declared, "but sometimes you have to point out to him what's happening outside the lab window, not to mention the rest of the world."[30]

And this, he thought, was one of those times.

11

The Rivals

THE SCIENTIST SPEAKS FOR HIMSELF" ended at 11:00 P.M. An hour later, Salk boarded a train for Pittsburgh, arrived at dawn, and went directly to the lab. A workaholic by nature, he rarely saw Donna and the three boys in these months, returning home to clean up and grab a few hours of sleep. Each day he would lay out precise instructions for his ever-expanding staff; each day he would push a little harder, feeling, he recalled, "like someone driving a team of wild horses and being whipped at the same time." Anointed a protector of children, a people's scientist, Salk had been given the green light—and virtually unlimited resources—to vanquish the nation's most feared disease. Do it right, but don't dawdle, he was told. Be careful, but hurry up.[1]

In January of 1953, the National Foundation for Infantile Paralysis gave him its largest annual grant ever—$255,472 including indirect costs—to continue his quest. Six months later, citing what he called "the open arrangement for handling our budgetary needs," Salk requested $145,000 more to cover "the remainder" of 1953. His lab now included two assistant research professors, eleven research assistants, seven technicians, an administrative assistant, and numerous "hourly hires." The monkey colony had reached 500, with 200 replacements arriving each week. "It was a factory," said one of the lab workers. "Communication was minimal." Salk "smoked cigarettes like a fiend," said another. He took to prowling the halls, peering over shoulders, consumed by detail, showing a tenseness carefully hidden from the outside world.[2]

What united the staff, beyond its obvious professionalism, was a palpable sense of mission. "Since we were in the same hospital with the polio victims," said Julius Youngner, Salk's top assistant, "the urgency was never out of anybody's mind." This was a group that loved what it did, but not always how it was treated. "There was no personal warmth— I mean none," Youngner added. "The first rule we learned was to call him 'Dr. Salk,' never 'Jonas.' He would speak to us through a wall of notes and memos. He refused to teach. We were the only lab that didn't hold a seminar, not even a bag lunch. Here was a guy who could always find an hour to brief some reporter at the local Chinese restaurant, but could never find the time to sit down with his own people."[3]

Once the goal was reached, the group would split apart amidst charges that Salk had not appreciated, much less acknowledged, the collaborative nature of his success. At this point, however, the vaccine was all that mattered, though personal slights and grievances were growing more intense. The worst one, according to Youngner, involved a paper he wrote with Elsie Ward about the vital color test he had developed to measure the amount of poliovirus in living tissue culture. "After I had what I considered to be a good draft," said Youngner, "I gave my copy to Jonas for his comments. It should be noted that this was 1954, the pre-Xerox, pre-word-processing era. I had made a working transcript of the paper for my own use and it was this copy that I handed to him. Also, it should be noted that the title page had the authors listed as 'J. S. Youngner and E. N. Ward.'"

A week later, according to Youngner, Salk returned from a trip with some troubling news. He had lost the paper. Fortunately, he said, he had jotted down "some notes" while reading it on the train. "I was incredulous," Youngner recalled. "If there were those who could be scatterbrained or disorganized enough to 'lose' a manuscript, Jonas was not among them. Quite the contrary; he was meticulous and disciplined and I knew of no instance in which he behaved in such an irresponsible manner. Holding my tongue, I waited to see what he would come up with."

A few days later, Youngner said, he was handed a "recognizable" draft of the paper. Attached to it was a long appendix with the data intact. How was this possible? Salk explained that he had found the tables but not the text. More disturbing, said Youngner, was the new title page. "The authors were now 'Jonas E. Salk, J. S. Youngner, and Elsie N. Ward.' When I questioned the change, [Jonas] said that since he had to reconstruct the entire paper it was only fair that his name go first. I was dumbstruck and realized that this was a substantive issue that would break our relationship if I carried the argument further and I did not pursue the matter. It was obvious to me then, and is more so now, that he considered the advance in this paper a major one and wanted his name associated with it, even though at the time he had done nothing in the lab (no kidding!) or of an advisory nature to initiate or carry out the work."

Project leaders often demand coauthorship, or even lead authorship, on work that emerges from their lab. Had that happened, had Salk simply pulled rank, said Youngner, "I would have understood it, although I wouldn't have liked it. I would have argued but not from a position of strength since I did not want to stop my work on the vaccine." But Salk chose a different route—a duplicitous route—Youngner added, and things between them would never be the same.[4]

AT THE NATIONAL FOUNDATION, meanwhile, it was full speed ahead. A major polio trial was now in the works, with a private philanthropy betting its reputation and a good chunk of the public's money on the outcome. Was the vaccine truly safe? Would it work well enough to justify the enormous effort involved? To Harry Weaver, there was but one way to find out. "These questions," he said, "can only be determined after injecting a relatively large number of human beings."

Weaver tapped Joseph A. Bell, from the National Institutes of Health, to oversee the trials as scientific director. On paper, it was the ideal choice. A physician with a PhD in public health from Johns Hopkins, Bell was as an expert on the immunization of children. He had won wide acclaim for improving the vaccines against diphtheria and whooping cough. His name brought instant credibility.[5]

But his personality brought instant trouble. Joseph Bell had his own agenda. He didn't much care what the public wanted, or what Salk wanted, or, for that matter, what the foundation wanted. He'd come to serve the cause of science and he'd settle for nothing less.

The first problem concerned the design of the trials. Basil O'Connor favored a plan based entirely on "volunteers" and "observed controls." In this model, several hundred thousand elementary school children across the country would be given the Salk vaccine in late winter or early spring of 1954, before the onset of polio season. Their rate of paralytic polio would then be compared to the rate among their unvaccinated classmates, the "observed controls." The plan seemed straightforward, economical, and fair. Expenses would be limited, record keeping relatively simple. There was no secrecy in the process, no need for random picking and choosing. Those who volunteered would get the *real* vaccine; those who didn't would be "observed."

The opposition to O'Connor's plan came from researchers and statisticians who questioned its scientific worth. "It was well known," said Salk biographer Richard Carter, "that families of superior education and economic standing were most likely to submit their children to experimentation of this kind. It also was well known that low-income families, living in inferior neighborhoods, were much less susceptible to paralytic polio, tending to contract the nonparalytic form of the disease in infancy and remaining immune for life. Thus, a project to vaccinate all volunteers would immunize the most susceptible children."[6]

Bell demanded additions. Besides observed controls, he said, there must be *injected* controls—children vaccinated with a liquid other than the Salk vaccine. Furthermore, the process must be "double-blind," meaning that neither the child getting the shot nor the person giving it could know which solution—the real vaccine or the look-alike placebo—was being used. All information would be carefully coded, known only to those who ran the trials and recorded the results.

There were obvious benefits to these measures. For one thing, injected controls allowed researchers to deal with the variables of age, sex, race, and class. For another, double-blind trials helped local physicians evaluate suspected polio cases without the added pressure and built-in bias of knowing which child had received which solution. Finally, since doctors would lack the code to tell one injection from another, they would not be tempted to cheat by making the "real" vaccine available to favored patients (such as their own children).

The greatest benefit, of course, was credibility. Scientists would be far more likely to accept the results of a double-blind trial with injected controls. Still, the drawbacks were considerable. Using injected controls—with half the children getting the Salk vaccine and the other half receiving a placebo—meant that twice as many subjects would be needed for inoculation. And employing the double-blind method for a trial of this size would require an unprecedented level of surveillance, record keeping, and evaluation.

There were ethical issues as well. Were injected controls really suited to a polio trial? Was it proper, in short, to deny someone access to a potentially lifesaving vaccine in the name of statistical accuracy? Thousands of parents were going to volunteer their children to receive an injection—all of them hoping it contained the polio vaccine, not the placebo. Yet one-half of this study composed of six- to nine-year-olds, the group most vulnerable to paralytic polio, would receive a *worthless* liquid. Some, including Salk himself, saw this as elite science at its worst, a cynical form of Russian roulette.

Bell understood. He took the ethical issue to heart. In a memo to the Vaccine Advisory Committee, he agreed that all "injected products" in these trials "must hold promise of benefit to the recipients, that is, no inert placebos [should] be used." His plan was to give half the children the Salk vaccine, and the other half a look-alike influenza vaccine. Doing so would defuse the ethical issue while leaving scientists free to run two separate experiments—one for polio, the other for flu. "[We must] be prepared," he said, "to take advantage of Unforeseeable Research Opportunities."[7]

But changing the trial design was not enough, Bell insisted. The vaccine itself would have to be changed. Unlike some researchers, who fretted about Salk's use of the virulent Type I Mahoney strain, Bell took aim at the dangers posed by Salk's mineral oil adjuvant. He wasn't alone. A number of virologists suspected that the occasional reaction experienced by small children following vaccination—swelling of the injected arm and painful sores—was caused by the adjuvant in the vaccine. Fears were being raised about long-term consequences, such as cancer. Why take the chance?

Finally, Bell urged that all vaccine in the trials be "triple-tested" to assure its safety and potency. These tests, he said, should be conducted by Salk's lab, by the commercial manufacturer, and by the Biologics Control Division of the Public Health Service—the sole mention of any government involvement in the coming trials. In fact, Bell's agenda was very much in step with the ideas already proposed by Tom Rivers and the Vaccine Advisory Committee. The main difference, it turned out, was the committee's insistence that a true placebo (a water-based solution) be used for safety reasons in the double-blind trials. Bell reluctantly backed off his plan for using influenza vaccine.

Expectations now were sky-high. There was no missing the impatience of a long-suffering public and no avoiding the scrutiny of the scientific elite. In June 1953, at a national meeting of pediatricians, Albert Sabin publicly positioned himself as the "anti-Salk" in a withering assault upon his rival's work to date. "Since there is an impression that a practicable vaccine for poliomyelitis is either at hand or immediately around the corner," he said, "it may be best to start this discussion with the statement that such a vaccine is not now at hand and that one can only guess what is around the corner." It took him fifteen typed pages to explain both the folly of Salk's endeavor and the lurking danger it posed to human health. "Unquestionably," Sabin concluded, "the ultimate goal for the prevention of poliomyelitis is immunization with 'living' avirulent virus which will confer immunity for many times or for life"—in short, Sabin's vaccine. Only then would the corner be turned.[8]

It was out in the open now, a bitter, widening free-for-all in which ego, careerism, and principle would become hopelessly blurred. Salk, hating direct confrontation, did not respond. He was confident that his vaccine worked, certain that the adjuvant was safe. What distressed him, far more than the public sniping, were the changes being demanded without his consent. "Jonas . . . felt that his baby . . . was being torn from his arms," Harry Weaver recalled. "He did not like this. Yet it couldn't be any other way. He couldn't take responsibility for the field trial himself. He could not be architect, carpenter, and building inspector—or judge, jury, prosecutor, and defense attorney all at once."[9]

On some points, Salk was willing to bend. He saw no problem in triple testing the vaccine. And he agreed to remove the adjuvant, despite the problems that would cause. Salk was well schooled in this field, having worked with adjuvants for most of his career. During World War II, he and Thomas Francis had found that a killed-virus influenza vaccine suspended in a mineral oil adjuvant significantly raised the antibody levels of the human volunteers. More recently, Salk had achieved similar results when testing his killed-virus polio vaccine on monkeys. The beauty of the adjuvant lay in its ability to shock the immune system. Salk believed that a single injection of his polio vaccine suspended in mineral oil would be potent enough to produce the antibody levels needed for permanent immunity. To remove the adjuvant—to use an aqueous or water-based vaccine—would likely require two or three carefully spaced injections to get the same result. This would complicate the process, but it certainly could be done. "Looking back," said Tom Rivers, "I would have to admit that I still don't know whether an adjuvant in Salk's vaccine would have caused the trouble that Bell described. . . . I can only say that at that time the Vaccine Advisory Committee was primarily interested in being bloody-well certain that the vaccine that the children got in the trial was as safe and nonirritating as could possibly be made."[10]

On the key point, however, Salk refused to budge. There must be no placebo. He could not deny his own product to those who volunteered to receive it. If thousands of children were going to be injected, then every one of them deserved the benefit of his vaccine. The object of these trials should be to protect as many lives as possible, not to run a textbook experiment. Given the stakes, Salk wrote O'Connor, "I would feel that every child who [gets] a placebo and becomes paralyzed will do so at my hands. I know this truthfully is not the case, but I know equally well that if the same child were to receive a vaccine that proved to be effective, then he might have been spared." It was enough, he said, "to make the humanitarian shudder [and] Hippocrates turn over in his grave."[11]

Though Salk no doubt believed this, he had other fears as well. He didn't fully trust the process under which his vaccine was likely to be tested. He felt uncomfortable with Joseph Bell. He thought the design changes, the new demands, the lack of communication were all setting him up to fail.

O'Connor was sympathetic. He, too, hadn't expected a blueprint quite this exacting. Less concerned with pleasing the scientists than with pleasing the public, he wanted trials that were uncomplicated, uncontroversial, and easy to promote. He had already endorsed the plan for observed controls because that's what people seemed to want. Double-blind? Placebos? Injected controls? O'Connor saw no need.

But Weaver did. As director of research, he couldn't simply disregard the wishes of the Vaccine Advisory Committee he himself had helped to form or the medical expert he had hired to plan the trials. It was one thing to ignore the broadsides of partisans like Albert Sabin, quite another to reject the counsel of advisors like Tom Rivers and Joe Bell. To do so, Weaver felt, would unleash a torrent of "expert" criticism against the trials, undermining the public confidence so vital to the vaccine's overall success.[12]

And here the matter stood. Having moved the vaccine project relentlessly forward over the years, Weaver found himself pushed aside at the moment he was needed most. In a bitter note to O'Connor, he complained of being denied access to meetings at which foundation bureaucrats were encroaching on his turf: "The staff must find it as difficult to understand the intricacies of research as a scientist finds it difficult to understand the nuances of fund-raising . . . public relations, etc." He spoke of the endless obstacles being thrown in his path: "I am disturbed that it has become progressively more difficult to obtain promptly the tools required to attain the goals I have set." And he dropped a desperate hint: "I have no desire of running out on you. [But] without the confidence and cooperation necessary to carry out the responsibilities assigned—I believe that I am wasting my time and yours, and that of many other individuals as well." The following day—August 30, 1953—Harry Weaver resigned.[13]

No one felt more vulnerable without him than Joseph Bell. Described by Tom Rivers as "a good fighter" and "a hard guy to get along with," Bell had already begun to antagonize O'Connor with his supposedly "inflexible" ways. In September Bell produced his "Tentative General Plans for an Epidemiologic Field Trial" that recommended a combination of observed and injected controls. Nothing happened. The Vaccine Advisory Committee was enthusiastic, but the foundation remained mute.[14]

On October 31 Bell followed Weaver out the door. His abrupt resignation and return to the Public Health Service was hardly a surprise. "He was a fine man," O'Connor grumbled, "but he wanted to retest everything from Year One, as if nothing had yet been tested." Bell's admirers disagreed, of course, calling him a martyr to science. Ironically, his tentative general plans would soon become the road map for the mass trials of 1954, with O'Connor reluctantly endorsing virtually all its major points. Like Harry Weaver, Joseph Bell had left his mark.[15]

THE LOW POINT HAD SURELY BEEN REACHED. These dual resignations shattered the National Foundation's carefully sculpted portrait of united purpose and unimpeded progress in the war against polio, offering instead a rare glimpse of the frictions and fissures that had been there from the start. The public had just heard a leading grantee, Albert Sabin, describe the Salk vaccine as unready for mass testing—perhaps, dangerously so. It had seen two top officials quit their posts in apparent disgust over O'Connor's intrusion into scientific affairs. Was the polio crusade in trouble?

Not, it seemed, to those who mattered most. On November 13 the Vaccine Advisory Committee voted unanimously to proceed with field trials, having "satisfied itself," Thomas Rivers wrote O'Connor, that the Salk vaccine was ready for testing "in a sufficient number of children." The committee did not recommend the kind of trial to be run, saying only that, in its view, "the *procedures* outlined by Dr. Salk provide exacting and adequate safeguards for the vaccine."[16]

Alarmed at the vote, Albert Sabin took to his typewriter. In two letters to Dr. Aims McGuiness, a leading pediatrician, Sabin blamed the foundation—not its grantees or scientific advisors—for the current state of affairs. Indeed, he wrote, "I wish to express my confidence in Dr. Salk. . . . He is highly capable, and the design of his experimental work to date seems sound and good. The direction of his experiment could not be in better hands, provided it *really is* in his hands."

The message was clear: bureaucrats had hijacked the scientific process, insisting *"there is a vaccine"* when, in fact, there was nothing of the sort. What Salk had produced thus far was "a proposed immunizing agent as yet untested," Sabin explained, a work in progress with "no published data" to guide the way.

Sabin listed the potential hazards—the most serious, he thought, being the inclusion of the virulent Mahoney strain in Salk's vaccine. "I do not like to be in the position of criticizing another person's experiment," he wrote without blinking, but there really was no choice. What was the hurry? Why rush into field trials with an unfinished product? "We have only just begun to learn, and it would be wise to make haste slowly. . . . The point . . . is that the time is not yet—perhaps soon, but not yet."[17]

Sabin circulated copies of these letters among his fellow grantees. The response was disappointing. Even old allies turned away. There was no support. John Paul warned Sabin that this was the wrong fight to lose; the foundation now had too much on the line. Howard Howe said much the same thing. "The tide has already been unleashed," he responded, "and the objector feels himself in the unfortunate position of a King Canute. It seems to me that to take a negative position now may very well lessen one's influence at a later date." Howe added, almost painfully: "I hope that you will not feel that I am in any way letting you down. . . . I value your friendship and the solidarity of our small group more than ever before. . . . But I must admit that after attending a meeting where the Foundation was pressuring the State Board of Health, I came away with the conviction that dragging the heels was not only useless, but actual folly."[18]

David Bodian took a more measured approach. Perhaps the most respected of all polio researchers, Bodian had steered clear of the politics and feuding so common to the field. He played no favorites and belonged to no camp. His response to Sabin was typical, telling him that the decision to go forward "*has been made*," that no one could seriously doubt "the competence and good faith" of the Vaccine Advisory Committee, and that there was, in truth, "a reasonably good chance for a favorable outcome." Harsh attacks at this point would be viewed as pure obstructionism, Bodian warned—and legitimately so. "My inclination is not to make the trial even more difficult by publicly reiterating criticisms which have already been put on record and which must be as obvious to those responsible for [it] as they are to us."

This was hardly what Sabin hoped to hear. And Bodian added a personal jab by reminding him that each minute spent on politicking meant a minute *not* spent on research. "We are continuing to do all we can to obtain new information [about] immunity," he said, "and hope that you will not be sidetracked from the important work in progress in your laboratory."[19]

An even harsher rebuke came from Thomas Francis. Fair minded but thin skinned, Francis admired Sabin the researcher a lot more than he liked Sabin the person, put off by a style than struck him as the epitome of naked self-promotion. Francis had his own ax to grind. He was Salk's mentor, after all, and a leader in the field of killed-virus research. To his thinking, the letters from Sabin to Aims McGuiness were slickly disguised attempts at sabotage. "I am afraid," he wrote, "that I shall have to reserve the right to disagree with some of your statements. In fact, one can support a very good position in complete contradiction to some of them. . . . Your appended note states that Paul, Melnick, Enders, Weller, Bodian and Howe have 'similar' views. I wonder on which points their views are similar, on which they are the same, and on which they are in disagreement." Enough was enough. "I believe research should be aided by scientific advice," said Francis, "but I also believe that the kind of comments I've been hearing from so many sides can be damaging to the entire field of scientific investigation. And I am opposed to them, and I shall not enter into any further argument on this subject until I feel I understand the objections in light of the personal interests involved."

Francis ended with a flourish. Did Sabin, he asked, really *want* "the responsibility of deciding when it is time for other people to believe it is time?"[20]

There was more to this than met the eye. Thomas Francis was not a disinterested observer, for he kept a secret inside. In November 1953, while vacationing in Europe, he had received a call from Hart Van Riper, the National Foundation's medical director. "Do you think the University of Michigan would accept a grant for you to evaluate the results of this [coming] field trial?" asked Van Riper. "I don't know, but I'm on sabbatical and I'm not interested," Francis replied. Van Riper urged him to give it more thought; Francis said he would. On December 5 the two men met over breakfast in New York City, joined by Basil O'Connor. After listening to the current plans, Francis recommended changes. Did that mean he would take the job? Perhaps, said Francis. He'd let them know.[21]

Francis was not their first choice. Others had already been offered the post that Joseph Bell had vacated in late October and all had turned it down. Francis was a gamble—a man of impeccable reputation, but a man with strong ties to Jonas Salk. The problem was one of perception. How would fellow scientists react to a mentor judging the work of a disciple?

Very well, it turned out. As word of the offer spread, colleagues besieged the notoriously cautious Francis to take the job. The pressure was ceaseless—and flattering. "I finally got home [from Europe]," Francis wrote a friend, "and have certainly walked into a whirlwind. You undoubtedly have heard that I am being importuned to undertake the job of conducting the evaluation of the vaccine trial—that is, the collection of data and analysis. I think I shall do it, although it is going to be a very difficult job to get organized."[22]

Still, Francis took a month to say yes. He laid out his conditions in meticulous detail, insisting that each one of them be met. The foundation, desperate now for a director, was in no position to resist. "I would think that [we] should yield to any reasonable request which . . . might influence his decision . . . ," Van Riper wrote O'Connor, "since at this late date I would be at a loss . . . to find someone who would be competent to do the evaluation." Put simply, Francis held all the cards.[23]

The foundation must give him complete freedom to run the Evaluation Center. Done. It must cover all physical improvements, salaries, supplies, and additional costs. Done. It must accept his timetable for analyzing and releasing the trial results. Done. It must continue to support his virus research at Michigan, no matter how these results turned out. Done.

Most important, it must accept *his* design for the trials. No reputable scientist, he said, would ever run an experiment of this magnitude based entirely on observed controls. To prove his point, Francis had the foundation host a meeting on the subject, attended by statisticians and public health officials from around the country. As he expected, the conclave strongly endorsed the use of injected as well as observed controls, encouraging him to proceed with both tests at once. Officials from the larger states—California, Illinois, Michigan, New York, and Ohio—all favored a double-blind process with injected controls.[24]

Francis got his way. Foundation officials agreed to both types of experiments, and so, too, did Jonas Salk. "For God's sake, he's been agitating against this for months," Van Riper told Francis, "Are you sure?" Francis was quite sure. He had just spoken to his protégé, and Salk was fully on board.[25]

But what about his pained letter to O'Connor? Whatever happened to humanity and Hippocrates? Salk, in truth, did not seem troubled by the switch, showing a part of him—some called it pragmatism, others opportunism—that would loom larger as the stakes increased and his celebrity grew. "I knew as well as anyone that a double-blind trial was preferable in many ways," Salk conceded years later. "But until it became possible to have a Tom Francis in charge, I had no confidence that the field trial could be conducted properly. Francis, I believed, would do it well or not do it at all."[26]

Actually, Salk had no other choice. Francis was his teacher. The two men approached immunization in exactly the same way. They had run mass trials together during World War II with influenza vaccine. Given this relationship, Salk's full cooperation was mandatory. Anything less would be seen as a slap in the face to Francis and—worse—a sign that Salk was afraid to have even his strongest supporter thoroughly test his polio vaccine.

LIKE JOSEPH BELL, THOMAS FRANCIS ENVISIONED a somewhat bigger field trial than the one the foundation had proposed. The objective was clear. Considering the incidence of paralytic polio among grade school children in the United States at this time—around 50 per 100,000—the sample, to be convincing, had to be very large. Suppose, said one statistician, that the vaccine was declared to be 50 percent effective. What would that mean? "With 40,000 in the [placebo] group and 40,000 in the vaccinated group, we would find about 20 control cases and 10 vaccinated cases, and a difference of this magnitude could be easily attributed to random variation. It would suggest that the vaccine might be effective, but it would not be persuasive. With 100,000 in each group, the expected number of polio cases would be 50 and 25, and such a result would be [more] persuasive." Big numbers mattered.[27]

So, too, did the selection of volunteers. Hard choices would have to be made, leaving many parents bitterly disappointed. These trials, after all, were never intended to immunize the entire juvenile population. That wasn't the point—nor was it possible. Commercial vaccine production had just begun. The plans for coding, transporting, and administering three doses of two identical-looking liquids were barely off the ground. Money was tight. As Hart Van Riper admitted, "we will have enough vaccine for between 500,000 and 1,000,000 children. It is, therefore, not feasible to go into every county in the U.S."[28]

Studies showed that five-year-olds had the highest incidence of polio, making them prime candidates for vaccination. The problem, however, was that the foundation hoped to run its trials through the local school systems, where good record keeping and regular attendance made for "maximum ease and convenience." This meant using slightly older subjects, starting logically with children in the first grade. But here, too, a difficulty arose. According to planners, the best model for a smooth-running polio trial showed second graders receiving the vaccination (real and placebo), with first and third graders acting as observed controls. In a memo, Van Riper explained why:

> By selecting children in the second grade, comparable pre-vaccination records are available in the schools for this grade as well as the first and third grades.
> By selecting the second grade, it is possible to compare the post-vaccination experience with the concurrent experience in the non-vaccinated children one grade before (first grade) and one grade later (third grade).
> Second grade children are better adjusted psychologically to school life than are first grade children and therefore offer less resistance and unfavorable . . . reactions to a three-dose vaccination procedure.[29]

In the end, a compromise was reached. County officials who endorsed the model originally proposed by Salk and the National Foundation would inject only second grade volunteers with the real vaccine, while using first and third graders in the same schools as observed controls. Meanwhile, county officials who supported the model proposed by Bell and Francis would inoculate volunteers from all three grades— first, second, and third—with half receiving the real vaccine and half getting a placebo. Should a vaccine shortage occur, priority would be given to the latter model, which Francis, and other researchers, saw as the more valuable of the two.[30]

The planners also wanted the counties to be widely spread across the national map, representing urban, rural, and suburban populations. The ideal size was between 50,000 and 200,000 people—large enough to reflect the region's diversity, yet small enough to be manageable and friendly. The feeling, said Thomas Dublin, an expert on statistical procedures, was that midsized counties would have "more community spirit than larger ones," offering "better cooperation when the vaccinations are to be done." Also, there was "less chance," he thought, "of having medical or other hierarchies who might throw a monkey wrench into the machine."[31]

The trials were going to need strong local support. Most of the work would have to be done by unpaid volunteers. The publicity, the training, the administration would fall to the National Foundation chapters, backed by professionals from the national office. What this meant, in practical terms, was that the trials would run more smoothly in places where the foundation was well entrenched, where fund raising and patient care were known to be successful, where "community spirit" might be easily tapped. The foundation couldn't really announce this policy without appearing to play favorites with children's lives. But all else being equal, it hoped to maximize what were euphemistically described as "advantageous situations."[32]

No factor, though, was more important in determining location than the *incidence* of polio among school children in the recent past. Working closely with state health officials, the foundation identified several hundred counties in the 50,000 to 200,000 population range with the most juvenile polio cases in the years between 1948 and 1952. By using these counties, the planners hoped to find the widest differences in "attack rates" between those who would get the real vaccine and those who wouldn't. Furthermore, if the vaccine proved to be even moderately effective, its use in high-risk counties would likely save more children from polio.

Over time, this list would be whittled down to 211 counties in 44 states—127 counties using observed controls and 84 using injected controls. The scope of these trials would be enormous. Almost 1.5 million schoolchildren would participate in what amounted to the largest public health experiment in American history. Even the statisticians would be impressed.

12

"The Biggest Public Health Experiment Ever"

THE SALK VACCINE TRIALS OF 1954 HOLD A SPECIAL, almost reverential, place in the annals of American medicine. Even the most recent articles, written three, four, and five decades after the event, carry titles such as "Making History," "The Shot Heard Around the World," and "The Biggest Public Health Experiment Ever." "The modern era of vaccine evaluation began with the landmark field trial of inactivated poliomyelitis vaccine," said one. "The polio vaccine field trials . . . are among the largest and most publicized clinical trials ever undertaken," said another.[1]

The view from 1954 reflected the same sense of historical excitement. National attention was riveted on the vaccine trials, with news coverage rivaling the other big stories from that remarkable spring—*Brown v. Board of Education*, the Army-McCarthy hearings, and the fall of Dien Bien Phu. Salk's likeness adorned the cover of *Time* magazine. A Gallup poll showed that more Americans were aware of the field trials than knew "the full name of the President of the United States." By one estimate, two-thirds of the nation had already donated money to the March of Dimes by 1954, and seven million people had volunteered their time. Never before, it appeared, had Americans taken such a personal interest in a medical or scientific pursuit.[2]

From a managerial standpoint, the field trials were divided into three parts: operational planning, vaccine production, and statistical evaluation. Part one involved a mobilization reminiscent of a country preparing for war. "Our basic problem," wrote Melvin Glasser, the man chosen to coordinate this herculean effort, "was to get three doses of [polio] vaccine or control solution into the arms of approximately 650,000 schoolchildren . . . and keep accurate records on all involved in the trial." Nothing like this had ever been tried before. There were no precedents to follow, no corporate donations to be tapped, no federal assistance. This was virgin territory, the biggest medical gamble in history. The National Foundation for Infantile Paralysis was completely—some thought distressingly—on its own.[3]

That, of course, was the way Basil O'Connor had envisioned it. Seeing polio as the exclusive territory of the foundation, he had fiercely opposed the "outside interference" of other groups, especially the government, which, he warned, would ensnare the polio crusade in a web of red tape and "socialist thinking." Unlike the American Cancer Society and American Heart Association, which strongly endorsed federal funding for cancer and heart research, the foundation had always lobbied *against* such funding for polio research, describing it, in words reminiscent of Senator Joseph R. McCarthy, as part of a "Communistic, un-American . . . scheme." So relentless was its message, so powerful was its voice, that others did step aside, leaving the foundation free to pursue its crusade as it, alone, saw fit. At a time when government support for science and medicine was becoming the norm, a top official at the National Institutes of Health told Congress: "We have felt for many years that [the foundation] supports research on such a scale that it would not be wise for us to direct our resources away from other important fields which are not so well covered to this one which is." In that year—1953—the foundation spent about $2 million on polio research; the National Institutes of Health less than $75,000.[4]

O'Connor never doubted the foundation's ability to run a major vaccine trial or the public's willingness to support it. Volunteers could easily be mobilized, he thought, and the money could be raised. Indeed, despite a record-breaking $55 million March of Dimes campaign in January 1954, the foundation would conduct its first ever warm-weather appeal in August, raising an additional $20 million to meet the ballooning cost of the trials. There would be some bad blood over this, with a number of cities denying the March of Dimes a solicitor's permit on grounds that it was siphoning too much money away from other worthy causes. O'Connor, naturally, was unmoved. Philanthropy was about choices, he would say. "The year the American people decide they don't want to give us what we need in order to do the job, we've got to close our doors! That's how democracy works."[5]

The vaccine trials would test the National Foundation as never before. Because millions of parents would be asked to risk their children in a potentially dangerous experiment they knew very little about, educating them and easing their fears would be essential. County health officials and school administrators would have to be involved; so, too, medical societies, newspapers, and PTAs. Tens of thousands of volunteers would have to be trained. The whole process "required infinite care in planning and execution," Glasser recalled. "We estimated that approximately 14,000 school principals, 50,000 classroom teachers, 20,000 physicians and 40,000 nurses would be needed. [We also required] somewhere between 200,000 and 250,000 active non-professional volunteers."[6]

Each of the 211 participating counties held a two-day workshop to plan for the trials. Doctors and nurses were briefed about running a vaccine clinic; school principals and teachers about record keeping and contact with parents; chapter volunteers about public participation, including ways to interest "the Negro population." The most delicate issue by far concerned how aggressively children were to be recruited for the trials. Or as the March of Dimes "Discussion Guide" aptly put it, "What pressure should be exerted on parents to get them to sign the request form?"[7]

There was no formal answer. Local counties were expected to meet their quotas with ease. On the one hand, recruiting children was not expected to pose a serious problem in 1954, given the widespread apprehension surrounding the disease. On the other hand, parents needed to know that the trials posed little or no threat, that the risks paled in comparison to the rewards. In the end, it came down to a contest between fear and faith. Americans had long supported the foundation in its effort to end the scourge of polio. Did they trust it enough to put their children on the line?

In a form letter to parents, O'Connor described participation in the trials as a moral act, benefiting not just the volunteers but generations to follow. "This is one of the most important projects in medical history," he wrote. "Its success depends on the cooperation of parents. We feel sure you will want your child to take part." Volunteering, therefore, was cast as a privilege bestowed upon youngsters special enough to be called "polio pioneers." On the parental consent form, the standard phrase "I give my permission" was changed to "I hereby request," implying that not every child would be fortunate enough to be picked.[8]

The potential risks were aired but quickly dismissed. The ominous-sounding "human experiment" was dropped in favor of "vaccine field study," which had the ring of a benign academic exercise. Parents were told that a killed-virus solution "cannot cause the disease," that the vaccine had been "used safely on over 5,000 volunteers, including Dr. Salk, his wife, and three young sons," that the placebo was a "harmless, but ineffective solution," and that the injections were "only slightly painful" with "no unpleasant effects." So confident was foundation that it claimed the sole purpose of the trials was "to determine whether the vaccine, *already proved safe*, will give adequate protection against paralytic polio."[9]

BEFORE LEAVING THE NATIONAL FOUNDATION in the fall of 1953, Harry Weaver had made a private deal. Plans for the vaccine field trial were just getting underway. In Toronto, Connaught Laboratories was cultivating large amounts of live poliovirus in a special solution known as Medium 199; in Pittsburgh, Jonas Salk and his staff were busy improving their vaccine. The problem was that Salk had neither the time nor the facilities to turn out the sheer volume needed for the sort of field trial the foundation had in mind. This level of vaccine production would require a commercial source.

In the spring of 1953, Weaver had asked Parke-Davis of Detroit, a major pharmacological house, about its interest in manufacturing Salk's polio vaccine. Parke-Davis was a logical choice. Founded just after the Civil War, it had a long list of credits, having isolated the first hormone, epinephrine, in pure form (Adrenalin), marketed the first antihistamine (Benadryl), and produced the first antibiotic by chemical synthesis (Chloromycetin). More important, it had a deep interest in the development of viral and bacterial vaccines. Weaver's understanding with Parke-Davis did not bind either party. It was an oral agreement, leaving the foundation free to pursue other options if it chose.[10]

For several months, Parke-Davis had the polio vaccine market to itself. Each week, Connaught Laboratories would send a station wagon filled with bottles of live poliovirus across the Canadian border to Detroit, where Parke-Davis had built a plant to manufacture the polio vaccine according to instructions provided by Salk himself. The process was complex and problems soon arose. Given the urgency, Parke-Davis felt great pressure to move things along. This led to production mistakes that the company blamed on Salk's faulty instructions, and that Salk, in turn, blamed on company error. To make matters worse, Salk was still refining his product, which meant that the advice he provided Parke-Davis was in a constant state of flux. "I [hadn't] time to advance my work to the point of deciding what combination of virus, formalin, temperature, inactivation time, acidity, and so on would yield a vaccine most suitable for the field trial," he said later, "yet I found myself . . . committed by Weaver to assist in the manufacturing process."[11]

It was a recipe for trouble. Lacking proper oversight, Parke-Davis found itself unable to reliably duplicate Salk's results. Live poliovirus was discovered in a number of its early batches, leading the foundation to quickly change course. In the fall of 1953 O'Connor invited other pharmaceutical houses to join the vaccine production effort, including Eli Lilly, Wyeth, Sharpe and Dohme, Cutter Laboratories, and Pitman-Moore. Though Parke-Davis didn't bow out of the process, its brief monopoly was gone.[12]

What O'Connor offered these companies was hardly risk free. They would have to build expensive production facilities; the field trials could easily fail; and the vaccine they manufactured would have to be sold at no profit during the length of the trials. Of course, if everything worked out—if the field trials proved successful and the government agreed to license the Salk vaccine for commercial production—these companies would enjoy a financial windfall in the future. The choice was theirs.

Tougher quality controls were also introduced. Each batch of polio vaccine would be triple tested—by the drug firm, by Salk's laboratory, and by the Public Health Service—to assure its safety and potency. In addition, O'Connor and Thomas Rivers prodded Salk to produce a set of *concrete* specifications for the manufacturers to follow. "You have to spell out everything and you can take nothing for granted," Rivers recalled, "because if anything later goes wrong you can't turn around and say to the commercial producer, 'Why any damn fool knows that you should have done thus and so.' Everything has to be put down, the i's dotted and t's crossed."[13]

But Salk kept procrastinating, overwhelmed by competing demands. As weeks turned into months, two government virologists, Joe Smadel and William Workman, agreed to draft the specifications from notes provided by Salk. Everyone was relieved. "It will be a big help to me," Salk told them. "I can't write specifications and do my own work at the same time."[14]

In the end, all of the polio vaccine used in the 1954 field trials was supplied by two pharmaceutical houses—Eli Lilly and Parke-Davis. The latter solved its production problems with the aid of more de- tailed specifications and more careful quality control. The four other companies—Wyeth, Sharpe and Dohme, Cutter, and Pitman-Moore— would enter the market in the following year, when the government gave the go-ahead for commercial licensing of the Salk vaccine.

That fall, on his thirty-ninth birthday, Salk received a telegram from the one person who had as much invested in the trials as he did. "You Connaught know life until you are one year older," it teased,

> Till then you have to rely on the sage of 120 Broadway and Albert (not Einstein) to see you through this adolescent period. Twenty years from now this will be Interesting But Good History and you will be a man. I'll be back on my regular job then. Best wishes from one who knows—Basil O'Connor.[15]

AT THE UNIVERSITY OF MICHIGAN, meanwhile, the man who would judge these field trials had begun to set up shop. In February 1954, Thomas Francis opened the Vaccine Evaluation Center in the medical school's old maternity hospital, a crumbling brick structure rendered obsolete by a new birthing facility a few blocks away. To Jonas Salk, it must have seemed like an omen. His vaccine, designed to save the lives of children, would be judged in the same building where two of his sons, Peter and Darrell, had been born.

Using foundation money, as promised, Francis went to work. His budget—a blank check, really—included line items for salaries, equip- ment, supplies, travel, communications, statistical operations, editing and coding, punching and tabulating, building alterations, and indi- rect costs to the university. Before long, however, Francis found him- self confronting the very safety concerns that the foundation had considered—and rather cavalierly dismissed. Queries poured into the Evaluation Center from people who had seen reports or heard rumors about the "hidden dangers" of the Salk vaccine. Several health depart- ments in California expressed concern about the inactivation process. Was Francis *certain* that there was no live virus in the vaccine? Perhaps he could fly out and address this issue in person. (He did.) Health officers in Erie County, New York, worried about "the possible presence of other viruses," unseen and untested, that might have entered the vaccine through the monkey kidney tissue used in production. (Francis sent them material about the sterilization process.) Officials in Michigan had heard that "a tuberculin-like reaction was encountered with one of the vaccine preparations." Was this true? ("I told them," Francis noted, "that it was one of those difficulties that nobody seemed to understand, and it was certainly unexpected.")[16]

Few doubted the independence or integrity that Francis brought to the job. But a number of health officers, seeing him as part of the larger foundation apparatus, sought other opinions as well. And this meant going outside the circle now drawn tightly around Salk. A Utah official contacted two likely sources: Sabin and Enders. "We are about to begin [the] immunization program," he wrote, and "your name has been associated with unofficial statements that there might possibly be some danger in this vaccine. Would you care to send us any information?"[17]

Sabin was blunter—hardly a surprise. He opposed "large scale tests on hundreds of thousands of children" and doubted whether the Salk vaccine, which used the virulent Mahoney strain, would ever be licensed in the United States. Enders was more diplomatic, though no less concerned. The vaccine should be "restricted to a relatively small number of subjects," he thought, "until all the technical procedures [can] be standardized and absolute assurance of their safety determined." In private, Enders went further. When a friend wrote to ask whether events were moving too quickly, he replied: "The question you raise about the polio vaccine is, of course, tormenting us all."[18]

The "us" no doubt referred to the church of live-virus believers to which Salk did not belong. But as Francis discovered, the apprehensions surrounding a trial of this size were bound to surface and had to be addressed. Thousands of children were about to be injected with a barely known vaccine. To ignore the doubters, to pass them off as quacks or rivals or complainers, could put the entire project in jeopardy.

The hardest blow, however, came from a bizarre and unexpected source. On April 4, 1954, Walter Winchell, the founding father of celebrity gossip, used his popular Sunday night radio show to attack the Salk vaccine, launching what one Winchell biographer described as his "most reckless charge yet"—no mean feat in a career like this one, spanning more than thirty years. "Attention everyone! In a few moments I will report on a new polio vaccine—it may be a killer!" he began in his dramatic staccato style. A commercial followed, and Winchell returned:

> Good evening, Mr. and Mrs. America, and all the ships at sea. . . . Attention all doctors and families: the National Foundation for Infantile Paralysis plans to inoculate one million children with a new vaccine this month. . . . The U.S. Public Health Service tested ten batches. . . . They have found (I am told) that seven of the ten contained live (not dead) poliovirus. . . . That it killed several monkeys. . . . The name of the vaccine is the Salk Vaccine; named for Dr. Jonas Salk of the University of Pittsburgh."[19]

Winchell had gotten the scoop from Paul de Kruif, the popular science writer who had worked for Basil O'Connor in the 1930s before losing his job in the wake of the Park-Brodie fiasco (see ch. 3). De Kruif had an obvious ax to grind; Winchell was probably looking for a headline. Together, they came close to sabotaging the trials.

Winchell's story had some merit if carefully told. De Kruif had learned from sources inside the National Institutes of Health (NIH) that traces of live virus had been detected in four vaccine lots recently produced by Parke-Davis and Eli Lilly, and that tests on monkeys had turned up spinal lesions suggesting polio. In response, a worried William Workman, who had coauthored the specifications for these companies to follow, had recommended that the field trials be postponed until the vaccine, in his words, met "acceptable criteria for safety." For the foundation, this was a nightmare come true. If the field trials were not up and running by the start of the 1954 polio season, they would have to be put off for a year, wasting all of the effort that had been expended and putting the nation's children at risk.[20]

A week of tense meetings followed at NIH headquarters in Bethesda. O'Connor and Tom Rivers represented the foundation. NIH Director William Sebrell and his chief assistant, James Shannon, sat in for the government. Salk had been invited, along with David Bodian, the world's leading expert on the pathology of polio. Having carefully examined the evidence, Bodian delivered his verdict. "That's not polio," he said "and that's not polio. And that's not polio. And that *may* be polio. We'd better do some additional tests."[21]

It was a masterful presentation, and it wound up saving the trials. All agreed that the problems encountered by Parke-Davis and Eli Lilly were fixable but that better safeguards were needed to insure consistent production of vaccine. The NIH representatives wanted to dramatically increase the size of the test sample, using several hundred monkeys for each vaccine lot instead of several dozen. The foundation people were furious. "Three hundred and fifty monkeys?" O'Connor shot back. "For every batch? Nobody in the country will have the money to buy a shot of the stuff." Rivers went further. "I've been making vaccines all my life," he said, glaring at James Shannon. "As far as I'm concerned, you can take your pencil and paper and shove them up your ass." At that, Rivers recalled, O'Connor sent him back to New York.[22]

With Bodian playing peacemaker, the two sides reached a compromise. The triple testing would continue. No additional monkeys would be sacrificed, and the existing specifications would remain in place. The new wrinkle, however, was that the manufacturers would now be forced to produce eleven consecutive lots of safe vaccine before a single lot could be cleared for public use. If even one of the eleven failed a tissue culture test, or caused polio in a monkey, then the other ten lots would have to be destroyed. Furthermore, at Workman's insistence, Salk would run a quick field trial on 5,000 children in the Pittsburgh area to make certain that the commercial vaccine was ready for mass testing. Both the NIH and the foundation's Vaccine Advisory Committee would reserve final judgment until the results were in.

Winchell's broadcast occurred a few days later. And it took a heavy toll. Local health officials started to have second thoughts about the field trials. In Michigan, the state Medical Society recommended against using the Salk vaccine "until we have further assurance . . . that it will not in any way damage our children." When Thomas Francis phoned the society to complain, he was told that Winchell's program "had caused a great deal of confusion and that many people had telephoned expressing great doubt re. willingness to proceed. . . . There had been a great change in public opinion."[23]

The foundation fired back. Yes, it admitted, several lots of commercially produced vaccine had failed to pass "the most rigid safety tests science has been able to devise." But that was a *good* sign, showing how well the triple testing process really worked. Salk had already inoculated hundreds of children in the Pittsburgh area, including his three sons, without a single mishap. He now was running further tests to ensure the vaccine's absolute safety. Asked for a comment by the press, Salk called Winchell a "sidewalk superintendent," adding: "He was wrong in his statistics and wrong about the danger. If [he] had called me I would have been able to explain. But the guy was just interested in creating a bit of a sensation."[24]

In mid-April, Salk reported the findings of his mini–field trial in Pittsburgh. Early results showed "no recognizable untoward effects" in any of the inoculated children. On April 25 the foundation's Vaccine Advisory Committee voted unanimously to endorse the larger field trials. A few hours later the Public Health Service concurred. Most parents seemed ready to move ahead. Most, but not all. The foundation later estimated that perhaps 150,000 children—about ten percent of the pool—had been lost to the field trials through Winchell's radio broadcast and the publicity surrounding it.[25]

On April 26, at the Franklin Sherman elementary school in McLean, Virginia, six-year-old Randy Kerr stood first in line, sporting a crew cut and a smile. A nurse rolled up his left sleeve; Dr. Richard Mulvaney gave him the injection. "I could hardly feel it," boasted America's first polio pioneer. "It hurt less than a penicillin shot."[26]

This procedure was repeated thousands of times in the coming weeks. Each participating school had been assigned a five-member vaccination team that included a doctor who gave the injection, a nurse, a clinic reporter, and two clinic aides. The children were taken to a holding area, where several volunteers (usually classroom mothers) were on hand to keep order. From there, the teacher walked each child to the vaccination room for identification. A clinic reporter entered the date of the shot, looked to see that a parental request form was on file, and checked the lot number of the vaccine. A clinic aide then prepared the child ("rolls up sleeve of left arm to expose triceps muscle; swabs site with an antiseptic on sterile cotton balls"), while the nurse opened the vials of cherry-colored liquid, filled the syringes ("5 cc. syringes will provide five inoculations"), and inserted a new needle after each shot. Before injecting the child, the doctor repeated the lot number to the recorder. A second aide was responsible for disposing of the used syringes, needles, and gauze patches. On the way out, a volunteer handed the child a lollipop.

In Lexington, Kentucky, dozens of children came for their first polio shot without a signed consent form. "Ignoring the rainstorms that blew up," a witness noted, "[four] mothers put on overshoes and raincoats, tramped over hills and back roads, calling on parents until every single child had been accounted for." In New York City, volunteers comforted foreign-born children and their parents by explaining the experiment to them in their native tongue. In Montgomery, Alabama, black children received their Salk shots on the front lawns of white public schools, summoned by their first name only, as southern racial etiquette demanded, and forbidden to use the rest rooms inside. "They didn't seem to be affronted by it. They expected it," a foundation official recalled. "That was the thing that was terrible. They just thought this was how it had to be for them."[27]

There was no better barometer for what went right and what went wrong in these trials than the diary kept by Thomas Francis, which spoke of triumph and frustration—and the endless problems to be fixed. For example: a child was accidentally given two vaccine doses in the first injection. Should his next shot be cancelled? (No, stick to the plan). A child received her first injection but missed the second one. Should she get the third? (Yes, two shots were better than one.) A child moved from one county to another. His parents wanted to continue the shots, but no one knew whether he had received the real vaccine or the placebo. Was it possible for local officials to be given the code? (Absolutely not; the code was sacred.)

Some problems defied solution. In Schenectady, New York, nurses carelessly reused syringes still wet with liquid, giving a "significant dose of immunizing vaccine to children supposed to receive the placebo" (and vice versa). In Davenport, Iowa, a school's entire vaccination records were stolen from the principal's unlocked office. In Guilford County, North Carolina, doctors "walked off with vials of vaccine and proceeded to give injections to their own children and to children of close friends."[28]

Each time an injected child took sick, suspicions arose. Had the placebo contained impurities? Had the needles and syringes been properly sterilized? Had the vaccine triggered an allergic reaction, or worse, a case of polio? Every child who showed the telltale symptoms of the disease was examined by a doctor and a physical therapist; blood and stool samples were sent to a regional laboratory, which rushed the results to the Evaluation Center in Ann Arbor. Whenever a death occurred, Francis was personally notified by telephone. On May 31, for example, Francis learned about "a boy named Lane, age seven, of Jackson, Mississippi," who had been part of the injected study. Lane had entered a hospital the previous day with a "severe headache and projectile vomiting." He died a few hours later. Francis spent hours piecing the story together. He phoned the boy's doctor, the local health officer, and the pathologist who had performed the autopsy. Suspecting head trauma as the probable cause of death, the pathologist had not bothered to take stool samples or to remove the spinal cord for inspection. Now it was "too late to go back for them," Francis noted bitterly. The body had been embalmed.[29]

But Francis tracked down other clues. He learned that those who had witnessed the autopsy were satisfied that Lane had died of "edema of the brain." And further, that the boy had been wearing a neck brace for a head injury suffered a few weeks before. From a medical standpoint, Francis saw this evidence as persuasive. Children died from many things, they took sick all the time. Perhaps the hardest part of his job, Francis realized, was separating the vaccine from the normal illnesses that might afflict a polio pioneer. A child died in Oklahoma, another in Iowa, yet another in West Virginia. All had taken part in the injected study; all had received their first and second shots. Were the inoculations responsible for their deaths?[30]

Francis ran down everything, hoping, in his words, "to forestall another Winchell." It was depressing, exhausting work. Of the more than 1,300,000 children who took part in the 1954 vaccine trials, several hundred would die—the leading causes being accidents, followed by cancer, pneumonia, and polio (at five percent of the fatalities). Each time a tragedy occurred, Francis got a call. He plowed ahead, case by case, knowing that public confidence in these trials might easily collapse under the weight of too many unexplained illnesses and deaths. In his gut, Francis believed the vaccine to be safe. He had trained Salk, after all, and devoted much of his own career to the inactivation of viruses, including the poliovirus. Still, the sound he dreaded most, Francis recalled, was the ring of his office telephone late at night, the ring of unspeakably bad news.[31]

THE FIELD TRIALS WERE OVER by late spring, just as the school year ended and the polio season began. And for all the problems encountered, the achievement was immense. More than 600,000 children were vaccinated at least once—two-thirds of whom were in the injected control design and one-third in the observed control design. The most striking statistic was that 95 percent of them had received all three vaccinations, a sign of the intense national publicity, the dedication of local communities, and the devotion of individual parents to this passionate crusade.

None of this would matter, of course, if the vaccine failed to work. So all eyes turned next to the cluttered Vaccine Evaluation Center in Ann Arbor, where Francis and his staff were busy collecting, processing, coding, and interpreting the data that arrived in bulging mail sacks twice a day. In our world of high-speed computing it is hard to imagine the magnitude of the task that lay before them. A record had to be created and maintained for every one of the 1,349,135 children in the trials. These records had to be updated each time a new piece of information arrived, and then checked and rechecked for mistakes. To help set up a working model, Francis recruited statisticians from the U.S. Census Bureau who were comfortable with high-volume studies. To edit and code the data, he hired dozens of Michigan graduate students at $1.25 an hour. Some of the data entry was done in longhand; some of it was put on punch cards and sent to IBM in Detroit, which tabulated the results on a "decimal, drum memory machine" that used a new programming language (soon to be known as FORTRAN). In all, Francis employed about 120 people, with the bulk of his budget going to salaries, tabulating expenses, and indirect costs to the university.[32]

Francis was not about to hurried. The job, he said, would be "finished when it's finished." He would hold no press conferences, provide no periodic updates, and tolerate no leaks from his staff. Everything would be done in private. He must be left alone.[33]

While O'Connor had agreed to these ground rules, he had never expected to be fully shut out. It not only seemed unfair to him, given his deep personal stake in the outcome, but it also restricted his ability to make future plans. O'Connor didn't want much; a hint or two from Francis would suffice. Instead, he got nothing.

What O'Connor did have, however, was confidence in Jonas Salk. As a result, he took a huge gamble that summer, betting that the polio vaccine would do well enough in the field trials to be licensed by the government and win wide popular support. In private meetings with six drug companies, O'Connor offered them $9 million of National Foundation money to manufacture the Salk vaccine at their normal markup, so that stockpiles would be available in 1955 if all went according to plan. For the companies, this was a win-win proposition. They stood to turn a profit regardless of how the trials came out. All six enthusiastically signed on.[34]

For Jonas Salk, these months of waiting were even worse. A perfectionist by nature, he kept tinkering with his vaccine. And what he noticed, with growing alarm, was that several of the lots he tested had lost their potency over time. Salk soon discovered why. On the eve of the trials, the NIH representatives had demanded that the preservative Merthiolate be added to his vaccine as a safety measure to prevent the possible growth of bacteria and molds. Salk had protested, to no avail, claiming that Merthiolate was only needed when a product sat in storage for long periods, which was not the case in these field trials, and—worse—that Merthiolate had the potential to ruin his vaccine.[35]

Salk had a point. The addition of Merthiolate appeared to reduce the effectiveness of killed Type I poliovirus. Salk wrote increasingly frantic letters to Rivers and Francis, listing the numbered lots that he knew to be seriously weakened by the preservative. He hoped that accommodations could be made, that Francis might either discard these lots or, at the very least, take note of this problem in writing his final report. But Francis remained noncommittal; the decision would be his alone to make. "The Merthiolate spoiled the vaccine," Salk bitterly recalled. "The field trial would have been close to 100 percent effective if the Merthiolate hadn't been rammed down my throat." It was a lesson he would not soon forget.[36]

IT TOOK ALMOST A FULL YEAR for Francis to evaluate the vaccine trials. In early March 1955, he told O'Connor that the work was largely done; he was ready to sit down and write his final report. It would take him about a month, said Francis, who offered no clues about the contents.

When should the announcement be made? Where should it be delivered? Polio season was rapidly approaching. If the Francis Report turned out to be positive, and the government moved quickly to license the vaccine, then the foundation might be able to release the lots it had stockpiled in time to do some good. O'Connor gave Francis four dates to consider—two in late March, two in early April. Francis naturally chose the last one. The date was April 12, 1955—the ten-year anniversary of Franklin Roosevelt's death. O'Connor called it a coincidence; critics called it a publicity stunt. The truth likely fell somewhere in between.

Selecting the venue proved an equally demanding task. Francis lobbied for a scientific conference, or perhaps a medical convention, where he could deliver his report to knowing colleagues, free from the pressures of the outside world. O'Connor hoped for a grander pulpit, celebrating both the scientific achievement *and* the March of Dimes. There was no point trying to contain this, he believed. "If Tommy were to announce his findings in a men's room, the reporters and cameramen would be there. This thing is bigger than us all."[37]

Salk had his own preference. He pressed for the National Academy of Sciences in Washington, the distinguished body that counted Francis, John Enders, John Paul, Albert Sabin, and most other polio researchers *except* Salk among its inductees. The National Academy oozed scientific prestige; its location guaranteed major press coverage. And a positive report by Francis might speed up Salk's nomination for membership. According to one Pittsburgh colleague, "Jonas ran around the lab like a little boy, smiling from ear to ear and telling us, 'It looks like we may get the Academy.'"[38]

No one else supported the idea. Foundation officials thought the notion too elitist, and the Academy shied away. When Salk next suggested the University of Pittsburgh, Francis intervened. If the report were to be delivered in an academic setting, it would have to be in *his* academic setting, where the evaluation itself had occurred. Officials at the University of Michigan were enthusiastic. They recommended Rackham Hall, an elegant structure, home to the graduate school, which contained an auditorium large enough for anything the foundation had in mind. Promises were made to accommodate the press and to maintain a proper sense of decorum. Ann Arbor it would be.

Donna Salk almost never traveled with her husband in these years. With young children to care for, she could rarely find the time. It seemed odd, therefore, that her husband asked her to come to Michigan with the boys. "We had no premonition, no idea of what was going to happen—and that includes Jonas—no idea whatsoever," she recalled. "Here we are, a couple of parents taking three kids on their first plane ride."[39]

The Salks stayed at Inglis House, a former estate near the campus that served as a guest residence for VIPs. By this point, rumors about the Francis Report were flying in all directions. The *New York World-Telegram* had just asserted that the Salk vaccine was "100 percent effective," adding (preposterously): "Not one child who received [it] during last spring's nationwide tests contracted the dread disease." In Pittsburgh, reporter John Troan learned that officials of the NIH had recently visited Salk's lab to discuss plans for licensing the vaccine. "It isn't perfect—no vaccine is," Troan declared , but "the word in drug circles is that the vaccine is 'terrific.'"[40]

On the morning of April 12, over breakfast with O'Connor, Salk, and others, Tommy Francis broke his formal silence. The field trial results were positive, he said, and his report would be favorable. Salk, though not exactly surprised, heaved an audible sigh of relief. The men shook hands and headed for Rackham Hall, where more than 150 reporters were crammed into a makeshift press room on the third floor. The plan called for reporters to be handed a packet of information, including a summary of the Francis Report, at precisely 9:10; as part of a gentleman's agreement, they had promised to withhold comment until Francis was scheduled to speak. It was, in retrospect, too much to ask. When aides from the University of Michigan press office fell slightly behind schedule, arriving at 9:17, a near-riot ensued. Fearing for their safety, the aides jumped onto nearby tables and began tossing the packets to the crowd below. A reporter likened it to "hungry dogs at a garbage pail."[41]

By 9:20, the verdict was out. The first to announce it to the world was Dave Garroway, host of NBC's infant *Today* show, his sidekick J. Fred Muggs, the lovable chimpanzee, grinning appropriately at his side. "The vaccine works," said Garroway, quoting the Michigan press release. "It is safe, effective, and potent." The suspense was broken. Schoolchildren and factory workers got the word over public address systems. Office workers heard it while huddling around radios. In department stores, courtrooms, and coffee shops, people wept openly with relief. To many, April 12 resembled another V-J Day—the end of a war. "We were safe again," recalled author Frank Deford, then a fourth grader in Baltimore. "At our desks, we cheered as if the Orioles or the Colts had won a big game. Outside we could hear car horns honking and church bells chiming in celebration. We had conquered polio."[42]

As Francis rose to speak, millions already knew his secret. The audience at Rackham that morning—five hundred dignitaries and fifteen camera crews—expected a short, crisp talk. What it got, instead, was a full-blown lecture, ninety-eight minutes long, delivered in numbing monotone, dotted with charts and slides. When the press took a friendly poke at Francis, comparing his performance to the sleep deprivation techniques of a torture squad, Basil O'Connor sent him a soothing note of concern. "Tommy, you did the right thing Tuesday morning," it said. "The very fact that you took so much time . . . helped forestall questions which might otherwise have arisen. Your presentation only underlined the validity and the integrity of the data."[43]

Francis made it clear that the vaccine, while safe, had varied widely in quality; some lots were more effective than others in preventing the disease. Then came the findings:

If the results from the observed areas are employed the vaccine could be considered to have been 60–80 percent effective against paralytic poliomyelitis, 60 percent against Type I poliomyelitis, and 70 to 80 percent effective against Types II and III.

Francis had never trusted this part of the trials. He believed that the cultural and economic differences between the parents who volunteered their children for inoculation and the parents who didn't would almost certainly skew the results. His own studies had shown that the families of "polio pioneers" had more education and higher incomes, lived in "better neighborhoods" and "better kept" homes—putting these mostly "middle-class" children at higher risk for polio than the mostly "lower-class" children in the observed controls. As such, said Francis, the Evaluation Center had "greater confidence" in the results obtained from the injected study areas, where the test populations receiving the vaccine and the placebo were "almost identical" to one another. "On this basis," he went on,

> it may be suggested that vaccination [in these areas] was 80–90 percent effective against paralytic poliomyelitis; that it was 60 to 70 percent effective against disease caused by Type I virus and 90 percent or more effective against that of Type II and Type III virus.[44]

The raw numbers broke down this way:

	Placebo Areas		Observed Areas	
	Vaccinated	Placebo	Vaccinated	Observed
Number of Children	200,745	201,229	221,988	725,173
Number of Paralytic Cases	33	115	38	330

One point was clear: the positive results that Francis presented did not quite match the boldness of the press release that had spawned the celebrations. Questions had been raised about the vaccine's consistency and overall power. "Indeed," a writer noted, "a 60–70-percent effectiveness against Type I, the cause of most paralytic polio, promises no great cure-all; turned around, it means 30–40-percent ineffectiveness."[45]

Salk, of course, had not seen the Francis Report in advance. As the next speaker up, he had a tough decision to make. How did he respond to a document that was clearly favorable to him on the one hand, yet filled with question marks on the other? Did he simply thank Francis for a job well done? Or did he try to answer the concerns? Was this the time and place for a defense of his work? Or only for celebratory remarks?

Salk tried both paths at once. Introduced to a standing ovation, he lauded Francis—"His kind of objectivity is rare, even among scientists"—and moved quickly down the list, thanking the departed Harry Weaver first (a loyal gesture), the scientists at Connaught Laboratories, Tom Rivers and the Vaccine Advisory Committee, the March of Dimes and Basil O'Connor (the "one person without whom all this would not have been possible"), the people at the D. T. Watson Home and the Polk School, and the various deans and trustees from the University of Pittsburgh. Salk seemed to recognize everybody that day—everybody, that is, except the people in his own lab. This group, seated proudly together in the packed auditorium, would feel painfully snubbed.[46]

Salk turned next to scientific matters, responding more aggressively, some thought, than the occasion required. In words that would come back to haunt him, he claimed that recent improvements to his polio vaccine had made it a different and *better* product than the one Francis had just tested—hardly a ringing endorsement of the trials. Salk emphasized two points that day: first, the removal of the preservative Merthiolate from the new vaccine had dramatically strengthened its potency; second, a wider spacing of the three injections had produced higher, more consistent, antibody levels, offering hope of long-term immunity. Where Francis had cautiously praised the Salk vaccine for being 60 to 70 percent effective, Salk himself seemed to be shooting boldly for the stars. "Theoretically," he boasted, "[my] new 1955 vaccine and vaccination procedures may lead to 100 percent protection from paralysis of all those vaccinated."[47]

NOT EVERYONE APPLAUDED Salk's presentation that day. The crowd at Ann Arbor had many faces, some angry, some jealous, some confused. The first category included Salk's coworkers from Pittsburgh, who had come expecting to be honored by their boss. A tribute seemed essential, and long overdue given the lingering tensions in the lab. Feelings were still bruised over the publication of Salk's "preliminary report" about the polio experiments of 1953, which had listed "Jonas E. Salk, M.D." as the sole author, and others, in smaller print, as mere collaborators. Julius Youngner already sensed a pattern of deception on Salk's part to take undue credit for the discoveries of others. But now, standing before the bank of microphones and cameras in Rackham Hall, Salk appeared ready to make amends. "The world is listening to [him]," a staffer recalled. "The *whole world* is listening. He seems about to give us credit for our work. But it never comes. The other shoe never drops!"[48]

Why it didn't is a matter of debate. Salk's defenders insist that he acted in the finest scientific tradition—by prefacing his *printed* remarks with the phrase, "From the Staff of the Virus Research Laboratory by Jonas E. Salk, M.D." If so, the gesture was too subtle to be appreciated. His staffers wanted an acknowledgment, name-by-name, of their contributions to a lifesaving vaccine—a minute of thanks to salute their grueling years of service. They felt more than ignored by Salk's omission; they felt betrayed. That evening Byron Bennett took the train home to Pittsburgh "and wept most of the way." Decades later, Julius Youngner still smarted from the slight. "Everybody likes to get credit for what they've done," he said. "[Salk] hid us. It took me a long time to catch on to that. It was a big shock."[49]

Others, meanwhile, were offended by what Salk *did* say that morning. By claiming that his new vaccine was better than the one that Francis had exhaustively tested, Salk appeared to dismiss the 1954 trials as ancient history. Why focus on the Francis Report, he seemed to say, when its findings were already old news? "After Jonas finished talking," Francis recalled, "I went over to him, sore. 'What the hell did you have to say that for,' I said. 'You're in no position to claim 100 percent effectiveness. What's the matter with you?'"[50]

Tom Rivers was furious. Having placed his formidable reputation on the line to get the polio vaccine tested, he could not believe that Salk, the major beneficiary of the trials, had the temerity to undermine the results. Rivers took the remark as a personal slap at himself and at Francis, who had devoted a year of his life to the project and deserved unqualified praise. "To my mind, it was an implied criticism of the way Francis had run the field trials," Rivers told his biographer, "and nothing should have detracted from the kudos that Tommy received that day." To another writer, Rivers was more explicit. "Salk," he said, "should have kept his mouth shut."[51]

As the session broke up and reporters fled to file their stories before deadline, a number of the scientific dignitaries on hand were hustled off to a meeting that would seem a lot more consequential in retrospect than it did on this raucous April afternoon. Because the federal licensing of vaccines fell within the jurisdiction of the newly created Department of Health, Education, and Welfare (HEW), officials from the Public Health Service—now an arm of HEW—had come to Ann Arbor to seek the advice of the assembled polio experts about the immediate licensing of commercially produced Salk vaccine. There was no reason to suspect trouble, given the findings of the Francis Report. The six vaccine manufacturers were well established, and their production records—or protocols—seemed impressive. Furthermore, no medical product had ever been as widely tested as this one. A great deal had been learned in a remarkably short time. Since the 1954 trials had shown the Salk vaccine to be safe, one could logically assume that the commercial version, carefully prepared, would be safe as well.

Speed was essential. The experts rushed through the Francis Report and the company protocols knowing that the public was clamoring for the vaccine. No one there was satisfied with the thoroughness of the effort, least of all Albert Sabin, who found himself in the awkward position of having to sign off on a product he didn't trust so as not be seen as a jealous obstructionist. It was over in less than two hours. From Washington, HEW Secretary Oveta Culp Hobby endorsed the group's unanimous recommendation to license the Salk vaccine. Nine million polio shots were ready for distribution, ordered and paid for by the National Foundation. "It's a wonderful day for the world," Hobby said. "It's a history-making day."[52]

IN HIS 1970 BOOK, *A History of Poliomyelitis*, Dr. John R. Paul noted his disgust at the circuslike atmosphere in Ann Arbor. "The information that had been gathered so painstakingly at the Evaluation Center, and at such an expense of time, money, and energy, did not deserve to be so cheapened by the outburst that ensued." Paul was not alone. "The bedlam was disgusting," a scientist recalled. "It was as if four supermarkets were having their premieres on the same day. . . . It was a souring experience and a black eye for us all."[53]

Privately, Paul expressed a deeper resentment, involving the elevation of one man at the expense of those who had done the pioneering research. In a letter to Nobel laureate John Enders, who had declined to attend the Ann Arbor event, Paul uneasily described the "thunder of applause" that had greeted Salk alone, as "flash bulbs popped away." Though Paul blamed the press and the foundation for these excesses, he did wonder if Salk had done enough to move the spotlight off himself. "I need not dwell on your stake in this," he told Enders. "I wish there had been a little more emphasis on placing credit where credit is due."[54]

Some went further, blaming the foundation for creating a "celebrity-scientist"—and Salk for acting the part. As Paul Clark wrote his good friend Tommy Francis: "I am deeply concerned, as are many others, with all the hysterical publicity—Polio is licked, Salk the miracle man stuff. The public is gullible. . . . There is so much anti-intellectualism . . . rampant today that the reaction is something to be feared. . . . I am tempted to get out my sharpest pen and stick it into the balloon as far as I can."[55]

In fact, Salk's triumph had begun a process now impossible to reverse. It was part of the expanding world of public relations and mass communications from which even the drones of laboratory science were no longer automatically immune. Anointed by the foundation, acclaimed by the press, Salk was handed a role virtually guaranteed to offend his colleagues and ensure his ostracism from their ranks. The nation needed a special hero, it was felt, someone to thrill the public that had supported polio research for so long. It needed a uniquely American story about individual grit and ingenuity, about a brilliant scientist using the tools of modern medicine to work wonders in the lab. It needed, above all, a single *recognizable* benefactor of mankind.

To scientists, inevitably, Salk became a figure of derision, an example—if one were really needed—of how America's new huckster class went about recklessly bending the truth. Since respect for Salk inside the academy had not been very high to begin with, the adulation suddenly showered upon him was bound to cause a stir. What had *he* done to deserve so much attention? Who was *he* to reap all these rewards? Some claimed later to have known what was coming—the proverbial train wreck, eerily preordained. "We could see that success . . . would make a public god of him," recalled a foundation insider, "distorting the meaning of his work, crediting him with achievements that belonged to Enders and Bodian and so many others, and lousing him up with other scientists. We could see . . . but it was not our headache."[56]

Salk, in truth, was more than an innocent bystander. Chosen early on by the foundation as the perfect scientist for its public relations campaign, he did all that was asked of him without appearing to revel in the process. One of his great gifts was a knack for putting himself forward in a manner that made him seem genuinely indifferent to his fame, a reluctant celebrity, embarrassed by the accolades, oblivious to the rewards. This was clear from his first major photo shoot in 1950, when he sat through a grueling all-day session for a national magazine and then modestly requested anonymity, so as not, he said, to bring undue attention upon himself. ("For some foolish reason I would prefer that you indicate these pictures as having been taken at the laboratory of a 'grantee.'") Thereafter, reporters and photographers would always find Salk grudging but available. He would warn them not to waste too much of his time; he would grouse about the important work they were keeping him from doing; and then, having lodged his formulaic protest, he would fully accommodate their needs.[57]

The reporter closest to Salk, John Troan of the *Pittsburgh Press*, saw his reluctance as genuine. "Salk was very private, very shy," he said. "He dealt with us because he had to, not because he wanted to. He'd much rather have been left alone." But others knew a different Salk, a man who cultivated the press with the same care he cultivated viruses, crafting his image with a film director's eye. Here was a new breed of scientist, Julius Youngner recalled. "All the photographs of Jonas 'in the laboratory.' All the shots of Jonas in his white coat, surrounded by lab equipment, microscopes; Jonas intently holding up and looking at culture bottles—all were set up either in his office or an empty room before the photographers came." No reporter ever left the laboratory without a story, Youngner said, though Salk used reliable favorites, John Troan included, for his more important scoops. "Jonas was his own press agent," Youngner added. "He leaked like a sieve."[58]

AMONG THE DIGNITARIES AT ANN ARBOR had been Edward R. Murrow, the father of modern broadcast news. Intense, chain-smoking, fearless, Murrow looked the part of the quintessential trench-coated foreign correspondent reporting live from faraway hot spots and battlefields—all of which he had done. His wartime broadcasts from Europe and his ability to spot new talent had made CBS News, his long-time employer, the leader in its field. All the big networks were represented that April day in Ann Arbor. But Murrow's particular presence there, covering a scientific conclave as if it were a national party convention or a major military campaign, spoke volumes about the event.

Murrow's credits included a nightly radio newscast and two weekly television shows—*See It Now*, a news documentary devoted to the "hard" issues of the day, and *Person to Person*, a popular though frequently awkward visit to the homes of celebrities such as Milton Berle and Marilyn Monroe. Murrow never much liked television. As a reporter, his strength lay in the power of his words. (He opened his first broadcast of *See It Now* in 1951 by admitting, "This is an old team trying to learn a new trade.") Murrow's jump to television reflected the enormous growth of the medium; no invention had ever reached American homes this quickly. In 1946 there were 17,000 TV sets in the United States. Three years later, the Sears, Roebuck catalogue advertised its first television—$149.95 with indoor antenna. By 1955 there was one set for every two households in the country, forty million in all. The Nielsen ratings now showed more Americans watching television than listening to the radio in the hours between 9 P.M. and midnight, what the networks called "prime time."[59]

Murrow's trip to Ann Arbor was due largely to Salk. The two had met a few months before, when Murrow took the overnight train to Pittsburgh to ask Salk to appear on *See It Now*. It hadn't taken much convincing. Murrow was a giant, after all, and *See It Now*, was television's most influential public affairs program, airing subjects that others instinctively avoided, such as the impact of Red-hunting Senator Joseph McCarthy, the security problems of atomic scientist J. Robert Oppenheimer, and the morale of U.S. soldiers in Korea. Salk was not just flattered by Murrow's attention, he was star struck, seeing the renowned journalist's interest in him as proof of his own importance in the larger world. Here, at last, Salk believed, was someone with the sensitivity and worldliness to understand the journey he had undertaken. "I had come to discover a trivial manner in so many journalists," Salk remembered. "Ed Murrow was not trivial. I found myself responding at the level I like to respond to. I found him introspective, meditative, with a purity of thought. He had true pitch."[60]

Salk's first appearance on *See It Now*—a full half-hour on February 22—had been a publicity bonanza, defining Salk, over his mild protests, as the focal point of the polio crusade. When Murrow, who had seen friends and family battle the disease, asked how the vaccine actually worked, Salk had responded with an explanation so carefully scripted as to include an "on-camera demonstration" of monkey kidney tissue being ground up like malt powder in a Waring blender. Murrow was impressed. A successful field trial, he thought, would transform this modest scientist into "a minor god."[61]

On April 12, at 10:30 P.M., Murrow hosted his live broadcast from the Vaccine Evaluation Center in Ann Arbor, seated next to Francis and Salk. "Today," he began, "a great profession made a giant step forward and the news that came out of this room lifted a sense of fear from the homes of millions of Americans." Exactly *how* giant a step was still unclear. When Francis, ever cautious, described the vaccine as having "a protective effect of no insignificant level," Murrow pressed him for specifics, something the public could understand. "Your figures go from sixty to ninety percent in effectiveness, depending on the type of polio. What about going to ninety-five or a 100 percent? What are the prospects?"[62]

Here was the nub of the debate—the difference between the results that Francis had reported from the vaccine of the moment and the results that Salk had predicted for the vaccine of the future. Francis stood his ground. Improvements were inevitable, he replied, "but when you talk about ninety-five to a hundred percent, there is no vaccine that really . . . reaches that point, except under very ideal conditions."

Salk didn't argue the point. There was no sense stirring the pot again. "Well, this may be so," he said, simply, but "I think [it's] one of the things that would be very interesting to try to do something about." It was a good answer, signaling his determination to keep improving the vaccine. And the night would soon get better, as Murrow shifted gears.

HOST: Who owns the patent on this vaccine?

DR. SALK: Well, the people, I would say. There is no patent. Could you patent the sun?

No remark Salk ever made would be as cherished or widely quoted as this one. Here, truly, was the people's vaccine, spearheaded by a charitable foundation, driven by the spirit of voluntarism, subsidized by millions of small contributions, aided by numerous scientists, tested on enthusiastic volunteers. Birthday balls, theater drives, fashion shows, marching mothers, poster children—all had played a role. Developed in the public interest, this particular vaccine belonged to everybody.

It was, as one writer noted, "a noble and generous answer," reflecting the highest values of laboratory science. What Salk didn't mention that night—and really wasn't obliged to—was that both the National Foundation and the University of Pittsburgh had seriously considered seeking a patent for the vaccine before finally abandoning the idea, and that a key reason for not doing so was Salk's own skepticism, as laid out in a frank meeting with patent attorneys who had visited his Pittsburgh laboratory in 1954. Initially, Salk had refused even to sit down with the lawyers, claiming he didn't have the time. "I know that [he] is carrying a terrific burden," the lead attorney had complained, but "I cannot do much more useful work . . . until he can spare a few hours for discussion." When the meeting finally took place, Salk readily acknowledged that his vaccine quest, like so many scientific endeavors, had been built on the ideas and techniques of others. As the attorney noted:

> One of the purposes of our visit to Dr. Salk was to get his views as to exactly what features of the processing were new and possibly patentable. Even before meeting Dr. Salk, it seemed very clear from his published articles that, as usual in such cases, much of what he had done was based on prior work by others, and this was readily confirmed by Dr. Salk. He disclaimed any novelty, as far as he was concerned, in tissue culture or the preparation of the virus . . . and I gathered that the use of formalin was an old technique which he had merely adapted to the particular requirements of the polio virus. If there were any patentable novelty to be found in this phase, it would lie within an extremely narrow scope and would be of doubtful value.[63]

In a sense, Salk was validating what his critics had been (and would be) saying for years: there was nothing really novel or dramatic about his vaccine. It was old science—a stopgap measure to be used until something better came along. To Salk, of course, this badly missed the point. He had never claimed to be charting a completely new course; his objective was to show that an inactivated vaccine, a well-established but heretofore limited commodity, could be made to induce long-term immunity against a viral disease. And in doing so, he had used the work of others to demonstrate a principle that most virologists, especially those involved in polio research, were loath to admit: that durable immunity did not depend exclusively upon a natural infection.

For the moment, the critics stood silent. Salk's vaccine had clearly exceeded their predictions. "I must confess that I was not surprised that [it] could be effective," John Paul wrote Basil O'Connor in a tepid letter of congratulation, "but I was surprised at the degree of effectiveness. My guess would have been that it would have been about 50–60% effective." Salk had good reason to be optimistic. The Francis Report had legitimized his vaccine, and the 1955 version looked even better. As a new summer approached, edgy parents had cause to feel relieved.[64]

At a party following the *See It Now* broadcast on April 12, Murrow put a fatherly arm around Salk. "Young man, a great tragedy has just befallen you," he said. "What's that, Ed?" Salk asked. "You've just lost your anonymity," Murrow replied.[65]

Actually, that process was well under way. Ann Arbor had dramatically raised the stakes, validating the potential of this gentle young scientist and his lifesaving vaccine. "When we got home [to Pittsburgh], the world had changed," Donna Salk recalled. "And I must say, from our point of view, not for the better. It started with us being met at the airport with a limousine [and a police escort]. The first thing that happened was that Jonathan, who was five at the time, walks into the house . . . goes over to the phone and calls his friend Billy. And both Jonas and I hear him saying, 'Hi Billy, I'm back from my vacation and I'm famous and so is my dad.' We thought, well, that just about says it."[66]

Tommy Francis spent the next few weeks decompressing from the tumult. He wrote to thank Ed Murrow: "I want to tell you in retrospect that what I had looked forward to with dread had a much more pleasant ending . . . owing to your staff and yourself." He wrote to thank Basil O'Connor: "It was a pleasure to have enjoyed the benefits of your integrity and firmness in supporting the independent character of the Center, thus removing anxieties and annoyances which otherwise might have arisen." Above all, he welcomed the peace and quiet that had returned to his life and to his campus, claiming that he had "expected the show [to] move on promptly," and comparing his role to that of "the boys in the small town who after the circus has left are still holding on to the bucket [they carried behind] one of the elephants."[67]

Truth be told, Francis had rather enjoyed his day in the sun. To friends who wrote him to complain about the circuslike atmosphere, he replied that what had happened was inevitable and not altogether bad. Everyone involved knew that "an emotional hailstorm" would erupt. The fact that "hucksters had a heyday" didn't really diminish the achievement. People had waited a long time for this moment. There was reason to celebrate—and room for a hero. Speaking for himself, Francis admitted, "it was a great experience."[68]

IN NEW YORK CITY THAT APRIL 12, a nine-year-old girl in a crowded hospital ward, paralyzed from the neck down by a polio attack the previous October, watched the televised images of a world celebrating the Salk vaccine through a mirror perched above her iron lung. The child's distraught mother sat nearby, weeping. "Seven months," she said. "Couldn't you have waited seven months?"[69]

For so many like them, the vaccine had come too late.

13

The Cutter Fiasco

THERE HAD BEEN CELEBRATIONS LIKE THIS for athletes, soldiers, politicians, aviators—but never for a scientist. Gifts and honors poured in from a grateful nation. Philadelphia awarded Salk its Poor Richard Medal for distinguished service to humanity. Mutual of Omaha gave him its Criss Award, along with a $10,000 check, for his contribution to public health. The University of Pittsburgh was swamped with thank-you notes and "donations" addressed to Dr. Salk. His lab was "knee-deep in mail," a staffer recalled. "Paper money [went] into one bin, checks into another, and metal coins into a third." (How much was collected, and who kept what, was never fully divulged.) Elementary schools sent giant posters—WE LOVE YOU DR. SALK—signed by the entire student body. Winnipeg, Canada, site of a major polio epidemic in 1953, sent a 208-foot telegram of congratulation adorned with each survivor's name. A town in the Texas panhandle bought him two heartfelt, if comically inappropriate, gifts: a plow and a fully equipped Oldsmobile 98. (Salk gave the plow to an orphanage and had the car sold so the town could buy more polio vaccine.) A new Cadillac arrived and was donated to charity. Colleges begged him to accept their honorary degrees. *Newsweek* lauded "A Quiet Young Man's Magnificent Victory," insisting that Salk's name was now "as secure a word in the medical dictionary as Jenner, Pasteur, Schick, and Lister."[1]

Hollywood wasn't far behind. Three major studios—Warner Brothers, Columbia, and Twentieth Century-Fox—fought for the exclusive rights to Salk's life story. Rumors flew that Marlon Brando was angling for the lead—an odd choice, most agreed, but a sure sign of box office pizzazz. Salk wisely told them no. "I believe that such pictures are most appropriately made after the scientist is dead," he remarked, "and I'm willing to await my chances of such attention at that time."[2]

Politicians embraced him. One senator introduced a bill to give the forty-year-old Salk a $10,000 annual stipend for life. Another proposed the minting of a Salk dime, just like FDR's. (Both ideas went nowhere.) Governor George Leader of Pennsylvania gave him the state's highest honor—the Bronze Medal for Meritorious Service—before a cheering joint session of the legislature (which soon created an endowed chair for Salk at the University of Pittsburgh Medical School with a princely stipend of $25,000 a year). On an even grander scale, the U.S. House and Senate began the bipartisan process of commissioning a Congressional Gold Medal, the nation's highest civilian award. Salk would become only the second medical researcher to receive one, joining Walter Reed of yellow fever fame. The two men were in good company. Previous honorees included Thomas Edison, Charles Lindbergh, General George C. Marshall, and Irving Berlin.[3]

Hundreds wrote President Eisenhower to request a special White House ceremony for Salk. Some urged the president to find him "big money" and "lots of cash" to help cure cancer and other deadly diseases. A New Jersey businessman put it well: "Medals and degrees mark respect and are fine, but if [Dr. Salk] could be completely relieved of any financial cares . . . there is no telling what he might accomplish for the good of mankind."[4]

"Big money" was not what the White House had in mind. On April 4 an aide to Sherman Adams, the president's chief of staff, circulated a memo suggesting that a Rose Garden ceremony for Salk might give Eisenhower a boost by showing that "he is just as interested as Franklin D. Roosevelt in polio, and [taking] away the perennial [Democratic] thunder." Adams replied: "this is already being set up."[5]

On April 22 Jonas and Donna Salk, their three young boys, and Basil O'Connor arrived at the White House to meet the president. J. Edgar Hoover had sent his usual note warning of the couple's leftwing past, but no one seemed to mind. Salk was now a bona fide hero, beyond even the FBI director's formidable reach. In the cold war crusade against communism, Salk's propaganda value was immense. Medical breakthroughs like this one showed the scientific prowess of the United States and the generosity of its spirit. The polio vaccine would benefit children everywhere. It was America's gift to the world.[6]

The Rose Garden ceremony that day would not soon be forgotten. Few had ever seen Dwight Eisenhower struggle with his feelings in such a public way. "No bands played and no flags waved," wrote a reporter who had followed Ike for years. "But nothing could have been more impressive than this grandfather standing there and telling Dr. Salk in a voice trembling with emotion, 'I have no words to thank you. I am very, very happy.'"[7]

Eisenhower promised to give the Salk vaccine formula to "every country that welcomed the knowledge, including the Soviet Union." His voice broke again as he described the millions of families who would be forever spared "seeing their loved ones suffering in bed." Dr. Salk was more than a great American, the president declared. He was "a benefactor to mankind."[8]

Originally, Salk had not been asked to speak. This may have been his moment, but it wasn't his stage. He was supposed to say, "Thank you, Mr. President"—and nothing more: that was the protocol for such events. Ike got the final word.

Not this time, however. Salk insisted on speaking, and the White House gave in. At the podium that afternoon, he took great pains to portray the polio crusade as a team effort, including, first and foremost, the members of his lab. His words were designed to make amends for the damage done at Ann Arbor, which would never fully disappear. "I couldn't just say thank you, as if I were entitled to the entire accolade," Salk said later. "If I was going to be mixed up at all in occasions of this kind, I at least had to make it clear that I wasn't the only astronaut, as it were."[9]

He had reached the summit. Nothing in his future would come close to matching the intensity or the satisfaction of his grueling four-year quest for the vaccine. And nothing could have prepared him for the bitterness and the disappointment that lay ahead.

THE BANNER HEADLINE in the *Pittsburgh Press* on April 12, 1955 had set the tone—POLIO IS CONQUERED. The stories that day spoke of mothers weeping, doctors cheering, politicians toasting God and Jonas Salk. There was a joyful piece about Salk's first human volunteer ("He's studying to be a doctor, too"), and a tearful one about a crippled local boy ("Vaccine Too Late to Save Bobby's Legs"). There was swelling praise for the medical school ("Pitt's 1–2 Punch Put Polio on Run").

And a strong belief that Salk's "miracle" would soon be made available to all ("Ample Supply of Vaccine Seen").[10]

As these stories made clear, the Ann Arbor extravaganza went much deeper than the Francis Report and the canonization of Jonas Salk. For millions of Americans, it meant *instant* access to the most heralded product in recent medical history, one that had been followed and dangled and promised for the past twenty years. Rumor had it that polio vaccine was sitting in warehouses across the country, waiting only to be licensed by Secretary of Health, Education, and Welfare Oveta Culp Hobby, who had the stamp of approval poised in her hand.

Mrs. Hobby was a woman of many talents, health administration not being one of them. The daughter of a Texas state legislator, the wife of a Texas governor-turned-newspaper publisher, she had spent a lifetime in the political trenches. During World War II, General George C. Marshall, a family friend, chose her to organize the Women's Army Corps, a force of 600,000 uniformed volunteers who worked in non-combat positions from secretarial work and kitchen patrol to truck driving and parachute folding. Retiring as a colonel—the first woman ever to hold that rank—Hobby returned to home to direct the family's growing media empire, which included radio, television, and the flagship *Houston Post*. She was widely respected for her ability to operate in the rough-and-tumble Lone Star world of business and politics. "In a Texas culture renowned for spawning strong, resilient women," it was said, "Oveta Culp Hobby was one of the strongest."[11]

The *Houston Post* strongly endorsed Eisenhower for president in 1952. And Hobby, a conservative Democrat, proved influential in helping him carry Texas. "Very soon after the election," Eisenhower recalled, "[her] name was suggested to me as a possible appointee to the Cabinet. . . . I was hopeful of finding a woman of proven ability for a high post in government, and none seemed better fitted . . . than she." Ike named Hobby to head the newly created Department of Health, Education, and Welfare (HEW), an enormous operation that combined the Social Security Administration, the Public Health Service, and the Office of Education into a single megadepartment. For the first time in her life, wrote one observer, "the proud, supremely confident [Mrs.] Hobby found herself overwhelmed."[12]

Ike took little interest in HEW. Indeed, he could barely remember the department's name, often calling it "Health, Welfare and What

Not." As a political moderate, the president endorsed many of the programs put in place by Franklin Roosevelt's New Deal. As a fiscal conservative, however, he wanted to rein in the costs and keep the government from expanding into areas where, in his opinion, it didn't belong, such as national health insurance and the allocation of drugs and vaccines. Mrs. Hobby leaned well to the right of the president on most issues, claiming she had come to Washington to "bury" the dream of socialized medicine.[13]

The licensing of biologics fell within Hobby's jurisdiction. Officials of the Public Health Service, anticipating a positive verdict in Ann Arbor, had certified the Salk vaccine for commercial production within hours of the Francis Report. About forty lots had been released in the next two weeks, equaling ten million doses. That was the good news, and it didn't last long. Virtually all of these lots had been stockpiled by the National Foundation and promised, free of charge, to the nation's first and second graders—the single highest risk group for polio—and to those children who had received placebo shots in the 1954 trials. What this meant, with summer rapidly approaching, was that most Americans under age 18 would remain unprotected. There simply wasn't enough vaccine to go around. The situation "is made to order for panic and hysteria," wrote *Business Week*, "especially if there are any major polio outbreaks."[14]

On April 13, 1955, Mayor Robert F. Wagner of New York City had wired President Eisenhower to URGENTLY REQUEST ESTABLISHMENT OF FEDERAL SUPERVISORY ALLOCATIONS OF SALK VACCINE SIMILAR TO THOSE SET UP IN THE EARLY DAYS OF PENICILLIN. The mayor wasn't alone. Even those who opposed a large government role in this matter were shocked to learn that the Eisenhower administration had made no plans for the distribution of polio vaccine, believing that the drug companies could best handle it on their own. When asked by a Senate committee whether this inaction had led directly to the current shortage, Mrs. Hobby gave a candid, if suicidal, response. "I would assume that this is an incident unique in medical history," she mused. "I think no one could have foreseen the public demand."[15]

The reaction was volcanic. Editorials mocked the secretary and demanded her resignation. So did the vast majority of letters and telegrams that poured into the White House mailroom. Some described her as "hopelessly incompetent" and prone to "stupid mistakes." Others called her heartless. "Seldom," said one, "have I seen such a *callous* disregard for human life in peacetime." Still others focused on Hobby's gender, demanding that Eisenhower replace her with "a capable man" or ship her off to an obscure location—the choices included "Ambassadress to Luxembourg," where "a lady" could do no harm.[16]

Hobby's days were numbered. She had made the mistake of admitting an obvious truth. The administration's lack of planning was a conscious decision, not an unfortunate oversight. Neither the president nor his advisors viewed the distribution of polio vaccine as a legitimate government function. At a time when the very hint of federal intervention raised angry cries of "socialized medicine," they fully expected the process to remain in private hands, with the vaccine going from the manufacturer to the wholesaler to the druggist to the local doctor, who would inoculate the child three times in three paid office visits. As one administration official put it, "an allocation program for the Salk vaccine would constitute an undesirable precedent."[17]

The drug companies agreed. They had been lobbying Congress and the White House on this issue for months. "The polio vaccine being produced by the licensed six firms is their own property," an industry spokesman insisted. "It belongs to them." If the federal government stepped in—"if the Salk vaccine is socialized"—the drug companies would have no incentive to develop lifesaving new products, with dire consequences for the nation's health and safety. The genius of private enterprise would be quashed. America would become like Soviet Russia, the ultimate symbol of socialism run amuck.[18]

In truth, it was the model of democratic Canada—not Communist Russia—that the drug companies feared most. To the north, the government had taken immediate control of the polio vaccine with overwhelming popular support. The job was easier; Canada had far fewer children to inoculate. But the government-produced vaccine would prove to be safe and cheap and plentiful—a testimony, it appeared, to months of meticulous planning by the Ministry of Health. In Canada, polio was viewed as a national crisis requiring an appropriate national response.[19]

In America, the reverse was true. The drug companies not only lobbied furiously in favor of free enterprise, they also sank millions into plant construction and worker training as a way of keeping vaccine production in their own hands. Profits aside, they feared the long-term consequences of allowing the state to take responsibility and credit for a medical milestone like this one. As the head of Eli Lilly put it: "If the vaccine wasn't available commercially, we knew people would demand it from some source, and we didn't want it produced by the government."[20]

The Eisenhower administration expected these companies to deal with any shortages that might arise. They were the ones who had taken the risks, and they were the ones who would reap the rewards. Early in 1955 Eli Lilly set the price of its vaccine at 80 cents per cc. wholesale— more than double the 35 cents per cc. it had been paid by the National Foundation a few months before. The other companies quickly followed suit, sparking rumors of collusion and price-gouging. The administration did not intervene; it seemed to view the increase as the best way to bolster supply. According to the minutes of a cabinet meeting that April, Hobby explained that she had kept the press from attending a session between the vaccine manufacturers and HEW officials because "there would be anti-trust aspects to a public discussion." She said the meeting was "a complete success."[21]

From the manufacturers' standpoint, it was that and more. The executive vice-president of Parke-Davis sent Eisenhower a personal note of thanks. "The consistent efforts of Mrs. Hobby," he said, "are heartening to all who look with alarm at the developments which will surely lead to the socialization of both the medical profession and the pharmaceutical industry." He also predicted that Parke-Davis could double its vaccine production in four months if the price stayed high and the government didn't intervene. But four months was a long time to wait. A new polio season was approaching, the demand for vaccine was enormous, and parents were up in arms.[22]

Most everyone blamed Washington for the mess. The lack of planning, the threat to children's health, the high price and short supply of vaccine—all made the government look incompetent and unfeeling. In a withering editorial, the *New York Herald Tribune*, a powerful voice in Republican circles, challenged the administration to exert its leadership by monitoring the Salk vaccine "from the producing laboratory to the person receiving the injection." Anything less would put the lives of America's children at risk, it said, adding: "This is an emergency answer to an emergency situation, not a step toward socialized medicine."[23]

The criticism clearly stung. Eisenhower had a personal stake in the polio crusade. The handwritten notes of cabinet meetings reflect his deep emotion when the topic came up. He would reminisce about his early army days, when yellow fever had ravaged his troops and "I near died myself." He would speak of the wonders of new vaccines, and the pride he took in having the "polio miracle" occur on his presidential watch. "I'm so glad my grandson has been inoculated," he would say. "I'm just waiting till my granddaughters are old enough."[24]

Among the letters in the president's polio file is one from a friend in Denver asking Ike to do a small favor for "a good looking, strapping young college football player" now "completely paralyzed" from the disease.

> As he lives about 100 yards off the Cherry Hills Golf Course—between the 13th and 14th holes—his chief high point last summer was in watching for your foursome to come into view. I thought perhaps during your game this year you might give a very special wave in his direction as you pass his house. He spends a lot of his time on the patio watching others play golf.

The letter worked its way up the chain of command. In the margin is the handwritten scribble of an aide: "Matter Dealt With. President Waved."[25]

What remained was the larger business at hand. At a meeting with Republican leaders, the president reluctantly changed course. Given public opinion, there seemed no other choice. "He was fully agreeable to large federal role in the distribution and financing of this vaccine," the notes read, "so long as it should be in short supply and there was a danger of public panic or a black market. He didn't want wealth to be the governing factor as to who would be inoculated. He said this may violate his philosophy, but he looked on this as a real emergency."[26]

In the following weeks his administration would confront the polio crisis head on with enormous consequences for the future. Ironically, though, its action would come in response to a *new* vaccine emergency, far grimmer than the problems of supply and demand.

IT BEGAN WITH A CALL FROM A DOCTOR in Pocatello, Idaho, to J. E. Wyatt, a public health officer in that region. It was Sunday morning, April 24. "I've just seen a youngster who seemed to have polio," the doctor reported. "Her mother says she noticed a little stiffness of the neck yesterday and she had a fever. Today her left arm became paralyzed. Her name is Susan Pierce. She's one of the first-graders we vaccinated last Monday."

Wyatt wasn't alarmed. Dozens of youngsters in the 1954 trials had come down with polio after receiving the Salk vaccine. In some cases, the child had been vaccinated too late; in others, the shots hadn't produced sufficient immunity. No one claimed that the Salk vaccine was perfect, but most everyone assumed it was safe—it couldn't *cause* polio.

"She must have been exposed before her vaccination and there wasn't time for the vaccine to protect her," Wyatt responded. "But I'm glad you called. We'll keep a close watch on things."

Susan Pierce died three days later. In those seventy-two hours, four more polio cases were reported in Idaho among recently vaccinated children. Was this mere coincidence? Not likely, Wyatt reasoned. Polio season had never come this early to Idaho, a cold weather state. Something was wrong.[27]

The cases began to pile up. In Chicago, an infant recently inoculated with the Salk vaccine was brought to a local hospital, suffering paralysis in one arm and both legs. In San Diego, two seven-year-olds came down with severe polio after receiving their Salk shots at school. Similar incidents were reported in Oakland, Napa, and Ventura.

There appeared to be a pattern. All of the cases had occurred within four to ten days of vaccination. All had involved paralysis of the inoculated arm, a telling point of connection, since polio normally affects the body's lower limbs. And all had been injected with vaccine produced by one company, Cutter Laboratories of Berkeley, California.

On April 26, several of the government's top scientists met in Washington to map a response. The session lasted through the night. There was agreement that the evidence against Cutter was suggestive, not conclusive. The company's paper work appeared to be in order. "I have no lack of confidence in Cutter's protocols," said Victor Haas, who headed the National Microbiological Institute. Eight or nine polio cases did not equal an epidemic. Asking Cutter to stop production now was like yelling "fire" in a crowded theater. Parents would panic. Vaccinations would stop. And millions of children would remain at risk for polio.[28]

Of course, the consequences of doing nothing might be even worse. If some of the Cutter lots contained live virus, a full-scale epidemic could ensue. And what about the other manufacturers? They, too, had relied on the same basic set of instructions. Were their vaccines any safer? According to one participant, opinions ranged from "Let's wait and see" to "Let's stop the [whole] program right now." Nobody knew quite what to do.

At around three o'clock that morning, the scientists phoned Leonard Scheele, the U.S. surgeon general, to tell him of the divide. Scheele ordered them to talk it over with some "polio experts" and get back to him at once. Mass inoculations were scheduled that very day in California, where Cutter vaccine was widely used.

Four experts were rousted from bed, hooked in by conference call, told of the problem and asked what, if anything, the government should do. The four were Thomas Francis, Salk's mentor who had headed up the evaluation of the field trials; Joseph Smadel of the Army Medical Center, a Salk supporter; William McD. Hammond, Salk's Pittsburgh colleague, who was critical of the vaccine; and Howard Shaughnessy, director of the Illinois Department of Public Health, another critic. The options included recalling the suspected lots of Cutter vaccine, recalling all Cutter vaccine, suspending the entire vaccination program, or simply monitoring it.

DR. HAMMOND: I think we ought to be very cautious about having any more Cutter material injected until further data are available.

DR. SMADEL: I don't see how you can pick out Cutter and stop all the injections; if you are going that far you have to stop the whole [vaccination] business. . . .

DR. HAMMOND: I don't think we have any right to penalize the other manufacturers at this time. I think everything should be directed toward this one.

DR. FRANCIS: I would be tempted to hold out any of the suspected [Cutter] lots, I think.[29]

To break the deadlock, Haas asked whether "anyone would raise serious objections if the Surgeon General decided . . . to discontinue all use of Cutter material immediately?" Smadel jumped in. "I think that is fairly stringent," he replied. Hammond remained neutral, while Francis—cautious as always—complained about the lack of solid information. "You are asking questions," he said, "on which you don't have enough data to permit anything further than a guess."[30]

In the end, the experts agreed, in Smadel's words, that the government "had better do something." But they refused to make a formal recommendation, fearing they would be held responsible for a crisis over which they had no control. Francis even insisted on anonymity.

DR. HAAS: Well, I am sure that the surgeon general would not take any position that would put the heat on you.

DR. SMADEL: I think, Tommy, that [Surgeon General Scheele] must be in a position to say that he consulted people familiar with the problem.

DR. HAAS: Would you accept that?

DR. FRANCIS: Okay.

DR. HAAS: . . . I am sure Dr. Scheele will be very grateful to you for your discussion on this.[31]

Leonard Scheele was no stranger to controversy. A career public health officer, he had led early efforts to link cigarette smoking to lung disease as head of the National Cancer Institute. Appointed U.S. surgeon general in 1948, Scheele was best known for his strong public support of fluoridation, a program seen by extremists as a "Communist plot" to poison the nation's water supply. A skilled lobbyist, he had helped win huge budget increases from Congress for the Public Health Service, particularly in the field of biomedical research. Many credited Scheele with lifting the formerly obscure position of surgeon general into the modern era by speaking forcefully on issues of public health and medical reform.[32]

Tackling the Cutter problem would not be easy. For one thing, Scheele had no authority to remove even suspected vaccine lots from the market. Cutter had been issued a federal license to manufacture the product. Its protocols and production facilities had (supposedly) been inspected. By law, it could keep distributing the vaccine until its license was suspended—a lengthy process involving proof that the company had failed to comply with the federal standards it already seemed to have met. Furthermore, an attempt by the surgeon general to single out Cutter could do irreparable damage its reputation. Who would trust any of its products after this?[33]

Cutter was a respected operation, a midsized, family-run business started in the back of a pharmacy in Fresno, California, in 1897. Moving to Berkeley six years later, it became a leader in the field of veterinary medicine, introducing the first successful vaccine for blackleg disease, a dangerous cattle infection, and developing improved vaccines for hog cholera and rabies. During World War II, Cutter signed a lucrative contract with the military to supply penicillin and blood products to the troops. By war's end Cutter was thriving, with a thirty-acre complex in Berkeley and smaller plants throughout the west. Its product list included drugs, plasma, and intravenous solutions; sterile bags, bottles, and tubing; vaccines for animals and for human beings.[34]

Cutter's record was not unblemished, however. In 1949 the company pleaded nolo contendere to charges involving the contamination of intravenous solutions. In 1954, as one of the manufacturers invited by the National Foundation to produce vaccine for the field trials, it had run into trouble when testing showed that its trivalent samples had failed to include Type II poliovirus—a serious mistake, no doubt, but the sort of thing that often occurred in the early stages of product development. Cutter was dropped from the program but encouraged to keep working on the vaccine, which it did. By 1955 the company was confident of its product—so confident that it began a program to vaccinate the children of Cutter workers free of charge. None got polio.[35]

More than 400,000 children had already been injected with Cutter vaccine. Another 400,000 doses were in the hands of distributors. There is no transcript of Scheele's conversation with company officials on the morning of April 27. By his account, he asked them to recall the unused doses, and they agreed. Cutter then called its distributors while Scheele notified the press. The company's action, he said, "does not imply that any correlation exists between the vaccine and the occurrence of poliomyelitis."[36]

Few believed him. No company would remove a wildly popular vaccine only two weeks after it had been licensed unless something had gone wrong. And public suspicion spread like wildfire amidst news of further trouble. Idaho reported 14 new polio cases in the last week of April, exceeding the normal total for an entire spring. To make matters worse, polio was widely reported among the family members and "community contacts" of these stricken children. Each case, it turned out, was Cutter-related.

Scheele moved quickly. He dispatched several scientists from the Epidemic Intelligence Service, set up during the Korean War as a defense against biological attack, to review Cutter's protocols with company officials in Berkeley. A sanitary engineer also went along to look for production problems, "such as air flow, piping, and ventilation." On April 28 the Public Health Service created a Polio Surveillance Unit to track down new cases among recently vaccinated children. The same day, random testing began at sixteen regional laboratories on all lots of previously licensed vaccine.

By this point everyone suspected the presence of live virus in the Cutter lots. Either it had survived the killing process, passing undetected through a battery of safety checks, or it had entered during the bottling process, after the testing was complete. Cutter was the only manufacturer to bottle the vaccine in the same building where live virus was inactivated, leading one analyst to question the air quality inside. "Two considerations would imply this," he said. "First, production workers in at least one other polio vaccine plant have been found to have very high concentrations of polio antibody in their blood, sure evidence of repeated exposure to the virus. Some of this was probably airborne. Second, accidental polio infections have occurred from time to time in diagnostic laboratories. Some of these are also thought to have been airborne."[37]

As the data poured in, Scheele formed an elite scientific committee to advise him what to do next. Dozens of polio cases had now been identified in Cutter-vaccinated children. And scattered reports from the field had begun to implicate the vaccines of Wyeth and Lilly as well. These numbers, though very small, raised the troubling issue of risk versus reward. According to an internal report, the new committee was split.

> All agreed that Cutter vaccine should continue to be withheld. Some felt that the national program of vaccination should be indefinitely postponed; others wanted to go ahead without interruption. A point of agreement was that, since several million children had been injected, it would be logical to wait at least a few days to see if any further incidents [occurred.]"[38]

Scheele waited. The news got worse. The number of incidents kept climbing. So, too, did the pressure to act. A majority of committee members were now urging postponement; Basil O'Connor disagreed. "[He] tried every which way to talk me out of suspending the program," Scheele remembered. "He called me at all hours of the night. He threatened to have me fired." This was no exaggeration. O'Connor was furious, believing that the live-virus lobby was using the Cutter incident as a pretext to undermine Salk's killed-virus vaccine. He made similar threats at a meeting with James Shannon, deputy director of the NIH. "O'Connor started out with the dire warning of what he was going to do to [us]," Shannon recalled. ". . . I had many sleepless nights."[39]

Scheele had to act. The vaccine had been licensed for commercial production with the federal government taking responsibility for its safety. This was no longer a private matter for the National Foundation to decide. On May 8, in a dramatic television address, Scheele ordered a halt to further inoculations pending a review of all six manufacturers. Emphasizing the positive, he noted that the incidence of paralytic polio among the five million children who had received "other than the Cutter vaccine" in the past month was about one in 700,000, making the reward far greater than the risk. "I know," Scheele said hopefully, "that [people] will fully understand and appreciate the reasons for this decision which has been taken . . . on behalf of the children of the nation. There will in time be ample safe vaccine for all who need it and wish it."[40]

If the people understood, they hid it rather well. Under the headline "Turmoil Over Salk Shots," the *New York Times* remarked on the lightning speed with which everything had gone downhill. In less than a month, it claimed, "the air of victory" surrounding the Salk vaccine had become a stench of "confusion, conflict, and doubt."[41]

Who was responsible? Democrats accused the Republican administration of "horrendous mistakes" bordering on criminal negligence. "Meat is tested and inspected more carefully in the big packing plants than Mrs. Hobby . . . permitted the polio vaccine to be tested by the Federal Government," sneered a U.S. senator, who urged her "to visit the hospital rooms of the boys and girls who have contracted this horrible disease." Jonas Salk claimed that his vaccine was perfectly safe when produced according his exact specifications—a clear slap at the drug companies. Meanwhile, Basil O'Connor lit into the government *and* the manufacturers for soiling his personal crusade. "So long as the Salk vaccine and its research were in the hands of the National Foundation," he said, "you had some intelligence, intellectual integrity, and total courage—and you had no politics whatsoever."[42]

At a press conference following the Cutter shutdown, President Eisenhower was asked for his opinion of what had gone wrong. It was an easy question to dodge. A "no comment," "I'm not an expert," or "We'll need time to get to the bottom of this" would have sufficed. But the president, saying he was "just speculating," claimed that government scientists may have tried to "short-cut a little bit" on safety tests in response to the unprecedented demand for this particular vaccine. Without being explicit, he had raised an issue that had been bubbling below the surface for years, an issue regarding the tactics of the National Foundation in its relentless crusade against polio.[43]

There had been numerous critics along the way. But their words had been muted by the foundation's impressive progress on the research front, culminating in the dramatic Francis Report a few months before. Now this euphoria was gone, replaced by a fear that the Salk vaccine was a potential killer and that its licensing had been premature. Some naturally blamed the foundation for pushing too hard and too fast, creating a sense of "breathless urgency" more suited to a mass advertising campaign than to a serious scientific quest. What it failed to understand, a skeptic noted, was that inside the laboratory, at least, "the customer isn't always right."[44]

Many of the top polio researchers agreed. They had long viewed the foundation with a mixture of awe and contempt, thriving on its generosity while looking askance at the fund raising and public relations so vital to its success. Some of them had resisted Basil O'Connor's grand vision for conquering polio, believing he hadn't a clue about how scientific progress really occurred. Others went further, seeing him as a regressive force, undermining the sanctity of the lab.

For these researchers, the Cutter incident was like an evil prophecy come true. In a letter to John Enders, John Paul claimed that the message of Cutter was painfully clear. "If we continue to allow publicity experts to take over our responsibilities, [we] are certainly an unworthy group. It seems possible today for an ambitious promoter to assume leadership in affairs of this kind far too easily. This is our challenge."[45]

Enders hardly needed convincing. "We must never again allow decisions about essentially scientific matters to be made for us by people without training or insight," he responded. "That is the real lesson to be learned and remembered."[46]

ALBERT SABIN COULD NOT HAVE SAID IT BETTER. April 12 had been a dreadful day in his life. Invited to Ann Arbor, he had listened to speaker after speaker hail the triumph of a rival vaccine. He had endured hours of ringing praise for almost every prominent polio researcher but himself. And he had heard his distinguished colleague David Bodian commend the "energy, fortitude, and *urgency*" of "one of the fastest working laboratory teams in history, led by Dr. Salk"—a bitter reminder, if one really were needed, of who had come in first.

Sabin was not used to being humbled. And certainly not by someone he saw as an intellectual lightweight—"a kitchen chemist," he thought—who did not belong in the same universe with research giants like Enders, Bodian, and, most obviously, himself. How had it ever come to this? Sabin had no doubt who was to blame. He had long resented the influence of Basil O'Connor, accusing him of favoring

Jonas Salk in order to give the public a quick fix in the war against polio. Following Ann Arbor, Sabin held his tongue. He knew it would be seen as spiteful, or worse, for him to criticize O'Connor or Salk in this time of national celebration. But he seethed at his powerlessness to change the course of events. When an author approached him for guidance about a book she was writing on the "story of polio," Sabin replied: "I cannot 'play ball' with you. Anything written [now] is obviously intended to take advantage of the tremendous publicity and advertising. The time to write a history, in my opinion, is *not* in 1955."[47]

Sabin had been among the scientific advisors at Ann Arbor who recommended licensing the Salk vaccine. But he had gone along reluctantly, as his correspondence makes clear. In a letter to William Workman, written several days before the Cutter incident became national news, Sabin complained that speed, not safety, had been the dominant concern. "During our hurried meeting at Ann Arbor on April 12," he wrote, "we had to decide as to whether or not there was any evidence that the polio vaccine used in 1954 may by itself have been responsible for a certain number of cases of paralysis. Like the others, having had no time to examine the report, I was willing to accept the interpretation of Dr. Francis that there was no evidence. . . ."[48]

Now, after reading the various appendices and attachments, Sabin had his doubts. At least ten cases of paralytic polio had been reported in the first month of the 1954 trials among children who received the Salk vaccine. This was troubling. A few days after the Ann Arbor meeting, when Cutter hit the headlines, Sabin wasn't surprised. He suspected there might be trouble and he thought he knew the cause.

Sabin had long been wary of the Type I Mahoney strain that Salk used in his vaccine. The choice was controversial; Mahoney was known for its virulence, which meant that it produced a strong antibody response. But using this strain also raised the risk of *causing* polio if the inactivation process went even slightly awry. What made Mahoney so dangerous was its phenomenal ability to multiply in non-nerve tissue. If live particles were injected into an arm muscle, the chances of paralysis were extremely high.[49]

For Sabin, the message was clear. He did not think that any of the commercially manufactured Salk vaccine should be returned to the market since all six companies had used the Mahoney strain. In the coming days, as polio researchers and federal officials scrambled to meet the crisis, Sabin went public with his views. America's children deserved a better, safer vaccine, he said, warning: "At all costs, we must avoid another Cutter incident."[50]

IN WASHINGTON, MEANWHILE, INVESTIGATORS PORED OVER the manufacturer's protocols in a frantic effort to discover what had gone wrong. The timing could hardly have been worse. With polio season approaching, a long-awaited miracle vaccine had just been pulled from the shelves. Any further delay would put millions of children at risk for another year. What had to be determined—and quickly—was how the Cutter lots had become contaminated, and what this meant for the five other companies producing the vaccine.

These issues were not exactly new. It was an open secret that the companies selected to produce the Salk vaccine for the 1954 trials had faced early problems in trying to inactivate the live virus. According to one report, government scientists "became concerned about the feasibility of producing safe vaccine on a large scale." This problem had led Jonas Salk to work closely with the drug companies and the NIH in establishing "minimum requirements" for the manufacture and testing of his vaccine. And it appeared to have worked. The companies reported no more trouble, and the success of the 1954 trials seemed to bear this out. The Salk vaccine had been safely mass-produced.[51]

Or so it appeared. During the 1954 trials, each lot of polio vaccine had been triple-tested for safety—by the NIH, by Salk's laboratory, and by the companies themselves. But then, in the rush following the release of the Francis Report, this system came apart. The NIH did very little testing, and the results it got are still shrouded in mystery. One of its top researchers claimed, years later, that safety problems surrounding lots of newly licensed polio vaccine were consciously ignored. "We had eighteen monkeys," said Dr. Bernice Eddy, an NIH staff microbiologist. "We inoculated [them] with each vaccine that came in. And we started getting paralyzed monkeys."

The infected lots belonged to Cutter, Eddy recalled. She reported these findings to her superiors, along with photos of the monkeys, but nothing was done. "They just went ahead and released the vaccine anyway, a lot of it," she said. "The monkeys, they just discarded."[52]

This was not an isolated story. Other recollections, with equally damning details, have surfaced in recent years. Julius Youngner, for

example, told of accepting an invitation to visit the Cutter vaccine factory in the days following the Ann Arbor announcement. "I was appalled," he said. "Tanks containing live-virus pools and other tanks
containing virus lots in various stages of formalin inactivation were kept
in the same rooms. Conditions were not neat or esthetically appealing.
There was a worrisome lack of attention to the most basic rules. . . .
They never let me look at their data, but it was obvious to me that they
were having serious trouble with their inactivation procedures."

"My plan," he noted, "was to return to Pittsburgh and immediately
warn the powers-that-be to hold off licensing Cutter or, if this was not
possible, to stop distribution temporarily of their vaccine. I was frightened to think of the sloppiness of their operation." According to
Youngner, he went to see Salk, told him "that the people at Cutter
didn't know what they doing," and said he was going to write a letter
"detailing my impressions" to both Basil O'Connor and the NIH.
"Jonas," he recalled,

> was unexpectedly calm through my recital. He agreed that it was a serious
> situation with terrible potential consequences. For this reason he suggested
> that it would be better if the letter came from him. . . . I was completely taken
> in—to my knowledge the letter was never written. Jonas never gave me a copy
> of it, and he never mentioned the matter to me again. . . .
>
> When the Cutter incident began to unfold . . . I was immobilized. I realized
> that Jonas probably had done nothing—but neither had I. My guilt at being
> taken in by him was oppressive, but what to do? Silence was my response.[53]

Whether one accepts the details of these stories or not, what is known
for certain is that the testing process for the first lots of licensed commercial polio vaccine in 1955 was close to nonexistent. Under enormous pressure to speed things along, the NIH relied heavily on the
Francis Report and the drug company protocols in declaring these lots
fit for public use. During the 1954 trials, it had taken an average of
four weeks for each lot of polio vaccine to be deemed safe for public
use; in 1955, it took less than a day. And the big problem, it turned out,
was that the manufacturers were now able to conceal their production
difficulties by submitting protocols for the vaccine lots that had *passed*
their safety tests while remaining silent about the lots that had failed.
As a result, harried NIH officials got only part of the vaccine production story—the successful part—which made it easier for them to ignore the suspicions that something might be wrong. In the case of
Cutter, for example, the company later admitted that it had found live

poliovirus to be present in about one-third of the vaccine lots it had produced for commercial use—a figure that would have raised red flags had it become widely known. Cutter's response had been to discard these bad lots without informing the NIH. The practice was deceptive but not illegal. Cutter had no obligation, under the prevailing guidelines, to submit the protocols for vaccine lots it did not intend to market.[54]

And there the matter stood.

THERE WAS A BIT OF GOOD NEWS. On May 13, following a plant-by-plant inspection of production facilities, the government recleared selected lots of Parke-Davis and Eli Lilly vaccine for public use. The risk in this seemed very low, since there had been few reported problems among the millions of children who had received Parke-Davis and Eli Lilly polio shots. In giving the go-ahead, Surgeon General Scheele hoped to restart the national vaccination program in a cautious, incremental way. He realized that the majority of American children would not be vaccinated in time for the 1955 polio season—and that many parents now preferred it this way. Public confidence in the Salk vaccine had plummeted. An article in *Business Week* framed it well: "'Should we go ahead with the children's inoculations?'"

> That was the question you heard everywhere—on commuter trains, in supermarkets, in executive offices. The nation, which mere weeks ago clamored with one voice for the Salk vaccine, now is skeptical. The faith of the reading, listening and watching public has been severely shaken. The delays in school inoculation programs, the starts and stops in vaccine production, the cloak-and-dagger meetings in Washington, the recurring rumors that Secy. Oveta Culp Hobby would resign—all this had raised doubts. Nobody seems to be giving straight answers. It has the look of a cover-up.[55]

On May 23 Scheele appointed another committee to review the data on the individual vaccine lots and make recommendations as to their release. But even this limited step brought quick criticism from the likes of Sabin and Enders, who opposed any move to inject children with the current Salk vaccine. Things got so heated that fifteen scientists representing all sides of the controversy were asked to testify at a special session on Capitol Hill. Observers described it as "one of the most learned Congressional hearings ever held." It was one of the more contentious as well.[56]

The panel included two Nobel Prize winners—Enders and Wendell Stanley, a biochemist who specialized in the purification of viruses.

Both were critical of the Salk vaccine. Both mocked Salk's theoretical margin of safety, claiming that no process could be foolproof when dealing with viruses of differing resistances and with particles of various shapes and sizes and degrees of aggregation. "This," said Stanley, "is a very tricky business."[57]

Then it was Sabin's turn. Polio research had come to a crossroads, he thought. It could proceed on its present course, manufacturing a vaccine of questionable safety, or it could postpone production until the "potential dangers" were examined and removed. Sabin favored postponement. "I want to stress here my belief that possibility of immunizing [against polio] does exist," he said. But not with the Mahoney strain in a killed-virus vaccine.[58]

Salk had his allies. Tom Rivers claimed that the vaccine itself was safe—the mass trials of 1954, the Canadian experience, and the record of drug companies like Parke-Davis and Eli Lilly had already proven that. "I think it would be a tragedy if we stopped," he said. Joe Smadel agreed, noting that scientists often faced the ticklish question of when to "start using the material you have already produced." Since nothing is ever beyond improvement, he said, "one is left, then, with the ultimate decision, 'Shall we use what we have now, or shall we wait an indefinite period—three months, six months, five years—until we have something which we think is perfect at that time, and then use it?'"

"In my opinion," he concluded, "we should not wait."[59]

The panelists were then asked to vote on whether the vaccination program should be continued. Salk wisely abstained; so did three others, including Wendell Stanley, the chemist, who claimed the matter should be decided by physicians. The vote was 8 to 3 in favor of continuation. Sabin, Enders, and Hammond cast negative votes. John Paul, the panel's moderator, tried to end the two-day slugfest on an upbeat note. The differences, he said, were "trivial matters in light of the possibility of controlling this disease, which is in sight." No one had the strength left to argue the point.[60]

In truth, the testimony of Sabin and Enders was hardly unexpected. Both men had legitimate concerns about the Cutter fiasco. Both had a strong preference for a live-virus polio vaccine. And both viewed Jonas Salk as the lap dog of Basil O'Connor and the National Foundation. The two scientists had long corresponded about these matters, especially the foundation's preference for a killed-virus vaccine. "You know, of course, that I agree entirely with the facts that you have expressed frequently to me," Enders wrote to Sabin in 1953. "We should keep hammering away . . . until [they] are gained."[61]

Unexpected or not, their testimony threw O'Connor into a rage. So much had gone wrong so quickly. And now this: a public assault on the Salk vaccine by scientists with strong ties to the National Foundation. O'Connor viewed it as the worst sort of treachery. And, confronted by reporters, he let loose on Albert Sabin, one of the prime beneficiaries of foundation largesse. "This is old stuff," said O'Connor. "[Sabin] used it in an attempt to stop the field trials of the Salk vaccine. Since then he's been using it on every possible occasion to stop the use of the Salk vaccine." This wasn't about science, he added; it was about rivalry and envy. "For years Sabin's been trying to get what is called a 'live-virus' polio vaccine [and] there are no present prospects of getting [one.]" Nevertheless, the foundation had "supported Sabin's work to the tune of eight hundred and fifty-three thousand, three hundred and fourteen dollars, and seventy one cents," making him, O'Connor strongly hinted, a major league ingrate.[62]

There was more. The difference between Jonas Salk and his opponents, said O'Connor, was that Salk hoped to save children while his opponents hoped to further their careers. And people that selfish, he went on, "must be prepared to be haunted for life by the crippled bodies of little children who could have been saved from paralysis had they been permitted to receive the Salk vaccine."

It was quite a blast. In public, Sabin kept his composure without giving ground. "I'm not against the vaccine program," he said. "I am against continuation of it with the present Salk vaccine." In private, however, Sabin sent O'Connor a letter that further fanned the flames. "We have known each other for 17 years and good as well as bad words have passed between us," it began. Calling O'Connor "a great humanitarian," it asked: "Would it not be better if you . . . observed a more impartial attitude regarding the contributions of all the scientists whose work is supported by the donations from the American people through the foundation which you so ably lead?"[63]

Sabin, as usual, had found the tender spot. Nothing rankled O'Connor more than the charge that he had misused the *public's* money in the war against polio by favoring one scientist over another. "It occurs to me," he fired back at Sabin, "that you are the one who should be asked whether [you] observed a more impartial attitude regarding scientific work of [others]." While O'Connor didn't threaten a cut-back in funding, he made it clear that Sabin's attacks on the Salk vaccine were doing him no good. The 8 to 3 vote before Congress showed where the majority stood. "This seems to me," said O'Connor, "to be carrying the right of scientific discussion and debate beyond the point where it can properly be described as such."[64]

Sabin was not about to back down. In a blistering four-page response, he claimed that he had been right all along in believing that a live-virus vaccine was the better way to go. As for the 8 to 3 vote, well, "yes, it is a fact, but what does it actually prove? Seven of the 8 are old friends of mine . . . but six of them have never actually worked in polio research; the eighth, a highly respected public health officer, also has no first hand knowledge of poliomyelitis." Predicting that there would be "other crises" in the future, Sabin warned O'Connor about burning his bridges behind him. "Please don't deprive yourself of the benefits of a loyal and respectful opposition."[65]

THESE HAD BEEN DEVASTATING WEEKS for Jonas Salk. He had begun his scientific journey with two goals in mind. One was to prove that a killed-virus vaccine against polio could be safe and effective. The other was to save children's lives. Both goals were now in question, under assault from all sides. Salk still believed in his product; that would never change. But he could hardly forget the Cutter victims whose lives had been devastated, or ended, by a vaccine that was meant to protect them—a vaccine that carried *his* name. "I know it's purely emotional," he told a friend, "but I cannot escape a terrible feeling of identification with these people who got polio."[66]

For Salk, the worst moment came in early May, as the Cutter incident was unfolding. At an emergency session at the NIH, he faced the wrath of the formidable John Enders, who had just returned from Stockholm with a Nobel Prize. Their relationship had been distant but cordial. Following a rare visit to Pittsburgh in 1953, Enders had written: "Jonas: your laboratory is indeed magnificent and the work going on worthy of the greatest praise." Now Enders told him: "It is quack medicine to pretend that this is a killed vaccine when you know it has live virus in it. Every batch has live virus in it."[67]

Salk was stunned. He could feel the disappointment of those around the table that day, as if they blamed him personally for what had occurred. "This was the first and only time in my life that I felt suicidal," he recalled. "There was no hope, no hope at all." Salk returned to

Pittsburgh exhausted, depressed. He tried to be philosophical about his wild ride through the alien world of celebrity, hoping the bottom had been reached. "You find yourself projected into a set of circumstances for which neither your training nor your talents have prepared you," he observed. "It's very difficult in some respects, but it's a transitory thing and you wait till it blows over. Eventually people will start thinking, 'That poor guy,' and leave me alone. Then I'll be able to get back to my laboratory."[68]

Wishful thinking, indeed.

14

Mission to Moscow

WHAT HAD GONE WRONG WITH THE CUTTER VACCINE? There was no definitive answer—there never would be one—though theories abounded. The most plausible explanation was that the virus mixtures sat too long in storage, allowing sediment to gather. This led some of the particles to clump together, shielding them from the formaldehyde. More than 200 polio cases were traced to six contaminated lots of vaccine. The victims included 79 vaccinated children, 105 family members, and 20 community contacts. Most were severely paralyzed; eleven people died.[1]

The rules for producing polio vaccine were quickly amended. To prevent clumping, manufacturers were required to filter the virus fluid just before the formaldehyde was mixed in. More sensitive safety tests were introduced, and record keeping was upgraded to prevent the burying of mistakes. All vaccine lots would have to be accounted for, not just the ones that passed the manufacturer's inspection.[2]

These additions proved remarkably successful. There would be no more Cutter incidents. The Salk vaccine was safe and would remain that way, though public confidence was slow to return. The summer of 1955 came and went with few children getting their shots. A number of state and local health departments declined to use the Salk vaccine, claiming that the Mahoney strain was too dangerous and that starting the process that far into the polio season was not worth the risk. As major epidemics flared in Boston and Chicago, it seemed like old times, with beaches and movie theaters once again deserted and people fleeing the cities to escape the evil germs. "Most of the kids who missed their shots will be back," said one health official, "though perhaps not as soon as they should be."[3]

The remark was prophetic. Studies in 1955 showed the attack rates for paralytic polio to be "from two to five times greater among unvaccinated children than among vaccinated children in the same age-groups." More than 28,000 cases were reported in the United States that year and most of those could have been avoided. The blunders of 1955 had proved costly indeed.[4]

THE POLITICAL FALLOUT from Cutter was enormous. In July 1955, Oveta Culp Hobby stepped down from her cabinet post and returned to Texas. "This is one of the hardest letters I have ever had to write," President Eisenhower replied in accepting her resignation. "History will hail you." Two weeks later, Hobby's special assistant for health affairs followed her out the door. Heads rolled at the NIH, starting with the director's. "The Cutter incident resulted in everybody up the line who had anything to do with it—very few people know this story—being dismissed," an official recalled. "All went out." The new NIH director, James Shannon, was one of the few government scientists who had protested the quick licensing of the vaccine.[5]

In some ways, the Cutter incident worked to strengthen the federal health bureaucracy. The Laboratory of Biologics Control was reorganized and expanded. Vaccine testing became a major function of the NIH. The success of the Polio Surveillance Unit in tracking down Cutter victims dramatically raised the profile of the Public Health Service's Communicable Disease Center (now the Centers for Disease Control and Prevention). Between 1955 and 1960, the NIH budget swelled from $81 million to $400 million, accelerating the pace of federal support that had begun in earnest following World War II. As one polio writer noted, "the testing of the Salk vaccine, the largest field trial ever conducted [within the United States], was also in all likelihood the last such trial that could ever be managed in its entirety by a private organization."[6]

The Cutter incident put a harsh spotlight on Basil O'Connor and the National Foundation for Infantile Paralysis. Some believed that their aggressive tactics had triggered the crisis by creating a public stampede for a poorly tested product. Others expressed bitterness at the National Foundation's ongoing appeals for money and volunteers, as if no hard lessons had been learned. A backlash was inevitable. And it struck the foundation at its most vulnerable point.

There was always a feeling, within the scientific community and beyond, that polio had been oversold as a menace to public health. This was a hard subject to broach, given the scenes of children struggling to walk in leg braces or lying flat on their backs in tomblike iron lungs. But the Cutter incident opened a window on the politics of polio that diminished its status as a privileged disease. Articles now appeared with story lines that would have been unthinkable just a few months before: "Polio Is First in Funds, Least Among Victims," "Polio Fight Sold Like Hucksters Sell Soap," and "Why The Dimes March On."[7]

One fact was indisputable. When it came to fund raising, there was but one bully on the block. In 1954 the eight major health charities had raised just over $140 million, with the National Foundation accounting for almost half.

Agency	Money Raised (in millions)	Number of Cases in 1954
National Foundation for Infantile Paralysis	$66.9	100,000
National Tuberculosis Assn.	24.7	1,200,000
American Cancer Society	21.7	750,000
American Heart Assn.	11.3	10,000,000
United Cerebral Palsy Assn.	8.2	550,000
Muscular Dystrophy Assn.	3.9	200,000
Arthritis Foundation	1.8	11,000,000
National Assn. for Mental Health	1.5	10,000,000

This imbalance was hardly new. What had changed was the criticism it now provoked. Tough questions were being asked. Had the National Foundation cynically exaggerated the dangers of polio? Was its fund raising too aggressive? Might a fairer distribution of charity dollars lead to quicker cures and remedies for other serious diseases? Why did one organization need all that money?[8]

The foundation did not lack for answers. It replied that most of its budget went to the victims, who received quality care regardless of their ability to pay. Polio was a special disease. The children it paralyzed often needed treatment for years. Furthermore, the concerns of other charitable foundations—cancer, arthritis, tuberculosis, cerebral palsy, muscular dystrophy—received millions in grants from the NIH to fund research efforts. The National Foundation asked for nothing. "Our polio fight," it said, "is being won by the finest kind of *voluntary* community effort."[9]

The critics were unimpressed. "Polio has so few patients and gets so much money," said one, "that it can afford to pay all or part of [every] hospital, doctor, nurse, drug and equipment bill." And its high-powered research effort, while no doubt successful, had focused on defeating a relatively rare disease. "A vaccine is a good thing to have. So is a bullet-proof vest," a newspaper noted. "Statistically, more than three times as many people in this country die of homicide as die of polio."[10]

In 1955 a vocal new critic of the National Foundation appeared: the American Medical Association (AMA). This was not entirely unexpected. AMA officials felt slighted by the foundation. In 1954 they had been denied a role in planning the Salk trials and testing the results. On top of that, their request for an advance copy of the Francis Report had been rejected, making the association and the thousands of doctors it represented look like ignorant spectators in their own field of expertise. "It was," said one, "that old irritation at having to read about medicine in the *Reader's Digest* in order to keep with your patients."[11]

Things had escalated from there. The Francis Report was issued on April 12, 1955, the tenth anniversary of Franklin Roosevelt's death. O'Connor claimed the timing was a coincidence, but the AMA among other groups saw an obvious political slant. "Many Republicans hit the ceiling," a doctor recalled. In the coming months, as the Cutter incident unfolded, the AMA lambasted the foundation, claiming its speed and showmanship had "violated traditional methods by which investigators . . . announce and critically review discoveries."[12]

There was truth to these charges. The National Foundation had ignored the medical establishment, staged a razzle-dazzle press production, and demanded that its vaccine be licensed quickly, leaving little time for study or reflection. Physicians who raised questions were told to read the Francis Report. What else did a general practitioner need to know? When asked about the AMA's escalating criticism of the foundation, O'Connor refused to give ground. "The AMA is jealous of any invasion of its prerogatives," he said. "It feels it has a prior right in anything relating to disease or the health of the people."[13]

There was more to this feud, however, than the arrogance of one party or the bruised feelings of the other. AMA officials believed that the mass trials of 1954 had set a dangerous precedent by providing vaccinations at schools and public clinics instead of in a doctor's office where such things belonged. And their suspicions increased the following year when the foundation distributed millions of vaccine doses to first and second grade children free of charge.

To these officials, it all smacked of "socialized medicine," one of the great bugaboos of the cold-war era. The AMA had raised this specter in helping to defeat a plan for national health insurance in 1948. It was not about to endorse a vaccination program intended to exclude both the profit motive and the family physician. "Does the Salk vaccine program constitute a brainwash, to condition Americans for the docile acceptance of regimented medicine?" wrote one doctor. "Many [of us] think that it does." The AMA mobilized its forces. Within weeks, President Eisenhower and congressional leaders were on record supporting the physician's primary role in administering the polio vaccine. The model of low-cost immunization for the masses didn't have a chance.[14]

The repercussions from the Cutter problem were also reached in the courts. An article in the *Yale Law Journal* published a few months after the incident had predicted that negligence suits against the company would fail because the vaccine appeared "to satisfy the standards of care to which the manufacturing druggist has traditionally been held." So the authors suggested another approach. Why not sue Cutter for a breach of an "implied warranty," meaning that those who used its product had reason to assume it was safe? There would be no need to prove negligence. Damages, though probably smaller, could be won without showing fault. And the drug companies would be put on notice to prevent such defects in the future.[15]

This was precisely what happened. In 1958 a California jury awarded almost $150,000 to the families of two young children who had contracted polio after taking the Cutter vaccine. Jonas Salk backed the victims in court, claiming that the procedures in place at the time of the 1955 incident were adequate to insure the manufacture of a safe polio vaccine. The jury was skeptical. While agreeing that Cutter had marketed a product "which when given to plaintiffs caused them to come down with poliomyelitis, thus resulting in a breach of warranty," it did not find the company to be negligent "either directly or by inference"— a verdict that stunned the children's flamboyant attorney, Melvin Belli.

"Had we not had your [support]," he wrote Salk, "I am sure [Cutter] would have gotten away with a [not guilty] verdict and not only slandered you and the program but proved that the children didn't get polio at all—it was just our imagination."[16]

All was not lost, however. In the coming decades, the company would pay out millions in damages to the polio victims and families, with Salk frequently testifying or giving depositions on their behalf. Cutter would survive the debacle, becoming a part of Bayer Laboratories in 1974. But it would never produce another drop of polio vaccine.

For polio researchers, the fallout from the Cutter incident affected both current reputations and future plans. Winners gained ground at the expense of losers; the spotlight shifted; new faces emerged. In May 1955 *Time* ran its first major piece on Albert Sabin, titled "Next: Live Vaccine?" It couldn't have been more flattering. A photo showed him in his starched white lab coat, looking sagely into space. "While virologists were still trying to decide whether Dr. Salk's killed virus vaccine was safe, or how it could be made safer," the article began, "other experts argued that the killed virus idea should be abandoned altogether. Leader of this school: Russian-born Dr. Albert Sabin, 48, director of Cincinnati's Children's Hospital. His alternative: instead of killing a virulent virus, use a living virus that is nonvirulent to begin with."[17]

To this point, Sabin's public exposure had been as a critic, offering grim assessments of the Cutter affair. Few people beyond the laboratory knew of his own research on polio, much less his work on a competing vaccine. Now that veil had been lifted. Debate over the merits of live and killed viruses, once confined to scientific meetings and esoteric journals, had moved into public view. Albert Sabin was anonymous no more.

In later years his friends would try to debunk the popular notion that there had been a head-to-head race for a polio vaccine, Salk vs. Sabin, no holds barred. According to Peter Olitsky, the thought had never crossed Sabin's mind. "In a race," said Olitsky, "one doesn't stop to admire the scenery." Sabin's work on polio, spanning twenty years, had been anything but a hurried pursuit. "Never [was] any time limit set for any experiment. Never did we consider ourselves as racing against others; we never mentioned who was in front, alongside, or in back of us. We often dropped work on polio to take up some new, more alluring subject, e.g., other viruses, etc." Furthermore, Sabin had generously shared his insights and findings with a legion of researchers, including Salk. "Would any track tout call this a race?" Of course not! "Whatever happened to our old apothegms hanging on our walls: 'You can't hurry microbiology?'"[18]

Olitsky had a point. There never was a race for the polio vaccine in terms of a wild sprint to the finish line; what emerged, instead, was a bitter competition between Salk and Sabin that began in the early 1950s and kept gaining momentum—a rivalry that defined and dominated both careers, outlived both men, and continues to this day. It's true that Sabin never put a premium on speed—with good reason. Salk had a simpler vaccine and bottomless funding. Everyone knew he would get there first, forcing Sabin to adjust his sights. "His first object," a contemporary noted, "was to prevent Salk from running away with the prize before anyone else had a chance to compete. The second was to prepare his own contender."[19]

The Cutter incident had worked in macabre fashion to slow the momentum of the Salk vaccine. Interest had now been aroused in an alternative, a live-virus version that might prove more effective. A contender!

SABIN BEGAN WORKING ON A LIVE-VIRUS VACCINE in 1951, after learning that others, including Hilary Koprowski, had started down that path. Sabin had spoken with John Enders about his plans and had sent an assistant to Pittsburgh to study Salk's tissue culture techniques. He also had gone to Lederle Laboratories to see his old colleague from the Rockefeller Institute, Herald Cox. While at Lederle, Sabin had stopped in to see Koprowski, who remembered the visit well: "I would say he came to let me know that he was entering the same turf I was on. He came to communicate, discuss the project, say we were in the same boat—that he too now believed in the live-virus approach. He said he had been doing some heavy thinking about it. . . . He wanted to bury the hatchet, exchange samples of viruses. So I sent him some of my samples. But I never received any of his samples from him."[20]

Like Jonas Salk, Sabin could count on significant support from the National Foundation. In 1949 his five-year grant included $89,500 for equipment, $60,000 for monkeys, and $8,200 for supplies (including animal food). It also paid the salaries of a virologist, a research associate, two animal caretakers, and four technicians, while subsidizing the University of Cincinnati's indirect costs. Sabin may not have been Basil O'Connor's favorite scientist, but he would never hurt for research money. In fact, Sabin noted, the foundation "provided all the funds for my studies."[21]

His staff was smaller than Salk's, partly because he hated to delegate any procedure, no matter how mundane, that he thought he could do better by himself. As Robert Chanock, chief of the NIH Laboratory of Infectious Diseases recalled, Sabin personally inoculated "each of the more than 20,000 monkeys studied during the development of [his] live oral poliovirus vaccine, and he evaluated their clinical status each day these animals were under study. . . . When tissue cultures came into routine use . . . he evaluated almost all of the critical cultures himself." The end result, said Chanock, was that Sabin's colleagues, confident of his results, proceeded to build upon "his research observations without seeking prior verification."[22]

Sabin faced a more formidable task than did Salk. Put simply, it's harder to attenuate a virus than to kill it. In the latter case, Salk could assume that the concentration of formaldehyde needed to inactivate the most virulent of the three polio strains would be strong enough to inactivate the other two. But live viruses take more care because they continue to grow and multiply inside the body. Each strain must be potent enough to produce a mild infection, yet docile enough to do no further harm. "It is the difference," a science writer noted, "between slaughtering an ox and breeding from it, between wringing a parrot's neck and teaching it to talk. You can standardize death in a way that you cannot standardize life."[23]

Was it worth the effort? According to most virologists of that era, the answer was yes. They agreed with Sabin that a live-virus polio vaccine had numerous advantages. Given by mouth, it followed the same path as naturally occurring poliovirus, moving down the digestive system, multiplying extensively in the intestinal tract, and reproducing the durable immunity that resulted from a routine infection. A single dose, it was believed, might well protect a person against polio for life. There would be no need for multiple injections or "boosters." A live-virus vaccine also appeared to work more quickly, within a matter of days not weeks, which meant that it could halt an epidemic already in progress. Most important, it offered the prospect of "passive vaccination" to the general public, since those who ingested the vaccine would shed the weakened virus back into the environment through their feces, thereby immunizing large portions of the unvaccinated population. As a result, a live-virus vaccine—*safely* produced—had the potential to wipe out polio completely.[24]

Attenuating three strains of poliovirus for an effective vaccine, Albert Sabin recalled, "was no job for someone in a hurry." His task, involving monotonous repetition, was to develop viruses that were capable of replicating easily in the alimentary tract "with little or no demonstrable viremia and with the least detectable alteration in neurovirulence of the virus excreted in the stools." Put simply, three strains that could multiply in the intestines without damaging the nervous system and then exit the body in a state no more potent than when they entered.[25]

Sabin attenuated his poliovirus strains by passing them through monkey tissue in rapid succession until the strains were sufficiently attenuated. ("I have come to the conclusion," he wrote a colleague in 1954, "that a poliomyelitis virus which does not produce paralysis after direct spinal inoculation in chimpanzees . . . may be regarded as safe for orienting studies in human beings.") In the winter of 1954–1955, Sabin tested his viruses on thirty adult prisoners at a federal prison in Chillicothe, Ohio, beginning a process that would culminate, less than five years later, in a field trial involving millions of children in a communist country thousands of miles away—the largest medical experiment in world history.[26]

Sabin's use of prisoners reflected a curious reversal in his thinking. At a National Foundation roundtable in 1951, Sabin had bitterly condemned Koprowski for secretly testing his live-virus vaccine on children at a New York mental institution. "How dare you," he had shouted, "Why did you do it? Why? Why?" (See ch. 8.) Yet three years later, Sabin tried to do the same thing himself. Early in 1954, on the eve of the Salk trials, he had approached New York state authorities with his own plan for human testing. "I am [hoping to enlist your help]," he wrote, "in a crucial extension of current studies on poliomyelitis. The work has reached a stage where further . . . progress can be made only by observations on human beings. . . . The viruses that would be used are [from] the same lots which have been tested extensively in monkeys and chimpanzees. Mentally defective children, who are under constant observation in an institution over long periods of time, offer the best opportunity for the careful and prolonged follow-up studies which [we need]."[27]

At least sixty children would be required. "It is highly desirable," he wrote, "that only [those] without antibody for any of the three types [of poliovirus] be used in this study. As a first step, therefore, it would be necessary to bleed 120 to 150 children in the age group of 1 to six years." Remarkably, Sabin spoke of using the virulent Mahoney strain in his vaccine. "I am ready," he declared, "to start any time."[28]

His plan was a close copy of the experiment that Koprowski had run in 1951. The only difference was that Sabin expected to test three types of attenuated poliovirus, while Koprowski had used only one. When word reached the National Foundation, the alarm bells went off. Henry Kumm, the new research director, warned Sabin against proceeding "with any human experiments prior to further review of your grant." That review came quickly. The Virus Research Committee turned him down.[29]

But Sabin persisted. Realizing that Plan A, the use of institutionalized children, had reached a dead end, Sabin moved to Plan B, the use of institutionalized adults. Months of intense lobbying did the trick. Sabin convinced Thomas Rivers and Henry Kumm to back a limited human trial with carefully selected volunteers. "I have reason to believe that the National Foundation will probably lend their support to my proposal to carry out certain studies on poliomyelitis on prisoners," he wrote a friend at the NIH. "I would appreciate it very much if you could let me know the precise names and addresses of the people with whom . . . to deal . . . at the federal prison at Chillicothe, Ohio."[30]

Sabin got the green light after meeting personally with James V. Bennett, director of the Federal Bureau of Prisons. He chose Chillicothe because it was close to his home base in Cincinnati. The volunteers were paid $25 apiece and promised "some days" off their sentence. Virtually every inmate over the age of 21 signed on. Blood samples were taken "to determine the immunity status for the three types of poliovirus." Thirty men were selected—"those without antibody."[31]

Sabin was frank with the authorities. This was virgin ground. "It must be said," he wrote a prison official, "that there is no telling what risk, if any, is involved in these studies. The decision to proceed with . . . human beings is based on the demonstration that in the chimpanzee, a primate most closely related to man, these strains are harmless." Fortunately, the Chillicothe trials went off smoothly. All thirty prisoners developed antibodies to the three virus strains, and no one took ill. "The smallest doses used," Sabin noted, "sufficed to produce an immunizing infection in the volunteers."[32]

Where did he go from here? This, indeed, was a problem. The National Foundation was not about to sponsor a second mass trial for a polio vaccine—not after the Cutter incident and certainly not for its most abrasive grantee. The logistics were daunting. How could Sabin find suitable volunteers in the United States when millions of children had already received the Salk vaccine, effectively immunizing them against the disease? And how could he be certain that his attenuated viruses wouldn't revert back to virulence, bringing polio in their wake? In fact, Sabin had run into problems here, with "virus in some of the [early] stool specimens," he noted, showing "a greater neurovirulence than the virus originally swallowed"—a troubling sign. As a result, the respected Thomas Rivers, who Sabin himself had described as "the eminent father of American virology," had advised him in 1955 "to discard the large lots of oral poliovirus that I had prepared into a suitable sewer."[33]

Sabin found the prospects depressing. He had always considered Rivers to be his strongest ally within the National Foundation, a man who supported his quest for a workable live-virus vaccine. And now this! "I might say that up to the present I have had all the financial assistance that I required," Sabin wrote a colleague in 1955. "I might, however, stress the word 'financial' because in every other respect it can hardly be said that the foundation [has] displayed any special interest in furthering [my] particular approach." To others, Sabin went even further. "Whatever progress I have been able to make," he told a British friend, "has been against the constant impediments that have been put in my way by the very foundation that provides me with the funds for doing my work. I do not think it is an exaggeration to say that the foundation seems to behave more like a commercial company with a vested interest in a certain patent than as a dispassionate scientific foundation intent on getting at all the truth."[34]

Sabin had reached a crossroads. There was no way, he realized, that he would ever be able to mass test his live-virus vaccine in the United States. He would have to find a more respectable setting. The big question was, where?

FOR A TIME SABIN CONSIDERED JOINING FORCES with Cox and Koprowski. He had approached the two men in 1955 about creating a committee of interested researchers to study the live-virus polio vaccine. At this point, Sabin had as much to learn as to share. Since Cox and Koprowski had been working on their vaccine for several years, their response was guarded, to say the least. The idea looked promising, they replied, so please count them in. Of course, there were strict rules regarding what Lederle could release to outsiders, so please don't count on much. The plan soon fell apart. As Henry Kumm wrote Sabin: "It seems to me that . . . we would be traveling down a one way street. . . . They would have access to everything discovered by you or by any other grantee of the National Foundation while they themselves would not be allowed to furnish [anything] to us."[35]

In truth, the vaccine quest at Lederle had not been going well. A management shakeup at the parent company, American Cyanamid, had demoralized those engaged in biomedical research. The bean counters were now in control, a scientist noted. "Their idea of a good product was mixing two toothpastes together. Our freedom was cut." In addition, a personality clash had developed between the older, more traditional Herald Cox and the brasher, risk-taking Hilary Koprowski. "He wanted his name to appear on all papers written by members of his virology section," Koprowski recalled. "So I worked apart, published by myself. We were in competition as though we worked for different companies."[36]

Something had to give. Koprowski, the junior member, knew his days at Lederle were numbered. "I have reached [a] decision after an earnest seeking of a solution to some disturbances noticed in my private universe," he told John Enders in 1954. "I am writing in order to ask you a favor in remembering my name in an *academic* field of my specialty [if] a position opens in Boston or anywhere else."[37]

Before departing, however, Koprowski got the break he'd been waiting for—the chance to mass test his vaccine. It came in the form of an invitation in 1956 from George Dick, a virologist at Queen's University in Belfast. An advocate of the live-virus approach, Dick hoped to organize the first significant field trial of this sort. "One of the big attractions of working in Northern Ireland," wrote a student of the ill-fated Dick-Koprowski collaboration, "was the autonomy it offered, for in those days the province had its own parliament, and thus enjoyed a degree of independence from the political and medical grandees in London. It also offered a discrete and stable population, and one that had a reputation of cooperating with medical researchers."[38]

Dick viewed the field trials as a gift to the city of Belfast and a boost to his own career. The plan was to vaccinate the investigators and their children, and then move slowly through the general population. But there was trouble from the start. Stool samples from the children (including Dick's four-year-old daughter) turned up virus particles that were less attenuated than those in the original vaccine. Even more alarming, these excreted particles caused paralysis when injected into monkeys. It appeared that the worst had come to pass: Koprowski's vaccine had reverted to virulence during its passage through the human intestinal tract. In Dick's apt description, it had "gone in like a lamb, but come out like a lion."[39]

Dick stopped the trials. "I felt incredibly let down by Koprowski," he recalled. "I felt that his data [were] inaccurate." Had the tests proceeded, he said, "I have no doubt at all that we could have paralyzed a number of children." Koprowski, in turn, accused Dick of exaggerating the problem out of personal pique. Always the gambler, he brushed off those who demanded absolute safety as the criterion for a potentially lifesaving vaccine. "Protection of man against disease is obtained at a price," Koprowski told a scientific conclave in 1957. "Nothing in nature is given free, and all efforts should be made to reduce the cost of this payment." But it was asinine, he said, to give "more importance to the fact that a monkey's paw became limp after an intraneural injection of human feces, than to the possibility of elimination of poliomyelitis." There was no such thing as perfection; "the only virus particles which will never mutate are those which do not exist." People needed "*a sense of proportion*" in these matters. The virus strains presently available—the ones he had used in Belfast—were "as good as they probably ever will be." Good enough, he insisted, to save thousands of children from the horrors of paralysis and death.[40]

But not good enough for the bean counters at Lederle. Koprowski left that year to become director of the then-moribund Wistar Institute in Philadelphia, taking a number of Lederle colleagues along with him. It was a bitter parting. Having spent millions of dollars on polio research with precious little to show for it, Lederle officials accused Koprowski of pilfering research notes and virus strains that belonged to the company—a charge Koprowski denied. The chief accuser was Herald Cox.[41]

Koprowski would continue his polio research at Wistar, seeking other places to test his live-virus vaccine. He would even reach out to Albert Sabin, hoping, it appears, to begin a partnership that Sabin no longer had the slightest interest in pursuing. "I should like to say," Sabin wrote his colleague John Paul following the Belfast disaster, that "I can see no useful purpose in trying to do anything together with Hilary Koprowski because I can neither rely on the very gracious statements and promises that he makes in my presence nor on the data that he reports or fails to report at conferences." In the field of live-virus polio research, it was now every man for himself.[42]

BY 1956 SABIN HAD MADE GIANT STRIDES in the development of his viruses. "I have already selected the optimum type 2 and 3 progeny [and] am now in the process of testing . . . two type 1 strains," he wrote to John Paul, adding, as usual, that "I have not had a Saturday or Sunday away from the laboratory during the period of these studies." In January Sabin got a phone call from the Public Health Service informing him that a group of Russian scientists would be coming to the United States to "study polio" and "the preparation of the Salk vaccine." Though Pittsburgh was their primary destination, the Russians hoped to meet with other polio researchers, including Bodian, Enders, Paul, and Sabin. Would it be possible for them to visit his lab in Cincinnati?[43]

It was more than possible, it was *essential*, Sabin responded. "I expect to arrange a program of conferences and demonstrations, and the Dean of our Medical School is contemplating having a private dinner." The visit went well. The Russians told Sabin about the recent spread of polio in the Soviet Union and their early experiments with the Salk vaccine. Sabin showed off his live-virus strains and expressed an interest in touring their country, the land of his birth. The Russians promised an invitation from their Ministry of Health.[44]

Sabin took it from there. Concerned, no doubt, about the cold-war implications, he contacted the surgeon general, the Public Health Service, and the State Department, seeking approval in advance. All responded positively. "In principle, the State Department favors visits of American scientists to the Soviet Union," wrote one of its science advisors. But another warned Sabin "to move reasonably rapidly" because the department "is dragging its feet in the matter of U.S. scientific travel and [Secretary of State] Dulles simply fails to provide a set of procedures to be followed in the matter."[45]

The invitation arrived a month later. The State Department granted permission following two lengthy FBI interviews, and Sabin flew to Leningrad that June. He spent a month in Russia, giving lectures, meeting with researchers, and lobbying nonstop for his vaccine. Upon returning to Cincinnati, he sought permission to send virus samples to the Soviet Union for testing. The State Department approved, ignoring a Defense Department warning about their "biological warfare applicability." Sabin had a foot in the door.[46]

The timing couldn't have been better. Relations with the Soviet Union had begun to thaw a bit following the death of Joseph Stalin in 1953. Meanwhile, increased federal support for scientific research had created a powerful bureaucracy in Washington that sought greater international cooperation in biomedical affairs. President Eisenhower had promised to share the "technical knowledge" of the polio vaccine with the people of the world. And no people, it turned out, needed that knowledge as badly as the Soviets.

Polio had come late to the Soviet Union. Until 1930, it had the lowest incidence in Europe—less than one case per 100,000, as compared with 6.3 in Denmark and 15.4 in Sweden. But as the nation industrialized and sanitation improved, polio began to spread. In 1955, a series of major epidemics forced the Russians to establish the Polio Research Institute in Moscow, headed by Mikhail Chumakov, a top-flight virologist who led the delegation that had visited Sabin's lab. The Communist government wanted to begin large-scale human testing as quickly as possible. The issue facing Chumakov was which vaccine to use.[47]

It was a tough decision. Chumakov went back and forth. Early experiments with the Salk vaccine had shown mixed results. Though polio had been reduced in the Soviet Union, the vaccine was expensive to produce, difficult to administer, and erratic in potency. After talking to Russian scientists, Sabin felt good about his chances. "They pointed out," he told John Paul, "that they would like to work along with me on the attenuated oral vaccine." Yet a Foreign Service officer in Moscow told Sabin a different story: "I questioned [them] on their polio plans. They haven't decided about a live virus, deferring judgment until more testing; however they intend to begin their program with a Salk-type vaccine using other than the Mahoney strain."[48]

One of the key factors in the decision would be the interest of the two American rivals. Sabin was anxious to please; Salk less so. Chumakov had invited Salk to the Soviet Union to inspect the production facilities and discuss plans for mass testing. Salk had declined. "I can remember how many times my father kicked himself for not going," said Peter Salk, the oldest son. "But my mother put her foot down. She told him enough was enough; he'd been removed from us for too long. She rarely put limits on my father, but visiting Russia was one of those times. It's amazing. It may have changed the course of history."[49]

Instead, a bond was formed between Chumakov and Sabin that matured into a lifelong friendship (an odd one, given that Chumakov never learned English and Sabin barely spoke Russian). Chumakov and his wife, Marina Voroshilova, had been part of the movement to free Russian medicine from its Stalinist past. Textbooks still carried statements reading: "In the Soviet Union, infection is successfully controlled owing to the very essence of the Soviet socialist system." Indeed, Sabin had been criticized at one of his Leningrad lectures in 1956 for ignoring the discredited theories of Lysenko, which, he was told, would "produce a perfect vaccine because Soviet principles of genetics permit for better methods of selection."[50]

Though Chumakov would soon provide Sabin with the chance of a lifetime, the truth was that each man offered something priceless to the other. "In my own field, at the moment," Sabin told a State Department official, "Soviet science has much more to gain from the United States than the United States can gain from the Soviet Union." In 1959, using the virus strains supplied by Sabin, the Russians vaccinated 10 million children. The doses were administered by medicine dropper or wrapped in candy. A small minority received a trivalent vaccine—all three strains at once. The vast majority got three separate doses—Types I, II, and III—spaced a month or so apart. An expert on the scene described these trials as akin to a military campaign. Vaccination centers were set up in "schools, nurseries, kindergartens, clinics, factories, and the like." Parents were told where and when to bring their children. Local officials made sure that everybody showed up. Pediatricians took care of the medical end. Meticulous records were kept, "giving name, address, age, type of vaccine administered, and date of vaccination." It was a tribute to Dr. Chumakov, to good planning, and to the coercive powers of a police state.[51]

The Sabin trials of 1959 were a world apart from the Salk trials of 1954. There were differences in the vaccines, the sample size, and the experiment itself. The Russians made no attempt to duplicate the double-blind model used in the United States. There would be no control groups, no placebos, and no children purposely denied vaccine. These trials would be based on the "humanitarian principles" that Salk himself had wanted and had been denied. The sole objective, said Chumakov, was to wipe out polio.

By year's end, the first results were in. "I am very glad to tell you," Chumakov wrote Sabin, "that your vaccine is winning new victories in our country. The number vaccinated is steadily increasing which reflects the . . . great advantages of the live oral vaccine over the killed one." Chumakov then dropped the bombshell. The Health Ministry had decided to vaccinate every person under the age of 20, 77 million in all. "I am taking some measures," he said, "for you to be elected an Honorary Member of our Academy of Medical Sciences."[52]

Sabin was elated. "At the rate you are going," he replied, "the USSR will probably be the first country in which the eradication of polio will be achieved." But a problem loomed as well. News this good was certain to be dismissed as typical Soviet propaganda. There had to be some sort of independent verification from the non-Communist West. Without it, Sabin told Chumakov, "people will say, 'Yes, but how much can we trust the Russian results?'"[53]

Fortunately, there were allies willing to help. The Belfast trials had been a clear setback for supporters of the live-virus approach. But a victory in the Soviet Union might turn things around, leading to the introduction of a Sabin-type vaccine in Western nations, including the United States. The impetus came from polio researcher John Paul, a close friend of Sabin's. Paul convinced the World Health Organization (WHO) to send a scientist to Russia to study the vaccine trials and write a public report. He recommended his Yale colleague Dorothy Horstmann as the right person for the job.[54]

The WHO was a natural choice. It had already endorsed the oral vaccine as the best means of eradicating polio around the globe. And Horstmann had impeccable credentials. Her thoroughness was legendary, her integrity unquestioned. Though close to Sabin, she could be counted on to write an objective report.

Horstmann spent six weeks in the Soviet Union in the fall of 1959. Her report to the WHO was impressionistic but favorable. Everything seemed in order, she wrote. "The standards of laboratory work in the areas evaluated are high. The facilities are adequate." Though much remained to be done and the *final* results would be "slow in coming," it was apparent, she concluded, that the Sabin virus strains were safe and effective. Indeed, "the marked reduction of cases in 1959 in orally vaccinated Republics suggests that the vaccine may have played a significant role in reducing the incidence of paralytic poliomyelitis."[55]

Were things really this good? Was it possible for one person, spending six weeks in a vast and regimented environment like the Soviet Union, to draw any conclusions at all? A look at Horstmann's correspondence in these crucial weeks is somewhat unsettling. There are hints, for example, that Sabin was communicating with her through John Paul, who wrote Horstmann in October 1959: "I am hastening to send you an abstract of comments which ABS [Albert Bruce Sabin] made when he was here last week. Possibly there is very little here which you do not know, but I thought that some of these points might perhaps be of help to you, provided you can check and agree with them when it comes to writing your report."[56]

More revealing are Horstmann's "casual notes" dated October 3, 1959, which described "the caliber of the work, largely done by Prof. Chumakov on live poliovirus vaccine in Russia." Her conclusions here were more guarded:

> General Comments: Actually the Chumakovs have been attempting so much and sending out people all over the country with vaccine in hand that precise data from many areas is lacking and work on the laboratory specimens has fallen behind. Although more data will be ready by January, it will take much longer than that to sift out all the aspects, statistical, epidemiologic, serologic, and virologic, for the present program to go forward in a kind of frenzy.[57]

In truth, Horstmann had done her best to write a report based on sketchy information—a fact she alluded to but did little to emphasize. And that report, she acknowledged, was absolutely essential "to the acceptance of the Sabin vaccine in the United States."[58]

IN 1960, AMIDST GREAT FANFARE, a Soviet delegation attended the Second International Conference on Live Poliovirus Vaccines in Washington, D.C. The members came in triumph, speaking of the "monumental advances" their country had made in eradicating the disease. Though the Horstmann Report had convinced many researchers of the legitimacy of these claims, an American scientist rose to express his doubts in a blunt, confrontational way. When he finished, a Russian delegate took the floor and said simply: "I would like to assure [you] of one thing, that we in the Soviet Union love our children and are as concerned for their well being as much as people in the United States, or any other part of the world are for their children."[59]

The delegates stood and applauded. A new era had begun.

15

Sabin Sundays

E VER SINCE THE 1930s, the National Foundation for Infantile Paralysis had used the war cry "Polio Can Be Conquered" to rally the troops and bring in the dimes. In 1956 a new slogan appeared, reflecting all that had changed. "Polio Isn't Licked Yet," it warned. "The Fight Goes On." But to many it read like an epitaph, the last gasp of a movement that had outlived its mission, a victim of its own success.[1]

The timing said it all. In 1956, the Salk vaccine came into its own, fulfilling the promise of the mass trials and the Francis Report, the promise of polio's demise. There would be 15,000 reported cases of the disease in the United States that year, half the number of 1955. And there would be but 7,000 cases in 1957, half the number of 1956. A majority of Americans under forty had received at least one inoculation against polio. The future looked good.

Swimming pools reopened in the summer of 1956, and the wild rumors petered out. A child with a fever or a stiff neck no longer sent shock waves through the neighborhood. Newspapers stopped printing the daily box score of polio victims on the front page. The media moved on to other things.

Polio hadn't disappeared, of course. But given the steep decline in numbers, the disease had lost its power to alarm. Fear had given way to complacency, leading some to worry that Americans, seeing polio as fully defeated, would forget how the war had been won. "Our main problem now," said Thomas Rivers, "is not that anything is wrong with the Salk vaccine, but that something is wrong with the people who won't take it."[2]

But others saw a greater problem based on factors such as income and class. To be adequately protected, a child had to get three Salk shots, properly spaced, and a recommended booster shot once a year. This meant multiple trips to a clinic or a local doctor. The shots cost money and parents had to be involved. Statistics showed that millions of children were still at risk, especially those mired in poverty. In the past, polio had been a disease of cleanliness, striking hardest at the middle class. Now it had become a disease of the unvaccinated, which struck hardest at the inner-city poor. In 1959 a National Foundation report had warned that "the gravest danger today is in the urban 'soft spots' of the underprivileged . . . fed by the apathy and ignorance of people who don't care enough or know enough to use the Salk vaccine."[3]

The new slogan was correct: polio *wasn't* licked yet. But the dwindling number of cases as well as the shift toward inner-city victims had put the foundation on shaky ground. Mothers stopped marching. Contributions slowed. Bowing to the inevitable, Basil O'Connor circulated a memo to the Board of Trustees in 1958 about plans to move the foundation "beyond polio." No one knew more than he did about mobilizing a volunteer army. "In the case of the Salk vaccine," he wrote, "a man whose life may be routine, but who participated in the March of Dimes, can say, 'This is something I helped bring about. Whatever else I have done, this was worth doing.'" The foundation would have to tap that special feeling again. First, however, it needed a cause.[4]

O'Connor ran down the options. The two greatest health concerns of the modern era, cancer and heart disease, already had philanthropies up and running. Mental illness and geriatrics were too vast, and neither held much interest for the foundation's top grantees. The March of Dimes had always focused on children. That's what had mobilized the scientists and the volunteers. It must continue down that road.

"After protracted discussions with specialists," O'Connor recommended juvenile arthritis, birth defects, and prenatal care. Given his power at the foundation, there was nothing more to discuss. "Infantile paralysis was our wonderful beginning, but only a beginning," he said. "As the time was ripe twenty years ago for [us] to fight a terrifying disease, so the hour is right now to enter the broader battle that lies ahead."

There were assurances as well. The foundation would never abandon the victims of polio, though funding would probably have to be cut. And it would continue the effort "to bring the Salk vaccine as near as possible to perfection." This was important, for a movement was growing, led by Albert Sabin and his supporters, to license a live-virus polio vaccine. It was an outcome O'Connor didn't relish: the reality of Sabin elbowing Salk aside.

In 1959, at the director's urging, the foundation approved Salk's final polio grant for a whopping $306,564, plus an additional $28,000 in indirect costs. The grant, reflecting the foundation's new direction, was only "for a period of one year." The days of long-term polio funding were over.[5]

JONAS SALK WAS NOT ABOUT TO ROLL OVER AND GIVE UP the fight. He had great confidence in his vaccine and in the killed-virus principle it represented. In the years since that magical day in Ann Arbor, Salk had worked on a host of problems related to the vaccine's potency, the substitution of different virus strains, the proper spacing of the injections, and the like. But he also had begun to tire of the technical aspects of vaccine research, the fiddling and tinkering. Over time, he recalled, his thoughts had turned to the larger mysteries of biological science. His aim, grandly stated, was to use the extraordinary advances in modern medicine as "the foundation for understanding human problems at all levels"—physical, mental, social, and ethical.

Salk had a vehicle in mind. He hoped to create an "experimental institute" on the Pittsburgh campus, similar to the renowned Institute for Advanced Study in Princeton, New Jersey. Salk had gone there to study the operation and confer with its director, J. Robert Oppenheimer, the brilliant and controversial nuclear physicist who had led the Manhattan Project that developed the atomic bomb. The Institute for Advanced Study had no formal connection to a university; it was financed entirely through private grants and donations. Salk took a somewhat different approach. He expected the University of Pittsburgh to cover most of his institute's expenses, with the National Foundation providing the largest private donation. Basil O'Connor was enthusiastic. Salk assumed that others would be, too.[6]

It didn't turn out that way. Reaction to the institute was decidedly mixed. Some critics took it as proof of Salk's celebrity status, his need for attention and acclaim. Others saw it as a cushy refuge for a spent force, a man with nothing of his own left to contribute. "There's no mystery about Jonas' long silence, no mystery about his refusal to discuss his work with people who used to be his friends," a colleague sniffed. "He's afraid."[7]

In 1957 Salk had approached Pittsburgh's new chancellor, Edward H. Litchfield. His goal, he said, was to gather "a select group of scientists and scholars" for the purpose of studying "the fulfillment of man's biological potential." The response was cautious. Litchfield wanted something "more concrete." He was unwilling to commit resources without a firm grasp of what it might cost him, and where the university fit in. "Between us," he told Salk, "perhaps through the years we can realize some of the things you have in mind."[8]

Litchfield was a dynamic personality with an ego to match. Born in 1914—the same year as Salk—he had earned his doctorate in political science at the University of Michigan, playing minor league baseball on the side. Arriving at Pittsburgh in 1956 from Cornell University where he had been dean of the Business School, Litchfield stunned the trustees by accepting a second job as chairman of the board of the Smith-Corona Corporation. "I must find my own ways of pursuing our objectives," he declared. "One of these includes the allocation of my own time."[9]

Litchfield kept both jobs, commuting from one to the other by private plane. His nonstop motor made him a national celebrity, with mixed results for the university. In an interview in *Time* magazine, he described it as "a mediocre place in danger of stagnation," adding: "Our teaching is not as good as it should be. In fact, some of it is poor. Our research is not as good as it should be." Litchfield had been chancellor for less than six months.[10]

But Pittsburgh's national standing rose dramatically under his direction. Fund raising exploded, student admissions became more selective, faculty salaries increased, and outside grant money poured in. The problems with Litchfield were personal. "His was the Imperial Presidency," a colleague recalled. "He lived in royal houses and private planes. Like Louis XIV he bordered on the obscene. But he was the guy who made this university go. He was the emperor with the vision to go with it. And his ambitions were what moved the medical school."[11]

Litchfield understood the value of Salk's proposed institute. It would surely bring the university some added prestige. The sticking point was jurisdiction. The institute would be in a Pitt building, on the Pitt campus, spending Pitt dollars, and consuming Pitt resources. That, thought Litchfield, meant a sharing of control.

Salk disagreed. A great institute needed absolute autonomy, he replied. "I must be allowed . . . to go about this with . . . the kind of freedom available to an individual who functions independently. I want to contribute all I can to the University, but I need the assurance that I will not encounter either minor or major frustrations . . . that cannot easily be overcome."[12]

Both men had a point, and neither would budge. Salk wanted carte blanche to pursue a grander, less structured form of scientific inquiry. Litchfield hoped to please him within the boundaries of fiscal and organizational restraint. As a compromise, the chancellor formed a committee to study the issue. He even made Oppenheimer a member, which proved to be a mistake. Taking Salk's side, as expected, Oppenheimer launched into a theatrical monologue about the evils of oppressive bureaucracy. "Dr. Litchfield, we don't need any table of organization," he proclaimed. "That's why the United States doesn't have any Sputniks in the sky!"[13]

The committee deadlocked. Privately, Oppenheimer encouraged Salk to look elsewhere for a site—an option both sides would soon embrace. While not yet giving up on Pittsburgh, Salk's patience was wearing thin. "I would like to look forward to a year less beset by frustrations of the variety that I have lived with this year," he told a colleague in 1959. "With tongue in cheek I say 'I've had it.'"[14]

Litchfield felt the same way. In a withering memo, he portrayed Salk as a prima donna unable to see beyond his own selfish needs. "We are all anxious to try to find some way of keeping [him] satisfied," wrote Litchfield, but there were limits to what could be done. Salk already enjoyed the highest salary in the university as well as a state-of-the-art laboratory in a building that bore his name. "The medical school has permitted [him] a freedom never previously enjoyed by any other member of the faculty. He has no teaching load and is asked to make no contributions of any kind to the work of the faculty as such. The University leaves him free to undertake such research as he may have in mind in such a way as he may have in mind. In the meantime, he enjoys all of the privileges of faculty status, including the availability of graduate students to undertake his research for him."[15]

There was real danger in Salk's proposal, Litchfield warned. An independent institute "sets a precedent which will not be lost on other parts of the institution and would make it virtually impossible for the University to deny similar powers to other individuals." This raised the obvious question: Was Salk worth all the trouble? Litchfield thought not. To cave in to a faculty member on the basis of his celebrity, he said, would be an awful mistake. Other universities were watching—especially those "with Nobel Prize winners, for example, *with far greater distinction than Dr. Salk has achieved*." Pittsburgh must stand tall against blackmail. "There is a basic principle of the integrity of the University which cannot and should not be abandoned."[16]

Within a year, Salk was gone. For Litchfield and his inner circle, there were few regrets. Many had come to resent Salk, viewing him as a new breed of academic, the pampered superstar. They endorsed Litchfield's tough position in the negotiations and claimed that most of Pitt's faculty felt the same way. One dean rather gleefully circulated a rumor that Salk had offended "important doctors" with his arrogant, temperamental demeanor. The dean had heard it from his barber.[17]

For Litchfield, a final problem remained: damage control. Jonas Salk had been Pittsburgh's most illustrious faculty member. He had put the medical school on the map and made an entire region come alive with pride. How would the university explain such a grievous loss? How would the public react?

Litchfield's great fear had been that another university would offer Salk the very deal that Pittsburgh had denied him, making the chancellor look short-sighted and vindictive. But that didn't happen. In 1960 Salk announced plans to establish an independent scientific institute in La Jolla, California, supported entirely by private funds. Pittsburgh was off the hook. "Our objective now," wrote Litchfield, "is to make certain that this is explained in such a way as to make it abundantly clear that he did not leave Pittsburgh for another university appointment but rather to go to an entirely different atmosphere in an entirely different kind of situation." Fortunately, Litchfield added, "Dr. Salk shares in our desire that it be explained in this way to all persons concerned."[18]

That was true. Salk hoped to exit gracefully. He wanted it known that he was leaving Pittsburgh with great reluctance—not over a petty feud with the administration but because of a unique offer "in a very special place." The relieved chancellor claimed to fully understand. "When a man seeks independence," said Edward Litchfield, "that's a good thing."[19]

Years later, Salk would blame Litchfield for forcing him out. "We could have created the institute here, absolutely," he declared. "But

Litchfield and I had different views of how to set up such an entity. I felt it had to be built around particular people. His view . . . was that one could administer a science institute as one did a prison, a university, a church, all the same way. Eventually, when it became clear that I could not succeed in a place that was already programmed, in a sense, that led to my leaving." But others disagreed. A fair number of Salk's colleagues at Pittsburgh had come to view him as "an independent operator," increasingly selfish and remote. Few, in truth, were sad to see him go. "We had a team [here] it was important that we held together to build the school without feathering our own nests," the chief of medicine recalled. "Jonas was more interested in his own nest than in building the school, but, of course, [that was] his privilege."[20]

Independence proved elusive. The West Coast beckoned Jonas Salk to a new life, a fresh beginning, but there was no escaping the past. Old wounds would soon reopen, old adversaries would reappear. The same battles would be fought again with fresh ammunition, leading this time to humiliation and defeat.

THE 1960s WOULD BELONG TO ALBERT SABIN, the way the 1950s had belonged to Salk. Armed with the results of the Russian polio trials, Sabin set out to sweep his rivals from the field. His strategy had two main objectives: first to show the superiority of his vaccine over those of his live-virus competitors, Hilary Koprowski and Herald Cox; then to demonstrate its mettle over the killed-virus version of Jonas Salk. "They were fighting likes dogs over a bone," a scientist recalled. "Salk, Sabin, Koprowski, Cox," said another, "I would have loved to have seen them tag-team wrestling."[21]

The battle for live-vaccine supremacy was a rout. Sabin had a huge advantage over Cox and Koprowski. He was viewed as an independent agent, toiling for the good of mankind; they were seen as commercial scientists, working for private gain. He had strong support from the giants of polio research; they had almost none. He understood the importance of publicity—good for himself, bad for opponents—and could generate either kind. To watch him in action, said one writer, was to glimpse "scientific generalship of the very highest order."[22]

All three had mass tested their vaccines. Koprowski had run trials in the Belgian Congo, Cox in the Andes. But both projects were miniscule compared to Sabin's Soviet extravaganza, and their results were unconfirmed. Koprowski had yet to live down the Belfast debacle; he was clearly running third. Cox was backed by Lederle Laboratories, which had invested more than $11 million in live-virus polio research and another $2 million for a production facility. But knowing Sabin from their days together at the Rockefeller Institute, Cox could sense the grind that lay ahead. "There has been many a time when I wish I had never attempted to go into this project," he confided to a friend, "but now that I am in it there is nothing to do but fight it through to a successful completion."[23]

Cox had good reason for concern. In 1959, as the battle heated up, Sabin had told Lederle officials of rumors circulating that the Cox vaccine was "only slightly attenuated," and probably dangerous, implying, it appeared, that Lederle was backing the wrong man. Cox angrily demanded a retraction from Sabin, in vain. "I am sure you are aware," Cox responded, "that [your] statement is a very strong and incriminating one. . . . As you should know, if I or my associates had the slightest reason to believe that our strains were causing either frank or suspected illness . . . we would be the first ones to say so. . . . Your [charge] has caused us great concern because it is in such direct contrast with the facts."[24]

In 1960 Sabin and Cox received permission to run vaccine trials inside the United States. Sabin logically chose Cincinnati and surrounding Hamilton County, Ohio. The community pitched in, knowing, as the major newspaper there put it, that "the whole nation is watching this experiment." Beginning on April 24 and continuing for several weeks, nearly 200,000 people, most of them young children, lined up outside schools, hospitals, and clinics on so-called Sabin Oral Sundays to receive vaccine hidden in sweet syrup and sugar cubes.

There was reason for community pride. Sabin was headquartered in Cincinnati, which, he vowed, would soon become America's first "polio-free" city. The problem, as usual, was that he wouldn't tolerate dissent. In a remarkable letter to the U.S. surgeon general, the health commissioner of Hamilton County complained of being "harassed and pressured" to participate in the trials. "Dr. Sabin has been most vigorous in his effort to gain local acceptance for his product," he went on, "and I think to such a degree that he is doing the public a disservice." According to the health commissioner, Hamilton County didn't need the Sabin Oral Sundays. It *already* was polio-free from the widespread use of the Salk vaccine. The truth, he said, was that Sabin had rekindled fears over a disease that no longer existed in the region, with the result that more pressing health issues were being sidetracked or ignored. "I feel this whole thing," he said, "is doing harm."[25]

Cox, meanwhile, ran his trials in Dade County, Florida, vaccinating more than 400,000 people. There was strong interest in his project because he alone had produced a trivalent vaccine—three strains in one—that could be given in a single dose. But the results proved controversial. Though the vaccine worked well in conferring immunity, six cases of severe polio were reported within seven to fourteen days of swallowing the cherry-flavored liquid, the exact length of time it takes for poliovirus to produce paralytic illness. There was no proof that vaccine had *caused* these cases, but suspicions abounded that another Cutter incident was at hand. Cox was through.[26]

In August 1960 Surgeon General Leroy E. Burney approved the Sabin vaccine for trial manufacture in the United States, the first step in the licensing process. The Cox and Koprowski vaccines were rejected on grounds of safety. Burney had been advised by a distinguished panel of polio researchers, a legacy of the Cutter affair. Within hours, four major drug companies announced plans to produce Sabin's vaccine. One was Charles Pfizer & Co., which had begun making the vaccine in England. Another was Lederle Laboratories, the employer of Herald Cox. A spokesman there said "business was business." Millions had been spent on research and development. Production facilities were already in place. It was time to ride the winner and get out a vaccine.[27]

IN HIS REGAL OFFICE at 120 Broadway, Basil O'Connor sat and stewed. Having financed Sabin's breakthrough with more than a million dollars in grants, he now expected some of the credit. Yet, despite all the money spent, he had prayed for Sabin to fail. The Ann Arbor announcement had been O'Connor's shining moment, the Salk vaccine his gift to the world. Now he could see his legacy crumbling under the weight of Sabin's success. And there was nothing he could do.

Salk's support had melted away. Former allies like Thomas Francis and David Bodian refused to take a public stand. Meanwhile, prominent medical experts such as John Paul and John Enders and Mikhail Chumakov were telling anyone who would listen about the superiority of Sabin's vaccine. They spoke at medical conventions, scientific conferences, and public health conclaves, often with Sabin at their side. A foundation official who attended a panel discussion in Boston sent this memo to national headquarters: *"Dr. John Enders, moderator. [Says]* polio problem not yet solved. Salk vaccine has now been under trial for five years. Protects a certain proportion of individuals for an unknown length of time. Evidence that it's not entirely satisfactory . . . Introduced [a panelist], asking: 'Why the Salk failures?'"[28]

Much of this anti-Salk ammunition was provided by a series of sporadic polio outbreaks in 1958 and 1959. Most experts agreed that the problem lay more with the vaccination process than with the vaccine. Studies done in major American cities concluded that perhaps half the population there under the age of forty had not been fully vaccinated against the disease. Indeed, evidence from Detroit showed that "only 12 percent of the paralytic cases [had] occurred in persons who received three doses of [Salk] vaccine, whereas 73 percent of such cases occurred in persons who had received no vaccine." According to Alexander Langmuir, chief of epidemiology at Health, Education, and Welfare, the problem was worst "in our lower socioeconomic and negro areas," where current polio rates, he suspected, were even higher than in the pre-vaccine era.[29]

The National Foundation naturally stepped up its publicity campaign to increase awareness of vaccination schedules for children. But O'Connor put some of the blame on Albert Sabin, claiming that his relentless attacks on the Salk vaccine were encouraging people to postpone their vaccinations until the new and supposedly better Sabin vaccine came along. Furious at what he believed to be a conscious effort to mislead the public, O'Connor turned to Tom Rivers, the foundation's most revered scientific figure, to put a stop to it.

Rivers was as much a part of the foundation as O'Connor himself. He had been there from the beginning, first as special assistant to the president, then as medical director, and finally, in 1958, as vice president for medical affairs. During his time as chairman of the Virus Research Committee, he had been a supporter of Salk's killed-virus research and a guiding force behind the mass field trials of 1954. Rivers had no ax to grind. He played no favorites in the contentious vaccine wars. (He even-handedly referred to Sabin as "the smart Jew" and Salk as "the young Jew.") His goal, quite simply, was the eradication of polio.

Like O'Connor, Rivers had been offended by Sabin's stepped-up assault on the Salk vaccine. He thought it unseemly for a scientist to promote himself and dismiss the work of a colleague in such an arrogant way. It hurt him to hear Sabin claim that Salk's vaccine was "only

60 to 70 percent effective," when the Public Health Service had put the figure at about 90 percent, or that "hundreds of children" would die if the Sabin vaccine wasn't licensed at once. "I think you are way off base," Rivers scolded him. "You are a good virologist but I believe you should have had a little more training in the field of statistics than you have had."[30]

Nevertheless, Rivers expected the foundation to steer a neutral course between the warring sides, guided not by past loyalty to Salk or to Sabin, but rather by the strength of their respective vaccines. And his public statements to that effect made a collision with O'Connor inevitable. It occurred in 1961, at a symposium on the two vaccines sponsored by the Centers for Communicable Disease in Atlanta. In a room filled with notables, O'Connor accused Rivers of undermining the foundation and its goals. The two men had to be separated. But they continued the jousting at foundation headquarters in Manhattan, where Rivers collapsed and began to hemorrhage from a duodenal ulcer, almost dying from the loss of blood.

In a letter to Bodian from his hospital bed, Rivers described the impossibility of dealing with O'Connor when it came to the subject of Sabin and Salk. "Everyone at headquarters has to speak about [their] vaccine work in whispers," he wrote. "Since I can't whisper, I am always in trouble." O'Connor's loyalty to Salk was admirable, even touching, Rivers said, but it also came at a price. "Nothing is sacred in science; you give up the old when you find something new that is better."[31]

Bodian understood. He had been there from the outset, one of the foundation's first grantees. Polio, he replied, "has been hard on both the victims and those who have led the fight. Your comment reminds me that there have been very few years since we first met without a crusade or a crisis! It must be especially difficult for those of you in the Foundation who would like to look forward but are forced to look back."[32]

IN 1961 THE AMERICAN MEDICAL ASSOCIATION got involved. Though normally avoiding such controversies, this one, said its president, could no longer be ignored. Doctors were confused about the competing vaccines; they needed guidance from an unbiased source. The AMA's Council on Drugs, therefore, would study the issue and report back on "the present state of polio vaccination in the United States."[33]

All momentum was now on Sabin's side. One observer portrayed him as "a cheshire cat riding a jet propelled steamroller." Congressmen demanded to know why Russian children had access to Sabin's vaccine and American children did not. Some spoke of a "vaccine gap" that rivaled the missile gap, making polio a matter of national security and American pride. Lederle and Charles Pfizer, meanwhile, were bombarding the public with radio and television spots about the miracle of Sabin Oral Sundays. Newspapers and magazines were asking, "What's Delaying the New Polio Vaccine?"[34]

The Council on Drugs, it turned out, was chaired by a former medical director at Pfizer, whose bias was undisguised. Indeed, the man he chose to write the report would correspond regularly with Sabin, asking for advice, information, and even a favor. "One of my colleagues is leaving next summer with his wife and three children for a year in India," he wrote. "Is there any way he can get some live polio vaccine for them?" Sabin was eager to oblige. He sent a vial directly from his lab.[35]

Salk, on the other hand, had to learn of the council's work through the newspapers. When he asked for permission to appear before it, he was told that "it would not be practical at this time." In July 1961 at its national convention, the AMA accepted the council's recommendation that the Salk vaccine be replaced when the Sabin vaccine became available. In doing so, a writer noted, "it committed an act unprecedented in the organization's colorful 114-year history. It voted approval of a commercial product that had not yet been licensed for public use—the Sabin vaccine."[36]

Salk was furious. "This was the only time I have ever seen Jonas get mad enough and *stay* mad enough to fight back," O'Connor recalled. At a hastily called press conference, Salk accused the AMA of scientific bias against a killed-virus vaccine. More personally, he charged that polio in the United States would have been eliminated already had the AMA shown as much enthusiasm for the Salk vaccine as it now displayed for a product "not yet in existence." The association, he implied, had blood on its hands.[37]

It didn't make a dent. The AMA's scientific director, John Youmans, fired back a prickly note, telling Salk that his "actions concerning the report were not, in my opinion, in keeping with either good taste or good ethics." When Salk then asked for advanced warning about any plans the AMA might have to "revise" its position, the response was pure acid. "[You] seem to imply that you are entitled to special consideration," Youmans wrote. "This I cannot accept, and I do not believe there is any more obligation to furnish reports to you in this manner than to Doctor Kaprowski [*sic*], Doctor Sabin, Doctor Cox, Doctor John Paul, or others in this field." Left unsaid, of course, was the fact that Sabin had been privy to this information from the start.[38]

The AMA's decision was both popular and defensible. There was much to be said for the oral vaccine in terms of effectiveness and application. And the live-virus principle had the overwhelming support of the researchers in the field, most of whom viewed the Salk vaccine as a relic of the past. It was the AMA's tactics that were disturbing—the favoritism, the hidden agenda, the loading of committees, the managing of information—all designed to achieve a predetermined result.[39]

Salk had only one avenue left. In August 1961 he met with the U.S. surgeon general and his staff, hoping to prevent the quick licensing of the Sabin vaccine. He reminded them that a revolutionary experiment had been undertaken in 1954 to determine if a killed-virus vaccine could eliminate a deadly viral disease. The experiment, he said, had yet to run its course. Having invested so much, the American people deserved to know whether the Salk vaccine was worthy. And they would never get that answer if a competing vaccine were allowed to enter the market prematurely and "becloud" the final results. Salk literally pleaded for delay.[40]

It wasn't to be. Less than a month later, HEW licensed Sabin's Type I live-virus strain. Within a year, it would license Types II and III. By 1963 the battle for supremacy was over. The Sabin vaccine was in, approved by the government and endorsed by the AMA. The Salk vaccine was out, a medical dinosaur apparently on its way to extinction.

A new celebrity-scientist had emerged, less likable than the one he had replaced. Albert Sabin would never be the cherished public figure that Jonas Salk had been. And he didn't seem to mind. A consummate insider, Sabin mainly sought recognition from his peers. There now were conferences held in his honor, rumors of prestigious job offers, and strong hints of a trip to Stockholm to accept the Nobel Prize. From Moscow Chumakov wrote: "I am glad to tell you that I [was] awarded the highest professional Prize—the Lenin Prize—for the work . . . on the study and use of your oral polio vaccine. I am sorry that for formal reasons it was impossible to nominate you . . . but I consider you to be one of the main heroes of this event. . . . Soviet virologists and with them millions of parents [are] eternally grateful to you."[41]

An obsessive researcher, intensely focused, Sabin had written his friend Peter Olitsky in 1958 that "I have worked hard all my life—and am still chasing tomorrow because I am not at all gratified with what I have achieved thus far." Two years later he told Olitsky: "I am really looking forward to 1961, when my work on polio will be at an end. The idea of exploring in a totally different field is most appealing." A year after that, with victory in his sights, Sabin spoke of longing "to get back to the bench and stay there," far removed from the controversies that he, in truth, had done so much to enflame. A day outside the laboratory, he often said, was a day that was lost to him forever. "How little we seem able to do in a lifetime—and how fast the years slip by."[42]

The losers were less philosophical. Herald Cox was known as a brittle man. "I mean the guy would ask the janitors, 'Do you think I'm doing a good job,'" a colleague recalled. Deeply depressed by Lederle's decision to produce the rival Sabin vaccine, Cox left Lederle soon after. He would not return to polio research. Koprowski, a tougher sort, claimed to be relieved. As director of the Wistar Institute, he could return to old projects such as rabies and move on to new ones like multiple sclerosis and cancer. It was enough, he said, to be remembered as the first researcher who had the courage to feed live poliovirus to humans, adding: "Sometimes I introduce myself as the developer of the Sabin poliomyelitis vaccine." He couldn't know it, but his connection to polio research had yet to run its course.[43]

Nor had Jonas Salk's. Though his laboratory days were now behind him, he would never accept as final the victory of Sabin's vaccine. "Normally, my father tried to let these things go. He absolutely hated confrontation," said Peter Salk. "But this one was so terribly painful, so personally insulting to him as a scientist, that he couldn't let go. It is no exaggeration to say that it haunted him for the rest of his life."[44]

IN 1961, THE LAST YEAR IN WHICH THE SALK VACCINE was exclusively administered in the United States, the number of reported polio cases dropped below 1,000, the lowest total ever. Few people seemed to notice. Polio in America had just about been licked.

16

Celebrities and Survivors

J. Robert Oppenheimer had first put the idea into Jonas Salk's mind. Ever since the collapse of his plans for a research institute on the Pittsburgh campus, Salk had traveled the country, often with Basil O'Connor in tow, searching for the perfect location. As Salk remembered, Oppenheimer "was the one who said to me, 'Did it ever occur to you to go to California, where you can do more unusual things than on the East Coast?'"[1]

"Unusual" was exactly what Salk had in mind. "The precise purpose of the Salk Institute is not easy to pin down," said a science writer who visited the facility in 1972, a decade after it opened its doors. The fundraising brochures had promised to create an institute to advance "the health and well-being of man." Salk himself had spoken of combining the hard sciences and the humanities in pursuit of "biology with a conscience." Unlike a traditional university, where faculty members were pigeonholed into specific departments, and where teaching loads and administrative duties ate up large chunks of valuable time, the Salk Institute would free the brightest minds in genetics, biology, philosophy, the visual arts, and other disciplines to collaborate on a blueprint for human health and advancement.[2]

Salk, in fact, had been mulling over this concept for years. It was a modified version of the one that Chancellor Litchfield at Pittsburgh had rejected following Salk's demand for full independence from university oversight. To some, Salk's utopian vision seemed to reflect the bitter conflict that had plagued his life since the heady days of Ann Arbor. He had done little serious research in his remaining time at

Pittsburgh. His attempts to refine his killed-virus polio vaccine had been overshadowed by the anticipation surrounding Albert Sabin's competing live-virus model. Occasionally, Salk would make news on another scientific front, as when he experimented with a line of monkey heart cells designed to create resistance to the growth of foreign (or tumor) cells when injected into the body. The very hint of Jonas Salk's moving into cancer research was bound to grab public attention, and it did. Responding to the queries, Salk declared, "We are not now working on a cancer vaccine. We are doing basic studies on the nature of cells. This has no practical significance at this time." There was, it turned out, good reason for his reticence. "The Salk theory of how to enhance tumor immunity in humans," a former colleague recalled, "had a quiet death and burial."[3]

His senior staff had also come apart. Julius Youngner left the fold in 1957, still bitter over Salk's failure to acknowledge his debt to those who had toiled so ably behind the scenes. Jim Lewis and Byron Bennett stayed on a bit longer, finding less and less to do. "Considering his eventual move from Pittsburgh and the redirection of his efforts," Youngner recalled, "Jonas no longer needed the skills these men possessed."[4]

Salk chose a stunning site for his Institute. In 1960, the voters of San Diego approved a ballot referendum giving Salk a parcel of coveted land on the Torrey Pines mesa overlooking the Pacific Ocean. With the National Foundation subsidizing most of the $15 million construction budget, Salk instructed architect Louis Kahn to create "a facility worthy of a visit by Picasso." The result, according to fellow architects, was Kahn's "first masterpiece," a series of stunning geometrical structures described by one critic as "the modern equivalent of a temple of Zeus beside the Aegean."[5]

The Institute opened in 1963. With generous stipends, state-of-the art laboratories, and lavish surroundings, Salk recruited extraordinary talent to the cliffside campus: physicist Leo Szilard, biologist Francis Crick, virologist Renato Dulbecco, and mathematician-philosopher Jacob Bronowski, to name a few. "I thought how nice it would be if a place like this existed and I was invited to work in it," Salk recalled years later. "I said, jokingly but not so jokingly, that if I had never created it I never would have been invited."[6]

The original plan had called for the National Foundation to provide most of the start-up money, plus an annual contribution of $1 million. In addition, Salk would use his fame to court new donors, while the

Institute fellows raked in grant money to fund their research. Early on, at least, the plan worked poorly. Fund-raising was haphazard, grant proposals were slow to develop, and the Institute spent far more than it took in, counting on the Foundation to make up the difference, which it did, but with growing unease. In 1965, Foundation treasurer H. E. White wrote Basil O'Connor: "I am reluctant to continue disbursements . . . without some indication of a determined effort to cooperate in containing costs and developing a source of income outside of the National Foundation."[7]

That same year, Salk stepped down as president of the Institute to become its director, concentrating on "research and academic development." But his penchant for spending continued to alarm. Even the fatherly O'Connor warned the Institute's Board of Trustees that "despite my wish to develop and maintain a scientific institution as we all envisioned . . . the casual and haphazard attitude towards the use of Foundation funds not only causes me the gravest concern, but also puts demands on the Foundation that threaten its own development and existence."[8]

O'Connor died in 1972. Fittingly, he was on the road, in Phoenix, conducting Foundation business when another heart attack struck him down. Though O'Connor had lived long enough to see polio almost entirely eradicated in the United States, he had also seen his daughter, Bettyann Culver, succumb to the disease in 1961, and had to witness the dramatic shift from the Salk vaccine to the Sabin vaccine—a shift he bitterly opposed. O'Connor's passing left Salk in a vulnerable position at the Institute. The new Foundation leadership demanded a change of direction, insisting that better management was needed at the top. Within months of O'Connor's death, a plan was devised in which Salk would retain his "highly visible and prestigious role" as director, while relinquishing all "duties and responsibilities in regard to the administration and direction of general research," becoming, in essence, a figurehead for the institute he had so lovingly created.[9]

Salk claimed to be relieved. A decade earlier, his talents in grant-writing and laboratory administration had been the envy of his peers. Now he saw a different role for himself—that of scientific impresario, bringing together great minds in a pressure-free setting designed to encourage the cross-fertilization of ideas. He had begun, as well, to reflect on the larger issues of human existence, sensing that a new phase

of evolution had emerged in which change was occurring more rapidly, and with greater consequence, than ever before. Salk wrote four
books explaining his philosophical insights (which often came to him
late at night as he gazed out at the Pacific). "We need to guide evolution consciously," he wrote, "relying upon some of the more highly
evolved among those with an evolutionary philosophy, for the purpose
of continuity and efficiency in improving the human condition."[10]

Pittsburgh seemed light years away. "The past decade has been a
long one and critical changes are taking place for me now," Salk wrote
Tommy Francis in 1965. "The shape of the future is becoming clear."
Salk had shed his white lab coat and dark tie for ascots, V-neck sweat-
ers, and silk jogging suits. With his three sons off to college—and eventually to medical school—his marriage fell apart. "There was no single
incident and no real bitterness," Darrell Salk recalled. "My parents
had been living parallel lives for years." The couple divorced in 1968,
with Donna Salk remaining in La Jolla to resume her career in social
work. A year later, Jonas met the French painter Françoise Gilot
through a mutual friend. News of their marriage plans in 1970 made
the front page of the *New York Times*: "Dr. Salk and Françoise Gilot,
Picasso's Ex-Mistress, to Wed." Following a small ceremony in Neuilly,
a suburb of Paris, the couple returned to California, where Gilot built
a studio to continue her work. "Françoise and I have the same world
view," Salk told a reporter. "There is art and style in all we do."[11]

FROM HIS PERCH IN CINCINNATI, meanwhile, Albert Sabin was methodi-
cally sweeping the board. His oral polio vaccine had now supplanted
the Salk vaccine in the United States and much of the world. Seen by
experts as the more effective product, easier to administer and cheaper
to produce, it was used in Australia, China, and Japan, large parts of
Central and South America, and most of Europe, East and West. (Holland and Scandinavia, which relied on government production and carefully supervised vaccination programs, stuck with the Salk vaccine.) In
1985, Sabin boasted that his vaccine had "probably prevented about five
million cases of paralytic poliomyelitis during the past 20 years (125 cases
per million total population per year × 20 years × 2 billion population)."[12]

The vaccine was not without its drawbacks, however. Following the
disastrous Cutter incident of 1955, not a single case of polio in the United
States had been attributed to the Salk vaccine. No one could question
its safety, if properly prepared. Unfortunately, the same could not be
said of the Sabin vaccine, which, studies showed, was responsible for

causing a tiny number of polio cases—about one per each million doses—with those at special risk being children with weakened immune systems. Put simply, a live-virus vaccine had clear advantages over a killed-virus vaccine—and one glaring fault. Everyone admitted this except Albert Sabin, who refused to give an inch. "There is no proof," he insisted "that cases of polio still remaining [are] vaccine-caused." As Joseph Melnick, a friend and colleague of Sabin's, put it: "He was so strong-willed, he thought he could will it away."[13]

In the late 1960s, researchers in Holland developed a more potent version of the killed-virus polio vaccine. Booster shots would no longer be needed, solving an enormous practical dilemma. Energized by this breakthrough, Jonas Salk and his son Darrell, a Seattle pediatrician, published a series of articles citing the superiority of the killed-virus approach. The plain fact, they wrote, was that polio in the United States had now been reduced to the point where the majority of remaining cases were directly related to the use of live-virus vaccine. It followed, therefore, that polio could only be eradicated if Americans abandoned Sabin's vaccine in favor of Salk's.[14]

The reaction, Darrell Salk recalled, was worse than disappointing. "There was no response, no debate, no interest—nothing. Complete silence." This should not have been a surprise. The government, the drug companies, and the medical establishment all felt comfortable with the Sabin vaccine. Tens of millions of children had been successfully vaccinated. By the mid-1970s, the annual rate of polio cases per 100,000 population in the United States had dropped below 0.1—the lowest measurement used by the Census Bureau. To switch vaccines at this point made little sense, the experts agreed. The risks were too low, and the costs were too high. Why do anything to lessen public confidence in a workable product? Why do anything to undermine the concept of vaccination itself?[15]

And here the matter stood. After 1980, almost every case of polio in the United States—about a dozen per year—would be attributed to the Sabin vaccine. Wild poliovirus, the cause of so much misery in the past, had been effectively eliminated. Noting these figures, Darrell Salk called once again for a switch to his father's killed-virus vaccine; the response once again ranged from indifference to derision. "He doesn't know what he's talking about," Albert Sabin sniffed. "[His work is] completely out of focus, distorted . . . erroneous information—just a chip off the old block."[16]

THE BITTER CHASM between Jonas Salk and Albert Sabin seemed only to widen over time. The two rivals enjoyed different reputations, had different supporters, and won different tributes for their work. Though both received the prestigious Lasker Award for Clinical Research—Salk in 1956, Sabin in 1965—it remained one of the few honors they would ever come to share. Sabin was a longtime member of the elite National Academy of Sciences, nominated in 1951 by fellow members Tom Rivers (1934), John Paul (1945), and Thomas Francis (1948). In the coming years, almost every prominent polio researcher would gain entrance to the Academy: John Enders (1953), David Bodian (1958), Thomas Weller (1964), Fred Robbins (1972), and Dorothy Horstmann (1975). Even the controversial Hilary Koprowski was elected to membership in 1976.[17]

The main exception, of course, was Jonas Salk. What he accomplished, his colleagues claimed, was simply not creative enough for serious consideration. He hadn't *discovered* anything. One scientist portrayed Salk's role in the polio wars as akin to that of a production manager, not a research pioneer. Others described him as old-fashioned and unoriginal, a man who had pandered shamelessly to the crowd. As one observer put it, Salk had broken "the unwritten commandments" of scientific research: "Thou shalt remain anonymous. Thou shalt give credit to others. Thou shalt discuss one's work in the medical journals and not in the newspapers."[18]

In 1970, Sabin received the National Medal of Science for his research in developing "the vaccine which eliminated poliomyelitis as a major threat to human health." ("You'll note that it says *the* vaccine," he would emphasize.) Sabin became president of the Weizmann Institute of Science in Israel, stepping down in 1972 following open-heart surgery. There had always been rumors that he or Salk might receive a Nobel Prize, but the rumors, in Sabin's case, lasted for most of his life. In 1976, Mikail Chumakov cabled Sabin from Moscow: "DEAR ALBERT: PLEASE SEND ME URGENTLY BY AIR MAIL YOUR CURRICULUM VITAE AND LIST MAIN PRAISE ON DEVELOPMENT POLIO VACCINE FOR NOMINATION IN STOCKHOLM." To which Sabin replied: "I [am] deeply moved by your kindness. . . . It may interest you to know, however, that at least for the past 3 years I have already been nominated for the prize by a number of people from different parts of the world—and thus far without any effect. Perhaps your recommendation will be the last straw—but I frankly do not expect it."[19]

His instincts were correct. That honor never came. There was talk that the endless carping over the polio vaccine had ruined chances on both sides. (Salk once joked that he didn't need the Nobel Prize because most people believed he had already won it.) In truth, the Nobel Committee in 1954 had recognized what most scientists considered to be key piece of the polio puzzle—the monumental discovery by John Enders, Fred Robbins, and Thomas Weller that poliovirus could be successfully cultivated in non-nervous tissue. There was no reason, it seemed, for a second award, although Enders would push hard for his friend's nomination, writing Sabin: "My admiration for you in all this [live-virus] work and the many other things you have done remains unbounded."

For Sabin's eightieth birthday in 1986, Dorothy Horstmann organized a scientific symposium in his honor at the National Institutes of Health in Bethesda. It was a gala event that included Nobel Prize winners like David Baltimore, leading government scientists such as Anthony Faucci, surviving polio giants Robbins and Weller, and the widows of John Enders and David Bodian. Salk wasn't invited. When Sabin died in 1993, the prestigious journal *Biologicals* devoted an entire issue to his life and career. Every contributor praised Sabin's live-virus vaccine for ending the scourge of polio in the United States and beyond. Every contributor ranked him among the world's greatest virologists.[20]

Praise for Jonas Salk came from very different quarters. Where Sabin had been a favorite of the academy, Salk was a favorite of the people. Where Sabin had been feted at scientific conferences and in prestigious journals, Salk's tributes included such things as the Harry S. Truman Good Neighbor Award or the Father Flanagan Award for Service to Youth (which Salk graciously accepted in a hotel ballroom in Omaha, Nebraska). Babies were named after him. "Airplane pilots would announce that he was on board," a writer noted, "and passengers would burst into applause. Hotels routinely would upgrade him into their penthouse suites. A meal at a restaurant inevitably meant an interruption from an admirer." Public opinion polls continued to rank Salk as the most famous of all medical scientists, along with Louis Pasteur. In 1985, President Ronald Reagan proclaimed May 6 as "Dr. Jonas E. Salk Day," urging Americans to organize "appropriate tributes" to the man who had saved so many young lives. A decade later, *Time* magazine would list Salk, alone among polio researchers, as one of the twentieth century's "100 Most Important Scientists and Thinkers," placing him on its cover with Albert Einstein and Sigmund Freud. "Salk's career stands out in at least two respects," *Time* noted: "the sheer speed with which he outraced all the other tortoises in the field and the honors he did not receive for doing so."[21]

THOUGH SALK NEVER WAVERED in his belief that the killed-virus vaccine offered the best hope of fully eradicating polio in the United States, his final scientific quest would move him in a different direction. By the 1980s, the Salk Institute had become a powerhouse in the fields of genetics, molecular biology, and neuroscience; gone for good was the grand design of combining basic scientific research with the humanities. As pure science came to dominate the Institute, attracting Nobel Prize winners and National Academy members, Salk closed down his laboratory and retreated to a suite of elegant offices, filled with sculpture and contemporary art, to ponder the social consequences of human evolution.

Then, suddenly, came the growing specter of AIDS. The more Salk learned about this disease, the more convinced he became that AIDS, like polio, could be treated with a vaccine. The main difference, as Salk saw it, was that a polio vaccine protected against a viral invasion that hadn't yet occurred, while an AIDS vaccine must protect against a viral invasion in those already infected. One vaccine was preventative, the other therapeutic. One aimed at stopping the virus cold, the other at keeping it dormant. But Salk believed the process in both cases to be largely the same: isolate the virus, inactivate it with formaldehyde, mix in an adjuvant for extra potency, and then inoculate the patient in order to stimulate the body's immune system to respond. "I began to look at the problem," Salk recalled, "from the point of view of how would I have approached it 40 years ago."[22]

For his many critics, of course, this was precisely the problem. "He's like Rip Van Winkle in a way. The Rip Van Winkle of Virology," said Joseph Melnick of the "new" Jonas Salk. "He came back after a long sleep. And when he came back, he thought science was exactly where he left it." Albert Sabin heard of Salk's AIDS work while confined to a wheelchair, suffering the effects of a stroke that had left him barely able to speak. Taking pen to paper, he fired off the final salvo of this bitter four-decade feud. "I see no scientific basis for Salk's tests of his AIDS vaccine," Sabin wrote, "and disagree with him scientifically on most other concepts."[23]

Some, however, were flattered and encouraged by Salk's interest. If nothing else, they believed, it would generate needed publicity for the cause. "Here's a guy who has enormous credibility with the public," said one AIDS activist. "He has a magical name and the word vaccine has a magical feeling to it." Salk himself invoked the symbolism of an earlier time, demanding a mobilization "equivalent in purpose to the March of Dimes for polio in the '40s and '50s."

He also co-founded a business called the Immune Response Corporation to produce and market his coming vaccine. This time, however, there was no talk of giving it to the world as a gift—no illusions about patenting the sun. Salk assigned the rights of his potential discoveries to the company, obtaining almost half a million shares of stock at the insider's price of $3,000. In 1990, when IRC went public, these shares were valued at more than $3 million.[24]

"Had Jonas Salk's life unfolded according to his own script," said the perceptive science writer Jon Cohen, "he would have coached the AIDS vaccine across the finish line, healing the world one more time, reinforcing his ideas about focusing on the Big Picture, and simultaneously deflating the Pooh-Bahs of science who had excluded him for most of his career from what he saw as their 'cabal.'" But unscripted endings are rarely this sweet. As Salk made little headway on the AIDS front, even those interested in a vaccine solution lost interest in his particular approach. Still, he pushed forward, scorning the critics who doubted his work. "There have to be people who are ahead of their time," he said. "And that is my fate."[25]

IN SEPTEMBER 1993, Salk returned to Pittsburgh to attend the unveiling of his portrait in the auditorium of the university's medical complex, a stone's throw from the hospital where he had done his historic polio research. Before the ceremony, Salk told Dean George Bernier that he wished to speak privately with his former assistant, Julius Youngner, now a distinguished service professor in the school of medicine. The two men hadn't talked or crossed paths since Salk's move to California in 1961. Salk saw the meeting as a courtesy to the only remaining member of his laboratory staff; Youngner had a different agenda. Speaking softly, he recalled, he slowly released the "hurt" he had bottled up for more than thirty years. "'Do you still have the speech you gave in Ann Arbor in 1955? Have you ever reread it?'" Youngner began. "'We were in the audience, your closest colleagues and devoted associates, who worked hard and faithfully for the same goal that you desired. . . . Do you remember whom you mentioned and whom you left out? Do you realize how devastated we were at that moment and ever afterward when you persisted in making your co-workers invisible? Do you know what I'm saying,' I asked. He answered that he did."

Youngner didn't stop there. "I [said] that I also was disturbed by his behavior [in] the Cutter incident and that I still had not forgiven him for this. Jonas was clearly shaken by these memories and offered little response. There is no doubt in my mind that he knew what I referred to."

The two men engaged in some uncomfortable small talk before Dean Bernier returned to escort them to the ceremony. Speaking later to a reporter, Youngner admitted, "I got a lot of things off my chest. I'm beyond the point where I pull my punches with him. I think it was the first time he ever heard it so graphically." Asked if he had any regrets about working for Salk, Youngner replied: "Absolutely not. You can't imagine what a thrill that gave me. My only regret is that he disappointed me."[26]

ALBERT SABIN DIED OF HEART FAILURE on March 3, 1993, at the age of eighty-six. His newspaper obituaries were respectful but hardly warm. "Throughout his long career," the *New York Times* wrote, "he was noted for diligence, hard work and long hours as well as brilliance in research." Jonas Salk died of heart failure on June 23, 1995, at the age of eighty-one. His obituaries, carried on the front pages of America's leading newspapers, were almost worshipful in tone. "Savior," "godsend," "humanitarian," "benefactor to mankind"—the words conveyed a deeply human bond. "One good way to assess the great figures of medicine is to see how completely they make us forget what we owe them," wrote *Time* magazine. "By that measure, Dr. Jonas Salk ranks very high."[27]

All the obituaries linked the two men, and most had a similar theme. "Jonas Salk was the hero," wrote the *Pittsburgh Post-Gazette*, "but in many ways, Albert Sabin was the victor." Both men died believing this to be true. Yet, amazingly, the entire landscape was about to change. In 1996, the Center for Disease Control's Advisory Committee on Immunization Practices offered a sweeping new recommendation. With wild poliovirus apparently eliminated in the Western Hemisphere— the last "natural" case of polio was reported in Peru in 1991—the committee members felt they could no longer ignore the dozen or so cases of vaccine-related polio that still occurred annually in the United States.

The logic was simple: the Sabin vaccine, so successful in disrupting the life cycle of poliovirus, had become the final obstacle to fully eradicating the disease.[28]

The committee's 1996 recommendation, which the CDC adopted, was a compromise measure designed to ease the nation into a new era of polio vaccination. It called upon pediatricians to begin a "mixed" program, with children receiving two doses of the killed-virus vaccine via injection (at two months and four months of age), followed by two more doses of live-virus vaccine given orally (at twelve to eighteen months and four to six years). Most pediatricians went along, accepting the CDC's explanation that the Salk shots would act to neutralize the minimal dangers presented by the Sabin vaccine. The "mixed" program did not work as well as expected; vaccine-related polio cases continued to appear, leading the CDC's advisory committee to conclude that the benefits of the live-virus vaccine no longer justified the risks. In 2000, the CDC endorsed a full return to the Salk vaccine in the United States, recommending that the Sabin vaccine be used only in special cases—among children, for example, who were visiting parts of the world where a polio outbreak was in progress.[29]

The vaccine war had come full circle. Though the Sabin vaccine would continue as a staple in much of the developing world, its thirty-year reign in the United States was over—at least for now. As Darrell Salk put it, simply: "My father would have been pleased."[30]

AT THE SAME TIME, however, new doubts about the safety of polio vaccination in general were starting to emerge. These doubts had less to do with the differences between the Salk and Sabin vaccines than with likelihood that *all* polio vaccine had contained harmful simian viruses in the early years of production, between 1954 and 1963. Though long debated in scientific circles, the danger of contaminated polio vaccine did not attract widespread attention until 1992, when *Rolling Stone* magazine published a piece entitled: "The Origins of AIDS: A Startling New Theory Attempts to Answer the Question, 'Was It an Act of God or an Act of Man?'"[31]

The "man" in question, wrote *Rolling Stone*, was none other than Hilary Koprowski, the former Lederle scientist, now at the Wistar Institute, who had pioneered the oral polio vaccine. The article implied that Koprowski—described as "a charming, deep-voiced man of seventy-five"—might have unwittingly transmitted the AIDS virus from monkeys to humans during his polio immunization trials in the Belgian Congo in the late 1950s, when close to a million people were given his oral vaccine. "Called by drums," wrote *Rolling Stone* journalist Tom Curtis, "rural Africans traveled to village assembly points. There they lined up and had a liquid vaccine squirted into their mouths." That liquid—like all polio vaccine—contained poliovirus grown in monkey kidney tissue. Curtis theorized that Koprowski's vaccine may have been cultured in a species of monkey known to be a natural host for HIV-1, the virus that causes AIDS in human beings.

The article created a sensation. But the evidence behind it was so slim, and the threat of a lawsuit so strong, that *Rolling Stone* was forced to publish a "clarification." The editors, it said, had "never intended to suggest [that] there is any scientific proof, nor do they know of any scientific proof, that Dr. Koprowski, an illustrious scientist, was in fact responsible for introducing AIDS to the human population or that he is the father of AIDS." Still, the issue wouldn't die. The timing and location of Koprowski's trials matched the timing and location of the world's first known AIDS cases. Was this merely a coincidence?[32]

The controversy took another turn in 1999 with the publication of *The River*, a massive tome by British journalist Edward Hooper, which suggested that AIDS had been transmitted to humans through contaminated chimpanzee tissue in Koprowski's oral polio vaccine. Koprowski vehemently denied ever using chimpanzee tissue, and the evidence collected in recent years has supported his claim. The charge that humans acquired HIV from these trials remains, for most experts, an empty accusation, made more improbable by recent studies that found no detectable traces of chimpanzee DNA in frozen stocks of Koprowski's vaccine. The results, said one group of researchers, "should finally lay the OPV/AIDS theory to rest."[33]

But AIDS was only part of this growing story—the lesser part. As early as 1954, the year of the Salk trials, researchers at Eli Lilly had begun to classify the different simian viruses they discovered in the monkey kidney tissue used for polio vaccine production, the first one being dubbed SV1. Over time, the numbers kept rising. In 1959, Dr. Bernice Eddy of the NIH injected a filtered extract of this kidney tissue into newborn hamsters, the majority of whom developed tumors and died. She had isolated SV40.[34]

Was this particular virus a threat to human beings? No one really knew. It was assumed, however, that any problems associated with SV40 would be limited to the oral polio vaccine—the belief being that the formaldehyde used to inactivate poliovirus in the Salk vaccine would work to kill the simian viruses as well. In 1960, Tom Rivers told Albert Sabin that traces of SV40 found in his oral polio vaccine had raised some concerns within the National Foundation. "I wish you would get together some convincing evidence," Rivers wrote, "that the vacuolating virus (i.e., SV40) now contaminating your vaccine will not infect human beings." Sabin had replied, with typical bravado, that his vaccine was safe, that the field trials just completed on eighty million Russian children had proved this beyond a reasonable doubt, and that no evidence existed to show that SV40 was dangerous to human beings.[35]

It soon became apparent that the Salk vaccine was contaminated as well. The formaldehyde had not been designed to kill monkey viruses that researchers didn't then know existed. This meant that close to 100 million American children had been inadvertently exposed to SV40 in the years between 1954 and 1963, when the government began to carefully screen all new lots of polio vaccine for simian virus. Sabin did not appear worried by this turn of events, and neither did Salk. Both men considered SV40 to be harmless to human beings. Theirs was the majority opinion, opposed by only a handful of scientists, including, it turned out, the iconoclastic Hilary Koprowski, who viewed the experiments of Dr. Eddy as too important to ignore.

Like polio and AIDS, the controversy over SV40 gained public attention through the press. Writing in the *Atlantic Monthly* in 2000, two enterprising journalists, Debbie Bookchin and Jim Schumacher, used the work of dissenting scientists to link SV40 to several deadly human diseases, especially mesothelioma, a form of lung cancer usually associated with smoking and exposure to asbestos. In a follow-up book, *The Virus and the Vaccine*, the writers accused the federal government, the drug industry, and individual scientists of ignoring the contamination of polio vaccine by a suspected—in their eyes, certain—human carcinogen, thereby perpetuating "one of the biggest blunders in medical history."[36]

In response, officials of the NIH and the National Cancer Institute have cited numerous studies done in Asia, Europe, and the United States that have found no correlation between human cancers, including mesothelioma, and exposure to SV40. "At this time," Dr. James Goedert of the NIH told Congress in 2003, "our opinion is that the body of evidence is inconclusive as to the role of SV40 in the development of [human] cancer." New experiments, he said, are presently under way.[37]

What is revealing, of course, is how dramatically the scientific debate over polio had shifted in recent years. "We're prisoners of our own success," a prominent researcher observed. "When formerly dreaded diseases are pushed into the shadows—or eliminated—questions about the vaccines themselves begin to spring up."[38]

SOMETIMES FORGOTTEN amidst these triumphs and controversies are the lives that were affected most by this devastating disease. Today, the word "polio" describes a vaccine to be taken, not a disease to be feared. "It's interesting," a polio survivor observed, "but even with my limp and all the braces I've worn over the years, people usually don't have any idea what's wrong with my leg." Another survivor recalled a young neighbor asking him whether his parents had practiced "a strange sort of religion" that didn't permit vaccination. "To her, and most others her age," the man added, "there had always been a polio vaccine."[39]

By conservative estimates, there are at least 400,000 survivors of paralytic polio in the United States. Some recovered much of their muscle function through a process of regeneration whereby surviving nerve cells developed extra branches, known as axonal sprouts, which reattached themselves to the orphaned muscle fibers. Others endured multiple surgeries to reconstruct a "dropped foot," realign a shortened leg, or straighten a badly curved spine—surgeries that required the stapling of bones, the lengthening of tendons, and the fusing of joints. Many still walk with the aid of canes and crutches, wear built-up shoes to compensate for a shorter leg, use motorized wheelchairs to move about, or need a respirator to help them breathe. What polio survivors have always had in common, however, is a drive to excel in the face of physical disability. Studies have compared them to the hard-driving, over-achieving individuals associated with Type A personality. In the words of one survivor: "We were [taught] to be tough and gritty. I did what was expected. . . . I needed to have a disciplined life with a no-quit attitude. That was what worked."[40]

According to Dr. Lauro Halstead, director of the post-polio program at the National Rehabilitation Hospital in Washington, D.C., most polio survivors developed "a special relation to their bodies unknown to able-bodied persons. They experienced a new mastery over their muscles and movements, an element of control . . . that carried over into other aspects of their lives and probably accounts for why so many . . . excelled at school and work." Surveys have shown polio survivors to be better educated than the general population, with higher incomes and marriage rates as well. "Don't let any [of us] tell you that they just want to be 'normal' like everyone else," a polio survivor wrote in a questionnaire. "We have to be better than everyone else just to break even . . . and that may not be enough."[41]

Following years of surgery, rehabilitation, and exercise, polio survivors came to regard their condition as stable. They saw polio as a static disease, unlikely to return or to worsen with age. But this comforting assumption was challenged in the 1980s, as polio survivors began to experience health problems eerily reminiscent of their earlier ordeal. The symptoms were alarming: joint pain, sensitivity to cold, difficulties in breathing and swallowing, progressive muscle weakness, and extreme fatigue. There were so many cases that polio survivors formed support groups to pool information and alert the medical community to their plight. Most American doctors of the post-Salk, post-Sabin era had never treated a case of polio. Their ignorance of the disease, beyond the importance of immunization, was distressing.[42]

In 1984, Dr. Halstead and others organized the first international conference on the delayed effects of polio. The idea was to increase public awareness and spur medical research. The organizers attached a handle to these multiple symptoms—Post-Polio Syndrome (PPS). "Without a name there was, in essence, no disease," Halstead recalled. "Having a name—even if imprecise and misleading as to causation—at least confers an element of credibility."[43]

In the past two decades, researchers have studied PPS at some length. Most believe that the fatigue and muscle weakness experienced by so many polio survivors are due to wear and tear on existing nerve cells— a theory bolstered by the three to four decades it took for these complaints to be voiced. According to researchers, the motor neurons that survived the initial polio attack and sprouted extra branches have degenerated over time. Part of this is due to the normal aging process, but a larger part, it appears, is caused by the heavy demand put on these remaining motor neurons. "It's as if you had a ten-cylinder car before you had polio and have a four-cylinder car afterward—a car that has driven just fine for forty years or more," a researcher explained. "At some point, the engine is going to break down."[44]

Though no conclusive diagnostic test yet exists for PPS, the percentage of polio survivors suffering from progressive muscle weakness and extreme fatigue is estimated to be as high as 50 percent. Moreover, those who endured the severest cases of polio and made the greatest functional recovery are the most likely to be affected. Dr. Halstead presents himself as an example. Contracting polio as a college student in 1954, he moved "from iron lung to wheelchair to foot brace and then to no assistive device at all." Though his right arm remained paralyzed, he sped through medical school, took up competitive squash and mountain climbing, and convinced himself that "polio is behind me. I have finally conquered it." But in the early 1990s, Halstead wrote, "I began developing new weaknesses in my legs. As the weakness progressed over a period of months, I went from being a full-time walker who jogged up six flights of stairs for exercise to having to use a motorized scooter full-time at work." Halstead had no doubts about his condition. It was the same one he had been diagnosing in other polio survivors for a decade.[45]

The recognition of PPS has had a powerful bonding effect on a group that showed great trouble acknowledging its past. "Until recently," a polio survivor noted, "most of us tended to avoid [each] other and polio help groups. We knew we weren't physically normal, but if we thought about it at all, we considered ourselves as inconvenienced, not disabled." Brought together by common fears and concerns, polio survivors began to relive the memories they had long suppressed: the splitting headaches and widening paralysis that signaled the disease, the excruciating spinal tap that confirmed it, the terror of the isolation ward, the grief-stricken parents, the long separation from family, the multiple surgeries, the months spent in a body cast, the feelings of helplessness, humiliation, and loss. Dr. Richard Owen, a polio survivor who founded the Post-Polio Clinic at the Sister Kenny Institute in Minneapolis, recalled that he and other victims were often treated at teaching hospitals, where, "clad only in little cloth things that barely covered us and our embarrassment," they became perfect subjects for clinical demonstration. "For many of us," Owen added, "the acute illness and convalescence was during adolescence with the impact of polio superimposed on all the usual stresses and strains of growing up. Barriers to buildings, activities, opportunities, and associations added to frustration and, in some cases, social isolation of young people with the residuals of poliomyelitis. Many barriers . . . were self-imposed.

Various coping mechanisms often covered true feelings of loss. Denial often led to a distorted reality."[46]

Those days are over. The concerns over PPS created a powerful network to deal with physical and psychological issues facing polio survivors, which in turn fueled a growing disability-rights movement across the United States. Polio survivors played a key role in lobbying for passage of the Americans with Disabilities Act of 1990, which prohibits discrimination against the disabled and requires physical access to most public spaces. More symbolically, they joined with disability-rights activists to protest a new memorial for Franklin Delano Roosevelt in Washington, opened by the National Park Service in 1997, which largely ignored the president's struggle with polio. The park service insisted it was only reflecting FDR's own desire to portray himself as able-bodied. "With the country ravaged by the Great Depression and yearning for strong leadership," it said, "Roosevelt realized the need to continue this façade." But polio survivors wanted Americans to remember him "as both heroic and disabled," arguing that his disability had been integral to his character, an essential part of who he was and what he accomplished. In the end, the park service reluctantly added a ten-foot statue of Roosevelt seated in his wheelchair. The concession spoke volumes to those who best understood the late president's dilemma. "Our national disability politics has come a long way since the 1930s," an activist explained. "Shouldn't our national aesthetics now take up the challenge to transform the meaning of disability?"[47]

IT HAS BEEN FIFTY YEARS since Thomas Francis mounted that podium in Ann Arbor and told the world what it so desperately wanted to hear: an effective polio vaccine had finally been produced. For most Americans today, the euphoria, the pure relief that greeted his announcement, is difficult to understand. They were not alive to experience the memories of polio summers before 1955—the images of shut down movie theaters and empty swimming pools, the panicked warnings of parents to their children, the daily counts of polio victims in the newspapers, the sight of toddlers struggling to use their leg braces and hospital wards lined wall-to-wall with iron lungs.

As polio has moved into the realm of history, its story has become a lens through which to study the culture of the mid-twentieth-century United States, the nation in which polio did its greatest damage and in which the tools of its destruction were so painfully forged. The battle was fought in a time before federal involvement in medical research and patient care became the norm. Bold leadership by a single philanthropy, the National Foundation for Infantile Paralysis, would turn the fight against a cruel, if relatively uncommon, children's disease into a full-fledged crusade against an insidious public enemy, with the Foundation employing the latest advances in advertising, fund-raising, and public relations to help guide the way. Bold leadership would bring together a band of contentious researchers, provide them with a plan of attack, subsidize their efforts, force them to pool their findings, and—yes—favor the one among them who showed the greatest urgency in working toward a vaccine. Bold leadership would direct the largest health experiment in American history, the Salk vaccine trials of 1954, involving almost two million children and several hundred thousand adult volunteers. Bold leadership would give the people what had been promised to them in return for their continued support: a nation free of polio, a safer place in which to live.

All of this was done in the spirit of voluntarism. And all of it reflected the steady faith of post–World War II American society in the progress of medicine and technology, and in the certainty of what one observer has called "the old Yankee virtues of know-how and can-do." In the strictest sense, these virtues were more generic than genetic, since Basil O'Connor was the son of Irish immigrants and Thomas Francis came from a Welsh steelworking family, while Jonas Salk, Albert Sabin, and Hilary Koprowski were the children of East European Jews. But all the more reason to view the conquest of polio as truly an American story.

Epilogue

POLIO STILL HAUNTS ISOLATED PARTS OF THE WORLD, despite persistent efforts to make it extinct. In 1987, amidst great fanfare, the World Health Organization launched a global initiative to wipe out polio within fifteen years. There was reason for optimism. Most nations had already interrupted the transmission of wild poliovirus through the widespread use of the Sabin vaccine. The 300,000 polio cases reported in 1987 were limited geographically to a number of Asian and African "hot spots." The WHO initiative had strong backing from the U.S. Centers for Disease Control (CDC), the United Nations Children's Fund (UNICEF), and other prominent bodies. The nations at risk for polio seemed anxious to cooperate.[1]

Most remarkable, perhaps, was the participation of Rotary International, which took up the cause of polio eradication with the same fervor shown by the National Foundation for Infantile Paralysis exactly a half-century before. Founded in 1905, RI emerged as the world's first service organization, allowing its individual clubs to pick and fund their own projects. Its collective interest in polio began in the 1980s, following a series of local vaccination campaigns in the Philippines and South America. Focusing on global health made good sense to Rotarians, many of whom lived and worked in Third World countries. And polio eradication seemed a plausible goal, given the availability of a successful vaccine.

Since 1987, Rotary International has raised $500 million to immunize the world's children against polio. (The Bill and Melinda Gates Foundation has contributed more than $1 billion to promote various child immunization programs, including polio eradication, in developing countries.) Working with the WHO, Rotarians helped to organize National Immunization Days that have vaccinated more than a billion people to date. "On these days," an observer noted, "Rotarians round up refrigerators to keep the polio vaccine cold, a challenge in countries with unreliable electricity or none at all. They find enough vehicles— Land Rovers, motorcycles, bicycles, even camels and canoes—to get the vaccine to remote villages. They staff immunization posts for hours." Without their help, said Robert Keegan, director of the CDC's polio effort, "we'd lose the heart of the program. What they have done is pretty monumental."[2]

By 2000, the promise of a world without polio seemed well within reach. The number of cases had fallen dramatically, from a thousand per day in 1987 to fewer than two thousand per year by century's end. Vowing to end polio by 2005, the WHO focused on the three countries that account for 95 percent of the remaining cases—Nigeria, India, and Pakistan. But the goal has proved elusive. Fresh outbreaks were reported in remote parts of northern India and northwest Pakistan, where logistical problems and cultural resistance to vaccination have put large populations at risk. Far worse was the situation in the northern Nigerian state of Kano, a largely Muslim area, where local politicians and clerics halted the immunization programs by claiming that the oral polio vaccine was purposely tainted to cause infertility and AIDS. Not only did new polio cases rise dramatically in Nigeria in 2004, but the disease spread to neighboring countries which had been listed as polio free, including Chad, Ghana, Ivory Coast, and Botswana. "Kano produced the spark," said a UNICEF worker, "and the region ignited."[3]

The WHO now sees eradicating polio as a goal to be reached before 2008. It has focused its efforts on what it calls the "political will, oversight, and accountability" of countries where endemic polio still exists, particularly Nigeria. In addition, it has urged polio-free nations to begin phasing out the live-virus Sabin vaccine in favor of the killed-virus Salk vaccine, noting that "the continued use of OPV for routine immunization could compromise the goal of eradicating all paralytic disease due to circulating polioviruses." The WHO sees its current initiative as the "best—and perhaps last—chance to stop polio forever." If the world "seizes this opportunity," it adds, "no child will ever again know the crippling effects of this devastating disease."[4]

Notes

Introduction

1. *San Angelo Standard-Times*, May 27, 30, 31; June 2, 6, 1949; Steven Spencer, "Where Are We Now on Polio?" *Saturday Evening Post*, September 17, 1949, 26–27.
2. *San Angelo Standard-Times*, May 28, 1949.
3. Ibid.; also Ralph Chase, "A Circle of Wagons," *West Texas Historical Association Yearbook*, 1990, 98–111.
4. *San Angelo Standard-Times*, June 3, 5, 6, 8, 9, 1949.
5. Ibid., June 4, 1949.
6. Ibid., August 7, 8, 1949.
7. Ibid., August 9, 14, 15, 1949.
8. Chase, "Circle of Wagons," 98.
9. Ibid.
10. U.S. Department of Health, Education, and Welfare, *Vital Statistics of the United States*, 1952, volume 2, Mortality Data, 50–94.
11. Helman, *Great Feuds in Modern Medicine*, 140–41.

Chapter 1

1. Paul, *A History of Poliomyelitis*, 1–9; Sass, *Polio's Legacy*, 1–20; Smith, *Patenting the Sun*, 34.
2. Crawford, *The Invisible Enemy*, 6; Oldstone, *Viruses, Plagues, and History*, 3–23; Simmons, *Doctors and Discoveries*, 270–74.
3. Dorothy Horstmann, "The Poliomyelitis Story: A Scientific Hegira," *Yale Journal of Biology and Medicine*, 1985, 79–90; Frederick Robbins and Thomas Daniel, "A History of Poliomyelitis," in *Polio*, ed. T. Daniel, 5–22; Joseph L. Melnick, "Enteroviruses," in *Virology* (2nd ed.), ed. B. N. Fields, 1990, 558–64; Karlen, *Man and Microbes*, 149–54; Lauro S. Halstead, "Post-Polio Syndrome," *Scientific American*, April 1998, 42–47; Richard L. Bruno, *The Polio Paradox*, 2002, 30–37.
4. Paul, *History of Poliomyelitis*, 12.

5. Ibid., 17–18.
6. Charles S. Caverly, "Preliminary Report of an Epidemic of Paralytic Disease, Occurring in Vermont, in the Summer of 1894," in *Infantile Paralysis In Vermont, 1894–1922*, State Department of Public Health, Burlington, Vt., 1924.
7. Paul, *History of Poliomyelitis*, 88–97; Saul Benison, "The History of Polio Research in the United States: Appraisal and Lessons," in *The Twentieth Century Sciences: Studies in the Biography of Ideas*, ed. Gerald Holton, 1972, 313–14.
8. Paul, *History of Poliomyelitis*, 98–106; Crawford, *The Invisible Enemy*, 105–8.
9. Tomes, *The Gospel of Germs*, 30–32, 92–96.
10. Corner, *History of the Rockefeller Institute, 1901–1953*, 22–29.
11. Lester King, "Medical Education: The Decade of Massive Change," in American Medical Association, *American Medicine Comes of Age, 1840–1920*, 1984, 83–87; Starr, *Social Transformation of American Medicine*, 116–27; Ludmerer, *Time to Heal*, 3–25.
12. Chernow, *Titan*, 468.
13. Burnow, *Organized Medicine in the Progressive Era*, 11–13; Brown, *Rockefeller Medicine Men*, 108.
14. Corner, *Rockefeller Institute*, 30–31; Chernow, *Titan*, 417–18, 471.
15. Benison, "History of Polio Research," 312–14; De Kruif, *The Sweeping Wind*, 12–15.
16. J. T. Flexner, *Maverick's Progress*, 8; J. T. Flexner, *An American Saga*, 218–35; Bonner, *Iconoclast*, 32–34.
17. Corner, *Rockefeller Institute*, 59–61; Flexner, *American Saga*, 440.
18. Corner, *Rockefeller Institute*, 60–61; Chernow, *Titan*, 478; Wall, *Andrew Carnegie*, 832.
19. Caverly, "Anterior Polio in Vermont in the Year 1910," in *Infantile Paralysis in Vermont*, 39; California State Board of Health, "Poliomyelitis," *Bulletin for Health Officials*, 1912; Robert Lovett, "The Occurrence of Infantile Paralysis in Massachusetts in 1910," *Monthly Bulletin of the Massachusetts State Board of Health for 1911*; F. G. Boudreau, "Acute Poliomyelitis with Special Reference to the Disease in Ohio," *Monthly Bulletin, Ohio State Board of Health*, January, February, March 1914.
20. Saul Benison, "The Enigma of Poliomyelitis: 1910," in *Freedom and Reform: Essays in Honor of Henry Steele Commager*, ed. Harold Hyman, 1967, 251–52.
21. Dorothy Horstmann oral interview, April 26, 1990, in Daniel Wilson File, Dorothy Horstmann Papers, Yale University Archives.
22. Williams, *Virus Hunters*, 136.
23. *New York Times*, March 9, 1911. Flexner's "discovery" of the nasal route is in Simon Flexner and Paul A. Lewis, "The Transmission of Acute Poliomyelitis to Monkeys," *Journal of the American Medical Association*, November 13 and December 4, 1909. He did not say flatly that this was the *only* route, although he clearly implied it was.
24. *Tom Rivers*, 192–93.
25. Horstmann, "Poliomyelitis Story," 81–82; Rogers, *Dirt and Disease*, 28.
26. Peter Olitsky to Albert Sabin, undated, 1936, File 6, Peter Olitsky Papers, American Philosophical Society. On the controversy at the institute over *Arrowsmith*, see Richard Lingeman, *Sinclair Lewis*, 2002, 206–9; Mark Schorer, *Sinclair Lewis: An American Life*, 1961, 366–67, 410–20; Charles Rosenberg, "Martin Arrowsmith, The Scientist as Hero," *American Quarterly*, Fall 1963, 447–58.

Sinclair Lewis had been aided in writing *Arrowsmith* by Paul de Kruif, a brilliant, eccentric researcher and science writer who had recently resigned from the Rockefeller Institute under pressure from Flexner. Not surprisingly, the book caused a stir there. "Of course there was a rush to see what *Arrowsmith* had to say about the Institute staff," a scientist friend wrote Flexner, adding: "The book annoys because of the false view it gives of science and the way to work at it. . . . It is, well—nauseating." Abraham Flexner called the portrait of his brother in the book "a travesty." See Peyton Rous to Simon Flexner, Spring 1925, Collection O, Peyton Rous File, 4; Abraham Flexner to Simon Flexner, June 13, 1925, Collection 1, Abraham Flexner File; both in *Simon Flexner Papers*, Rockefeller Institute. For de Kruif's role in polio research, see 55–60.

27. A good description of the 1916 epidemic can be found in Gould, *A Summer Plague*, 3–28; Rogers, *Dirt and Disease*, 30–71.
28. David Rosner, "Introduction," 7–15, and Gretchen Condran, "Changing Patterns of Epidemic Disease in New York City," 30–37, both in *Hives of Sickness*, ed. D. Rosner.
29. Alan Kraut, "Plagues and Prejudice: Nativism's Construction of Disease in Nineteenth and Twentieth Century New York City," 71–75, in Rosner, *Hives of Sickness*; Markel, *Quarantine*, 15–39.
30. Rosner, "Introduction," 14–15.
31. Kraut, *Silent Travelers*, 109; *New York Times*, July 8, 1916.
32. Naomi Rogers, "Dirt, Flies and Immigrants: Explaining the Epidemiology of Poliomyelitis, 1900–1916," in *Sickness and Health in America*, ed. Judith Walter and Ronald Numbers, 1997, 543–54.
33. *New York Times*, July 26, 1916; Rogers, *Dirt and Disease*, 54.
34. *New York Times*, July 14, 1916.
35. Rogers, *Dirt and Disease*, 53.
36. Rogers, "Dirt, Flies, and Immigrants," 543.
37. Ibid., 544.

Chapter 2

1. Goldberg, *The Making of Franklin D. Roosevelt*, 26–27; Cook, *Eleanor Roosevelt, 1884–1933*, 267–71, 305–6; *New York Times*, July 23, 1921.
2. Gallagher, *FDR's Splendid Deception*, 9.
3. Davis, *FDR: The Beckoning of Destiny*, 647–51; Anna Roosevelt, "How Polio Helped F.D.R.," *The Woman with Woman's Digest*, July 1949, 54.
4. Eleanor Roosevelt, *This Is My Story*, 330; Cook, *Eleanor Roosevelt*, 308; Cohn, *Four Billion Dimes*, 12.
5. Davis, *FDR*, 651.
6. Ward, *A First-Class Temperament*, 586–589. Eleanor Roosevelt well describes the events of these early days—the polio attack, the doctor's visits, the family's reaction, FDR's state of mind—in a long letter to James "Rosy" Roosevelt. See Eleanor Roosevelt to "Rosy," August 14, 1921, "Family and Personal Correspondence," 1894–1957, Box 2, "Condolence Letters After FDR's Polio Attack," Eleanor Roosevelt Papers, FDR Library.
7. Ward, *A First-Class Temperament*, 589; Paul, *A History of Poliomyelitis*, 337–38; R. W. Lovett, *The Treatment of Infantile Paralysis*, 1916.

8. Goldberg, *Making of FDR*, 44.
9. Though he did not specifically blame Dr. Keen for worsening his condition, Roosevelt agreed, in retrospect, that Keen's regimen had been a mistake. "What is considered the best treatment over here," he wrote a fellow patient, "is to allow absolute rest and quiet until such period when all soreness has disappeared from the muscles. Absolutely no massage is given until this takes place. Thereafter light massage and exercise are given to bring back the use of the muscles." See FDR to G. S. Barrows, October 31, 1921, "Family, Business, Personal," Box 23, Subject File: Infantile Paralysis, Franklin Delano Roosevelt Papers, FDR Library.
10. Cook, *Eleanor Roosevelt*, 308–10; Anna Roosevelt, "How Polio Helped F.D.R.," 54.
11. Goldberg, *Making of FDR*, 43.
12. Ward, *A First-Class Temperament*, 187–88, 203, 368–69, 407–10.
13. A good summary of the latest medical theories on chilling can be found in Abigail Zuger, "'You'll Catch Your Death!' An Old Wives' Tale?" *New York Times*, March 4, 2003; Ward, *A First-Class Temperament*, 595. One doctor later speculated that the removal of FDR's tonsils, twenty-one years before the polio attack, may have been a contributing factor. Researchers did believe that tonsillectomies should not be performed during the summer—or polio season—because the operation exposed nerve endings to poliovirus. But there is no evidence that a previous tonsillectomy would make someone susceptible to polio. See *Eye, Ear, Nose and Throat Monthly*, June 1957, 348–49.
14. See Armond Goldman et al., "What Was the Cause of Franklin Delano Roosevelt's Paralytic Illness?" *Journal of Medical Biography*, 2003, 232–40; also Associated Press wire story, November 3, 2003.
15. Hoy, *Chasing Dirt*, 3–27; Tomes, *The Gospel of Germs*, 1–20; Vinikas, *Soft Soap, Hard Sell*, ix–xix.
16. Ziporyn, *Disease in the Popular American Press*, 9–14; Tomes, *Gospel of Germs*, 26–47; Brandt, *No Magic Bullet*; Walzer, *Typhoid Mary*.
17. Starr, *The Social Transformation of American Medicine*, 180–97; Andrew McClary, "Germs Are Everywhere: The Germ Threat as Seen in Magazine Articles, 1890–1920," *Journal of American Culture*, Spring 1980, 38–39.
18. McClary, "Germs Are Everywhere," 37.
19. Tomes, *The Gospel of Germs*, 10.
20. Ibid., 249–50.
21. Vinikas, *Soft Soap, Hard Sell*, 28–44.
22. Ibid., pp. 43, 79–94; Martin, *Flexible Bodies*, 23–33.
23. *New York Times*, September 16, 1921; Ward, *A First-Class Temperament*, 600–603.
24. Ward, *A First-Class Temperament*, 595.
25. Gallagher, *FDR's Splendid Deception*, 28–33.
26. Lily Norton to Helen Whidden, November 14, 1921, Eleanor and Franklin Roosevelt, Small Collections, "Reminiscences by Contemporaries," Subject File: Lily Norton, Franklin Delano Roosevelt Papers, FDR Library.
27. Dumas Malone, *Jefferson and the Rights of Man*, 1951, 267; Allan Nevins, *Grover Cleveland: A Study in Courage*, 1932, 530–33; Edwin Weinstein, *Woodrow Wilson: A Medical and Psychological Biography*, 1981, 348–70; John Morton Cooper, Jr., *The Warrior and the Priest*, 1983, 335–42.

28. Ward, *A First-Class Temperament*, 781–83; Lewis L. Gould, *The Modern American Presidency*, 2003, 82–83.
29. Gallagher, *FDR's Splendid Deception*, xiii–xiv.
30. Franklin Roosevelt to Thomas C. Whitlock, March 23, 1923, Box 23, "Family, Business, Personal," Subject File: Infantile Paralysis, Franklin Delano Roosevelt Papers, FDR Library.
31. Goldberg, *Making of FDR*, 80; Ward, *A First-Class Temperament*, 657.
32. Walker, *Roosevelt and the Warm Springs Story*, 40–42; Dorothy Ducas, "Unto the Least of These . . . The Story of Basil O'Connor," *Sigma Phi Epsilon Journal*, February 1941; Frank Freidel, *Franklin D. Roosevelt: The Ordeal*, 119–20, 143.
33. Smith, *Patenting the Sun*, 54–55; Goldberg, *Making of FDR*, 81.
34. "George Foster Peabody," and "The Peabody Awards," in www.peabody.uga.edu; "George Foster Peabody," *Dictionary of American Biography*, 1958, 520–21. Each year, in his honor, the University of Georgia hands out the internationally known George Foster Peabody Awards for excellence in broadcasting and journalism.
35. Lippman, *The Squire of Warm Spring*, 32–34.
36. Nathaniel Altman, "Hot Springs and Mineral Spas in North America," in *Healing Springs: The Ultimate Guide to Taking the Waters*, ed. N. Altman; Ward, *A First-Class Temperament*, 645. "During the past six weeks," Roosevelt wrote his doctor, "I have been swimming three times a week—first in the Astor pool and lately in the pond on our place. The legs work wonderfully well in the water and I need nothing artificial to keep myself afloat. As a matter of fact, I see continuous improvement in my knees and feet." Franklin Roosevelt to Dr. George Draper, August 10, 1922, Box 23, "Family, Business, Personal," Subject File: Infantile Paralysis, Franklin Delano Roosevelt Papers, FDR Library.
37. Lippman, *The Squire of Warm Springs*, 31–43; Walker, *Roosevelt and the Warm Springs Story*, 3–16; Roosevelt Warm Springs Institute for Rehabilitation, "A Brief History of the Springs," http://www.rooseveltrehab.org/history.htm.
38. Walker, *Roosevelt and the Warm Springs Story*, 13–14.
39. Roosevelt, *This I Remember*, 26–27.
40. Walker, *Roosevelt and the Warm Springs Story*, 25.
41. Ibid., 28; Lippman, *The Squire of Warm Springs*, 33.
42. Walker, *Roosevelt and the Warm Springs Story*, 28; Ward, *A First-Class Temperament*, 707; Freidel, *Franklin D. Roosevelt: The Ordeal*, 193.
43. Davis, *FDR: The Beckoning of Destiny*, 767–68.
44. Cleburne Gregory, "Franklin Roosevelt Will Swim to Health," *Atlanta Journal*, October 26, 1924.
45. Walker, *Roosevelt and the Warm Springs Story*, 76–78; Noel Burtenshaw, "Warm Springs and Its Magic Waters," *Georgia Bulletin*, February 4, 1982.
46. Eleanor Roosevelt to Marion Dickerman, quoted in Davis, *Invincible Summer*, 61.
47. Ward, *A First-Class Temperament*, 728. For a full accounting of the sale, complete with legal documents, see Roosevelt, *This I Remember*, Appendix II.
48. Roosevelt Warm Springs Institute for Rehabilitation, "Our History . . . 75 Years of Commitment to Service," http://www.rooseveltrehab.org/history.htm; Gallagher, *FDR's Splendid Deception*, 45.
49. Jean Schauble, "Roosevelt and Warm Springs," *Columbia Library Columns*, February 1973, 3–9; Dr. George Draper to Franklin Roosevelt, July 25, 1925; Roosevelt to Draper, July 27, 1925, Box 23, "Family, Business, Personal," Subject File: Infantile Paralysis," Franklin Delano Roosevelt Papers, FDR Library.

50. Walker, *Roosevelt and the Warm Springs Story*, 31–117; Gallagher, *FDR's Splendid Deception*, 56.

51. Lippman, *The Squire of Warm Springs*, 50; Ward, *A First-Class Temperament*, 709. Though Franklin and Eleanor remained close and spoke frequently about political and family matters, the time they spent together had greatly diminished by 1924. "Their lives simply went in different directions," wrote Eleanor's biographer, Blanche Wiesen Cook. "They were pulled by different interests, attracted by different people." Mrs. Roosevelt, no doubt, was content to spend as little time as possible in Warm Springs. Her role as hostess and confidante there was filled by FDR's devoted secretary, Missy LeHand. See Cook, *Eleanor Roosevelt*, 314–17.

52. Quoted in Smith, *Patenting the Sun*, 56.

53. David Kennedy, *Freedom from Fear: The American People in Depression and War, 1929–1945*, 1999, 94–97; Mark H. Leff, "Franklin Roosevelt," in *The Reader's Companion to the American Presidency*, ed. Alan Brinkley and David Dyer, 2000, 369–71; Cook, *Eleanor Roosevelt*, 302–37.

54. Roosevelt returned the check, telling Raskob that his generosity might be called on in the future. It was. In the coming years, Raskob gave more than $100,000 to the Warm Springs Foundation, making him one of its largest donors. See Friedel, *Franklin D. Roosevelt*, 255.

55. Gallagher, *FDR's Splendid Deception*, 72–74; Freidel, *FDR: The Ordeal*, 257–69.

56. Ward, *A First-Class Temperament*, 794.

Chapter 3

1. Gould, *Grand Old Party: A History of the Republicans*, 256; Kennedy, *Freedom from Fear*, 91–92; McElvaine, *The Great Depression*, 52.

2. Black, *Franklin Delano Roosevelt: Champion of Freedom*, 211.

3. Gallagher, *FDR's Splendid Deception*, 81–82.

4. Ibid., 87.

5. Daniel J. Wilson, "A Crippling Fear: Experiencing Polio in the Era of FDR," *Bulletin of the History of Medicine*, 1998, 490. One historian, in particular, has emphasized the way FDR carefully blurred the critical distinction between "illness" and "disability." See John Duffy, "Franklin Roosevelt: Ambiguous Symbol for Disabled Americans," *Midwest Quarterly*, Autumn 1987, 113–35.

6. See Amy Fairchild, "The Polio Narratives: Dialogues with FDR," *Bulletin of the History of Medicine*, 2001, 488–534.

7. *New York Journal-American*, January 17, 19, 20, 21, 1938.

8. Wilson, "A Crippling Fear," 487–88.

9. Ibid., 483–84.

10. Ibid., 495; also Daniel J. Wilson, "Crippled Manhood: Infantile Paralysis and the Construction of Masculinity," *Medical Humanities Review*, Fall 1998, 9–27.

11. Alice Heaton, "A Friend—and Partner," *Good Housekeeping*, July 1953, 209.

12. David Sills, *The Volunteers*, 42.

13. Cutlip, *The Unseen Power*, 531–52; "Carl Byoir: A Retrospective," Museum of Public Relations, 2002.

14. Cutlip, *Fund Raising in the United States*, 361; Walker, *Roosevelt and the Warm Springs Story*, 229–31. For the career of Henry Doherty, see Rose, *Cities of Heat and Light*.

15. "Letter Number One to Town Publishers," December 13, 1933, in Basil O'Connor Vertical File, FDR Presidential Library, Hyde Park, New York. Byoir wrote these letters, but they were signed "Henry Doherty, National Chairman."

16. "Letter Number Two, December 22, 1933; Henry Doherty, National Chairman, to His Honor, The Mayor, January 5, 1934, ibid.

17. Cohn, *Four Billion Dimes*, 43; Dorothy Ducas, "Crusader-By-Accident: The Biography of Basil O'Connor," unpublished manuscript in Basil O'Connor File, March of Dimes Archives, White Plains, N.Y. (hereafter cited as MDA).

18. Byoir, "Organizing Suggestions," in Basil O'Connor Vertical File, FDR Presidential Library; Cutlip, *Fund Raising in the United States*, 366; for Wiley Post, see B. Sterling and F. Sterling, *Forgotten Eagle: Wiley Post*.

19. "Whole City Joins in Tribute To President on 52nd Birthday: New York Scene of 40 of 6,000 Balls to Benefit Warm Springs," *New York Times*, January 31, 1934; press release, "Birthday Ball for the President," Basil O'Connor Vertical File, FDR Library.

20. Walker, *Roosevelt and the Warm Springs Story*, 229–31; Cutlip, *The Unseen Power*, 558–59.

21. Carter, *The Gentle Legions*, 77; "Christmas Seals Celebrates 90 Years of Holiday Giving and Tradition," American Lung Association Web site.

22. Cutlip, *Fund Raising in the United States*, 129; Carter, *Gentle Legions*, 38–62.

23. Cutlip, *Fund Raising in the United States*, 242–91.

24. Heaton, "A Friend—and Partner," 209–10; Cohn, *Four Billion Dimes*, 39.

25. Cutlip, *Fund Raising in the United States*, 367–68.

26. Cohn, *Four Billion Dimes*, 44.

27. *New York World-Telegram and Sun*, January 27, 1938; *New York Post*, January 25, 1938.

   Roosevelt's attempted purge was remarkably unsuccessful. Almost all of his targets survived. It was ironic, to say the least, that one of the Democrats FDR did manage to unseat in 1938 was Congressman John J. O'Connor, a cantankerous Tammany Hall loyalist described by *Time* magazine as "one of the most unpopular members of a supposedly popular House." O'Connor, chairman of the Rules Committee, was Basil O'Connor's older brother. See James Patterson, *Congressional Conservatism and the New Deal*, 1967, 53, 278–87.

28. "Cripples' Money: Who Gets the Proceeds of the Presidential Birthday Balls?" 48 pp. Copy in author's possession; *Chicago Tribune*, December 21, 1938.

29. National Foundation for Infantile Paralysis, "Organization Chart," MDA; Cohn, *Four Billion Dimes*, p. 57.

30. Goldman, *Banjo Eyes*, 194–96; The Eddie Cantor Appreciation Society, "The Eddie Cantor Story," http://www.eddiecantor.com.

31. Goldman, *Banjo Eyes*, xiii.

32. Cutlip, *Fund Raising in the United States*, 385.

33. Ibid.

34. Ibid. Also Ira T. Smith, *"Dear Mr. President . . ."*: The Story of Fifty Years in the White House Mail Room*, 1949, 157–61.

35. Smith, *"Dear Mr. President . . . ,"* 159.

36. Ed Reiter, "Franklin D. Roosevelt: The Man on the Marching Dime," June 28, 1999, Professional Coin Grading Service Web site. A recent attempt by congressional conservatives to replace FDR on the dime with Ronald Reagan met stiff resistance. Nancy Reagan opposed the change, saying: "I do not support

this proposal, and I'm certain Ronnie would not." See Robert Scheer's column in the *Los Angeles Times*, December 13, 2003; and *USA Today*, December 5, 2003.

37. Simmons, *Doctors and Discoveries*, 401–4; Paul, *A History of Poliomyelitis*, 305; Benison, *Tom Rivers*, 182.

38. Paul de Kruif, "De Kruif Emphasizes Mystery of Infantile Paralysis," *New York World-Telegram & Sun*, January 24, 1948; Benison, *Tom Rivers*, 183–84.

39. Maurice Brodie and William H. Park, "Active Immunization Against Poliomyelitis," *Journal of the American Medical Association*, October 5, 1935, 1089–93.

40. "Specter of Paralysis Stalks Carolina," *Literary Digest*, July 1935.

41. Benison, *Tom Rivers*, 185.

42. H. V. Wyatt, "Provocation Poliomyelitis: Neglected Clinical Observations from 1914–1950," *Bulletin of the History of Medicine*, 1981, 550–55; Paul, *History of Poliomyelitis*, 255–60.

43. Lederer, *Subjected to Science*, 107; Benison, *Tom Rivers*, 189.

44. "William Hallock Park," *Medical Violet* (NYU Medical School yearbook), 1939, 43, 163; Altman, *Who Goes First*, 126–28; Hooper, *The River*, 198; Paul, *History of Poliomyelitis*, 254–61, 270–72. The notice of Brodie's death can be found in the *Canadian Medical Association Journal*, 1939, 632.

45. For de Kruif's explanation of the Park-Brodie fiasco, see President's Birthday Ball Commission for Infantile Paralysis Research, "Progress Report," March 28, 1937, 11, FDR Presidential Library; Carter, *Breakthrough*, 24–25.

46. "Biographical Sketch of Thomas M. Rivers, M.D.," Thomas Rivers File, MDA.

47. Ibid. Also Benison, *Tom Rivers*, 67–225; Smith, *Patenting the Sun*, 147–48.

48. Benison, *Tom Rivers*, 232.

49. Howard Howe to David Bodian, January 24, 1942, in Folder 1 (unprocessed), David Bodian Papers, Chesney Medical Archives, Johns Hopkins Medical School.

Chapter 4

1. Hawkins, *The Man in the Iron Lung*, 67.

2. Ibid., 66–70.

3. In a recent article, David Rothman, a leading medical historian, writes that the development of the iron lung "became the occasion for Americans to express and absorb the values that would continue to influence national attitudes and practices decades later. . . . It is here," he notes, "that we find the origins of the ethic that lifesaving technologies had to be available to everyone, that the prospect of benefit, however slim, outweighed the costs, however substantial."

From the very outset, he adds, doctors used the iron lung for desperately ill patients who had little chance of surviving. As a result, the mortality rate was very high, giving the machine a reputation as both a lifesaver and a death trap, combining "durability and awesome power" with "dread and revulsion." See Rothman, "The Iron Lung and Democratic Medicine," in *Beginnings Count: The Technological Imperative in American Health Care*, ed. D. Rothman, 1997, 42–66.

4. "Life in a Respirator," *Time*, June 14, 1937, 32; "Iron Lung: Metal Prison for a Traveling Paralysis Patient," *Newsweek*, June 12, 1937, 21.

5. Ibid.

6. "Snite at Lourdes," *Time*, June 12, 1939; 55.

7. Dorothy Corson, "Frederick Snite: The Man in the Iron Lung, a Legend at Notre Dame," in *Notre Dame Legends and Lore*, http://www.nd.edu.

8. "Married," *Newsweek*, August 21, 1939, 9; "The Man in the Iron Lung," *Time*, November 18, 1946, 68–69; "A Man Without Worries," *Time*, November 22, 1954, 59–60; Hawkins, *Man in the Iron Lung*, 243.

9. Hawkins, *The Man in the Iron Lung*, 174; Howard Markel, "The Genesis of the Iron Lung," *Archives of Pediatric Adolescent Medicine*, 1994, 1179.

10. Sills, *The Volunteers*, 116–48.

11. Ibid., 134.

12. Gould, *A Summer Plague*, 79–80.

13. "Remarks of Franklin D. Roosevelt at Tuskegee Institute, March 30, 1939"; "Statement at the Dedication of the Infantile Paralysis Unit at Tuskegee in Alabama, January 15, 1941"; in "The American Presidency Project: Public Papers of the President, Franklin D. Roosevelt, http://www.presidency.ucsb.edu.

14. Gould, *A Summer Plague*, 81–83; McMurry, *George Washington Carver*, 252–55; "World's Great Men of Color: George Washington Carver," in http://www.marcusgarvey.com.

15. National Foundation for Infantile Paralysis, "The Tuskegee Institute Infantile Paralysis Center, n.d., 10 pp. For Tuskegee's role in training nurses for the disabled, see Kimberly Carter, "Trumpets of Attack: Collaborative Efforts Between Nursing and Philanthropies to Care for the Child Crippled with Polio, 1930 to 1959," *Public Health Nursing*, July–August 2001.

16. Harry Weaver to Thomas Francis, December 6, 1946, "Weaver Correspondence," Box 51, Thomas Francis Papers, Bentley Library, University of Michigan.

17. On the racial issue in the 1916 epidemic, see Gould, *A Summer Plague*, 8; for the 1946 survey, see "The Incidence of Poliomyelitis and Its Crippling Effects as Recorded in Family Surveys," *Public Health Reports*, March 8, 1946, 345–46.

18. Francis to Weaver, December 10, 1946, "Weaver Correspondence," Box 51, Thomas Francis Papers, Bentley Library, University of Michigan; Weaver to Francis, February 6, 1947, "Weaver Correspondence," Box 51, Thomas Francis Papers, Bentley Library, University of Michigan.

19. "Fund-Raising," Box 1, Campaign Materials, 1939, 1944, March of Dimes Archives, White Plains, N.Y. (hereafter cited as MDA); Smith, *Patenting the Sun*, 83.

20. Franklin Roosevelt to Basil O'Connor, November 10, 1942, in Basil O'Connor File, MDA.

21. "Fund-Raising," Box 1, 1944, 1945, ibid.

22. See especially "Motion Picture Campaign Book," and "Motion Picture Industries Campaign," ibid.

23. National Foundation for Infantile Paralysis, "Facts and Figures About Infantile Paralysis," Publication No. 59, 1947; Sills, *The Volunteers*, 128–30.

24. "Infantile Paralysis, *Life*, July 31, 1944, 25–28.

25. Sink, *The Grit Behind the Miracle*, 115–19, 139–42.

26. Ibid., 53–61.

27. Ibid., 68.

28. Ibid., 35–36, 41; "Infantile Paralysis," *Life*, July 31, 1944, 25–28.

29. National Foundation for Infantile Paralysis, "The Miracle of Hickory," n.d., MDA; Rose, *Images of America*, 24–25.

30. *Greensboro Daily News*, August 9, 1944, quoted in Sink, *The Grit Behind the Miracle*, 69–70.

31. Ibid.
32. Ibid., 117.
33. Ibid., 121, 149.
34. Elizabeth Kenny, *And They Shall Walk*, 23; Robert Yoder, "Healer from the Outback," *Saturday Evening Post*, January 17, 1942, 18–19, 68.
35. Victor Cohn, *Sister Kenny*, 38–50.
36. Sonda Oppewal, "Sister Kenny, an Australian Nurse, and Treatment of Poliomyelitis Victims," *Image: the Journal of Nursing Scholarship*, 1997, 83–87; Naomi Rogers, "Sister Kenny Goes to Washington: Polio, Populism, and Medical Politics in Postwar America," in Robert Johnston, *The Politics of Healing*, 2004, 102–3.
37. Walter I. Galland, "The Post-Paralytic Treatment of Poliomyelitis from the Orthopedic Standpoint," reprinted in *Archives of Physical Medicine and Rehabilitation*, September 1969, 525–30; Paul, *A History of Poliomyelitis*, 338–40.
38. "Verdict on Sister Kenny," *Newsweek*, June 26, 1944, 77–78; Gould, *A Summer Plague*, 96, 108; Margaret Denton, "Further Comments on the Elizabeth Kenny Controversy," *Australian Historical Studies*, 2000, 157.
39. Cohn, *Sister Kenny*, 127; Benison, *Tom Rivers*, 282. In response to testimonials from physicians and family members of polio victims, Rivers did recommend to O'Connor that the foundation not close the door entirely on Sister Kenny, but seek, instead, to find some "ethical doctors" who "would be willing to investigate [her claims] without bias." See Rivers to O'Connor, March 4, 1941, Basil O'Connor File, Thomas Rivers Papers, American Philosophical Society.
40. Gould, *A Summer Plague*, 96; Marvin Kline (former mayor of Minneapolis), "The Most Unforgettable Character I've Met," *Reader's Digest*, August 1959, 205.
41. Cohn, *Sister Kenny*, 83–84.
42. Kline, "Unforgettable Character," 205; Miland E. Knapp, M.D., "The Contribution of Sister Elizabeth Kenny to the Treatment of Poliomyelitis," *Archives of Physical Medicine and Rehabilitation*, August 1955, 510–17.
43. Cohn, *Sister Kenny*, 147.
44. Yoder, "Healer from the Outback"; Lois Miller, "Sister Kenny vs. Infantile Paralysis," *Reader's Digest*, December 1941, 1–6; Lois Miller, "Sister Kenny vs. the Medical Old Guard," *Reader's Digest*, October 1944, 65–71; Cohn, *Sister Kenny*, 192–93; "Movie of the Week: Sister Kenny" and "A Doctor Comments on 'Sister Kenny,'" *Life*, September 16, 1946, 21.
45. Cohn, *Sister Kenny*, 172.
46. Ibid., 173, 213
47. Ibid., 151–52; "Verdict on Sister Kenny," *Newsweek*, June 26, 1944, 76–78.
48. Cohn, *Sister Kenny*, 206–7.
49. Ibid., 234.

Chapter 5

1. Walker, *Roosevelt and the Warm Springs Story*, 301.
2. Fund Raising Records, Series 7, 1944, "Motion Picture Campaign Book," March of Dimes Archives, White Plains, N.Y. (hereafter cited as MDA).
3. 1946, Motion Picture Industry Campaign, MDA.
4. Fund Raising Records, Series 8, United Funds, "Memoranda and Reports, NFIP," MDA.

5. Ibid.
6. Fund Raising Records, Series 7, Policy and Procedures, "History and Responsibilities of the Fund Raising Department, NFIP, 1943–1955," MDA.
7. Publications Collection, Series 2, Periodicals; Medical Programs Documents, Series 15, Box 15, Public Relations Department, 1937–1949; and Science Writers, 1946–1964, MDA.
8. Seavey, Smith, and Wagner, *A Paralyzing Fear*, 74.
9. Fund Raising Records, Series 4, Poster Children, "Donald Anderson—1946 March of Dimes Poster Boy," MDA.
10. Memo: Joe Kievit to Trudy Whitman, December 15, 1949; "Donald Anderson—1946 March of Dimes Poster Boy," MDA.
11. "Report on Donald Anderson," n.d., MDA.
12. Memo: Felix Montes to Trudy Whitman, December 3, 1948, MDA.
13. Future poster children would generally be photographed on crutches or in their leg braces, or sometimes using both. But the message was always optimistic, with the smiling child on his or her way to recovery. Indeed, by the late 1940s, the March of Dimes supplemented these posters with pamphlets titled "Look, I Can Walk Again" and "I'm Walking Because of You." See especially "Publications Collection: Series 2—Periodicals, Series 3—Poliomyelitis," MDA.
14. Black, *In the Shadow of Polio*, 39–42; Mee, *A Nearly Normal Life*, 3–13.
15. Black, *In the Shadow of Polio*, 40.
16. Davis, *Passage Through Crisis*, 37.
17. Black, *In the Shadow of Polio*, 47.
18. Spock, *The Common Sense Book of Baby and Child Care*, 419–20.
19. "Polio Panic," *Time*, August 5, 1946, 55–56; "The Polio Scourge," *Newsweek*, August 19, 1946, 22–24.
20. Fund Raising Records, Series 8, United Funds, "Memoranda and Reports," MDA.
21. Sills, *The Volunteers*; Nancy Weiss, "Mother: The Invention of Necessity: Dr. Benjamin Spock's *Baby and Child Care*," *American Quarterly*, Winter 1977, 519–46.
22. Annual Programs for "Fashion Show"; Miss Whitelaw to Miss Kay, January 11, 1945; in Fund Raising Records, Series 3: Fashion Show, MDA.
23. "Fashion Show, Program Scripts," MDA.
24. John Clifford to Elaine Whitelaw, November 27, 1946, MDA.
25. See 1949, "Jewel Tour" (The Court of Jewels; Harry Winston Collection), MDA.
26. Fund Raising Records, Report: 1950, "Mothers' March on Polio, Maricopa Chapter, NFIP," MDA; "March of Dimes Promotional Film," MDA; Sills, *The Volunteers*, 158–59.
27. "Chronological Outline of Mothers' March," MDA; also *Phoenix Gazette*, January 2, 1950; *Arizona Republic*, January 17, 1950.
28. "Foreword" of "Chronological Outline of Mothers' March," MDA.
29. "March of Dimes Promotional Film," MDA
30. Mothers' March Folder (including "Plan Book" and "Rural Supplement to Plan Book"), in Series 4, Institutional History, Box 8, MDA.
31. Sills, *The Volunteers*, 160.
32. Ibid., 184–85.
33. Ibid., 158; Joanne Meyerowitz, "Beyond the Feminine Mystique: A Reassessment of Postwar Mass Culture, 1946–1958," in Meyerowitz, *Not June Cleaver*, 229–62.

34. Fund Raising Records, "History and Responsibility of the Fund Raising Department," MDA.

35. Allan Brandt and Martha Gardner, "The Golden Age of Medicine?" in Cooper and Pickstone, *Medicine in the Twentieth Century*, 21–37; Brandt, *No Magic Bullet*, 40–41; Tomes, *The Gospel of Germs*, 254.

36. Simmons, *Doctors and Discoveries*, 256–60; Brandt and Gardner, "Golden Age of Medicine?" 26.

37. *National Vital Statistics Reports*, vol. 51. no. 3, December 19, 2002, 29; David Cutler and Ellen Meara, "Changes in the Age Distribution of Mortality Over the 20th Century," National Bureau of Economic Research Working Paper No. 8556, October 2001.

Chapter 6

1. See "Grant to National Foundation, 1941–42," and draft of article on Francis by Paul Ellis, January 7, 1947; both in National Foundation File, Box 51, Thomas Francis Papers, Bentley Library, University of Michigan (hereafter cited as Francis Papers).

2. Thomas Francis to Hart Van Riper, August 28, 1947, "Van Riper Correspondence," Box 51, Francis Papers.

3. See David Bodian, "Poliomyelitis and the Sources of Useful Knowledge," *Johns Hopkins Medical Journal*, 1976, 131.

4. A sampling of Sabin's correspondence on these matters can be found in Correspondence 1935–39, Box 3; Correspondence, 1946–47, Box 4; General Correspondence, 1950, Box 4: General Correspondence, 1953, Box 5; Albert Sabin Papers, University of Cincinnati Medical School (hereafter cited as Sabin Papers, UC). For Peter Olitsky, see Correspondence with Public, Peter Olitsky Papers, Archives of the Rockefeller Institute, Sleepy Hollow, New York (hereafter cited as Olitsky Papers). Also Dr. J. Plesch to Dr. Hart Van Riper, August 26, 1946, "Van Riper Correspondence," Box 51, Francis Papers; Albert Sabin to George Lyon, December 4, 1940; Sabin in "Science Service," June 6, 1940; "Mothers' Milk Has Chemicals to Kill Viruses," *New York Herald-Tribune*, May 29, 1951.

    According to the National Foundation, the most common misconceptions about how one contracted polio included bathing in polluted water, eating crops on which poliovirus had settled, and consuming lots of "sugar drinks," especially Coca-Cola, a rumor most widely believed in the South. See "Sources of Incorrect Information Which Have Recent Wide Circulation," Medical Program, Box 14, March of Dimes Archives, White Plains, N.Y. (hereafter cited as MDA).

5. Jonas Salk to W. S. McEllroy, December 9, 1947, Box 4, Folder 7, Jonas Salk Papers, Mandeville Special Collections, University of California, San Diego (hereafter cited as Salk Papers); W. H. Bradley, "Meteorological Conditions in Relation to Poliomyelitis in England and Wales, 1947–1952," *Monthly Bulletin of the Ministry of Health*, January 1953, 2–14.

6. "Resumes of Grantee's Progress Reports," Box 9, Medical Program, 1944; Box 12, Medical Program "Chemical Research," 1948; Box 15, Medical Program, "Research Program," 1951; all in MDA. Also "Polio Snake Venom" file, in *Newsweek* Morgue, Center for American History, University of Texas, Austin.

7. Paul, *A History of Poliomyelitis*, 412–13; Aaron Klein, *Trial by Fury*, 45–46.

8. Carter, *Breakthrough*, 57.

9. Bodian, "Poliomyelitis and the Source of Useful Knowledge," 131.

10. In the 1940s, the National Foundation bankrolled a number of projects designed to "wash" the spinal fluid of polio patients and to find a chemical solution for the disease. See especially Berg, *Polio and Its Problems*, 1947 (ch. 7, "A Pill for Polio,"), 60–77.

11. Dowling, *Fighting Infection*, 212–13; Robert Coughlin, "Tracking the Killer, *Life*, February 22, 1954, 121–25; Williams, *Virus Hunters*, 251–69.

12. Lee Salk, *My Father, My Son*, 10.

13. Interview with Jonas Salk, May 16, 1991, in "Hall of Science and Exploration," www.achievement.org; author's interview with Darrell Salk, February 19, 2003.

14. Ibid.

15. "New Townsend Harris High Keeps Old Goals," *New York Times*, June 10, 1985; "Our History," *Townsend Harris Online*; Traub, *City on a Hill*, 32.

16. S. Willis Rudy, *The College of the City of New York: A History*, 1949, 294.

17. Traub, *City On A Hill*, 9, 34; CCNY Alumni Association, "Facts on City College" and "City's Nobel Laureates of the Twentieth Century," in www.alumni associationccny.org.

18. Jonas Salk college transcript, Jonas Salk File, CCNY, Division of Archives and Special Collections, Morris Raphael Cohen Library.

19. *Microcosm 1934* (CCNY Student Yearbook), 60–63; Howe, *A Margin of Hope*, 61–89.

20. *Microcosm 1934*, 120.

21. Interview with Jonas Salk, May 16, 1991.

22. Alan Dumont and Claude Heaton, *The First One Hundred and Twenty–Five Years of the New York University School of Medicine*, 1966, 3–40; Thomas Francis Jones, *New York University: 1832–1932*, 1933, 281–304.

23. Gerard Burrow, *A History of Yale's School of Medicine*, 2002, 107, 143–44.

24. "New York University College of Medicine, Schedule of Exercises" (1935–1936, 1936–1937, 1937–1938, 1938–1939); "Third Year Class Section Lists" (1937–1938); "Fourth Year Class Section Lists" (1938–1939), NYU Medical School Archives.

25. *The Medical Violet 1939* (NYU School of Medicine Student Yearbook), 93.

26. Author's interview with Darrell Salk, February 19, 2003.

27. Carter, *Breakthrough*, 37.

28. Ibid., 41.

29. Author's interview with Darrell Salk, February 19, 2003.

30. Federal Bureau of Investigation, "Subject: Jonas Salk," File 161-22356.

31. Jonas Salk to Thomas Francis, September 20, 1941, Jonas Salk File, Francis Papers; John R. Paul, "Thomas Francis Jr.," *Biographical Memoirs*, 1974, 57–91.

32. Thomas Francis to Jonas Salk, December 18, 1841, Jonas Salk File, Francis Papers. The main roadblock at the Rockefeller Institute was Thomas Rivers, the chief virologist. A well-known anti-Semite, who also vetoed a permanent appointment for Albert Sabin at the Institute, Rivers would later play a key role in the development of the Salk polio vaccine.

33. Thomas Francis to Francis Blake, Chairman, National Research Council, January 17, 1942, Jonas Salk File, Francis Papers. Francis and Blake were longtime friends.

34. Col. S. J. Kopetzsky to Jonas Salk, March 13, 1942, Box 5, Salk Papers.

35. Thomas Francis to Selective Service Board 45, February 13, 1942; Thomas Francis to Col. Samuel Kopetzsky, March 24, 1942; Jonas Salk to Thomas Francis, April 8, 1942; all in Jonas Salk File, Francis Papers.

36. Paul, "Thomas Francis Jr.," 69; Benison, *Tom Rivers*, 256.

37. Benison, *Tom Rivers*, 257.

38. Kolata, *Flu*, 3–33; Crawford, *The Invisible Enemy*, 96–98; Crosby, *America's Forgotten Pandemic*, 203.

39. *Flu*, 6–7, 16; Crawford, *Invisible Enemy*, 97; Grob, *The Deadly Truth*, 224–25.

40. Susan Plotkin and Stanley Plotkin, "A Short History of Vaccination," in Plotkin and Mortimer, *Vaccines*, 1–7; Dowling, *Fighting Infection*, 197–200.

    Just prior to leaving Mount Sinai for Ann Arbor, Salk wrote Francis: "At present we have a patient with the clinical picture and clinical course that our [staff] say they saw in the 1918 epidemic. We've not been able to discover any bacterial pathogen and I believe she may die very shortly." See Jonas Salk to Thomas Francis, February 7, 1942, Jonas Salk File, Francis Papers.

41. Author's interview with Darrell Salk, February 19, 2003; Carter, *Breakthrough*, 45; Federal Bureau of Investigation, "Subject: Jonas Salk."

42. Thomas Francis Jr., "Draft of Grant Proposal to the National Foundation," n.d., Box 51; Henry Vaughan to Basil O'Connor, June 26, 1942; Basil O'Connor to Alexander Ruthven, President, University of Michigan, April 8, 1943, both in Box 51, Francis Papers. The grant was for $200,000 over three years, one of the Foundation's largest in those years.

43. On Salk's rise up the academic ladder, see Dean H. F. Vaughan to Jonas Salk, June 10, 1943; Vaughan to Salk, October 16, 1944; Thomas Francis to Provost James P. Adams, June 26, 1946; Herbert G. Watkins (University Secretary) to Salk, July 29, 1946. On military deferments, see Francis G. Blake Affidavit, October 21, 1943; Henry F. Vaughan to Clarence Moll, June 14, 1944; Thomas Francis to Clarence Moll, January 18, 1945; all in Jonas Salk File, Francis Papers. Salk's quote can be found in Carter, *Breakthrough*, 48.

44. Carter, *Breakthrough*, 51; Hershel Griffin, "Thomas Francis Jr., MD: Epidemiologist to the Military," *Archives of Environmental Health*, September 1970, 252–55; Cohen, *Shots in the Dark*, 26; Carter, *Breakthrough*, 48.

45. Dowling, *Fighting Infection*, 200; Williams, *Virus Hunters*, 223–27.

46. Williams, *Virus Hunters*, 225; Brian Murphy and Robert Webster, "Orthomyxoviruses," in *Virology* (2nd ed.), ed. Bernard N. Fields, 1116–20; Crawford, *Invisible Enemy*, 92, 229; Thomas Francis to Carolyn Kingdon, November 1, 1947, Box 51, Francis Papers.

47. Carter, *Breakthrough*, 51.

48. Ibid.

49. Ibid.; Benison, *Tom Rivers*, 258; Williams, *Virus Hunter*, 212.

    When Francis was elected to the National Academy of Sciences in 1948, Salk, who by then had moved to Pittsburgh, sent him this note of congratulations: "I think this is splendid, and it might convince you that you have not been wasting your time and energy about which you sometimes have some doubt." See Jonas Salk to Thomas Francis, May 17, 1948, Box 5, Salk Papers.

50. Carter, *Breakthrough*, 51.

51. Paul Stumpf to Jonas Salk, n.d., Box 4, Folder 8, Salk Papers.

52. Thomas Francis, "Memorandum: Concerning Doctor Salk and Parke-Davis & Company," September 1, 1945, Jonas Salk File, Francis Papers.

53. Jonas Salk to Thomas Francis, December 26, 1945, Jonas Salk File, Francis Papers.

54. Max Lauffer to Jonas Salk, June 30, 1947, Salk File, Edward Litchfield Papers, University of Pittsburgh Archive; Carter, *Breakthrough*, 53.

55. Jonas Salk to Thomas Francis, August 25, 1947, Jonas Salk File, Francis Papers.

56. Willard Glazier, "The Great Furnace of America," in *Pittsburgh*, ed. Roy Lubove, 1976, 23.

57. Michael Weber, *Don't Call Me Boss: David L. Lawrence, Pittsburgh's Renaissance Mayor*, 1988, 202–3; Lubove. *Pittsburgh*, 196.

58. "Pittsburgh's New Powers," *Fortune*, February, 1947, 69–74; Jonas Salk to Stella Barlow, n.d., Salk Papers.

59. Weber, *Don't Call Me Boss*, 228–76; Robert C. Alberts, *Pitt: The Story of the University of Pittsburgh*, 1986, 204–9.

60. Alberts, *Pitt*, 207.

61. Barbara Paull, *A Century of Medical Excellence: A History of the University of Pittsburgh School of Medicine*, 1986, 99–100; Julius Youngner, unpublished autobiography, 39, copy in author's possession.

62. Paull, *Century of Medical Excellence*, 145–50, 172–74.

63. Ibid, 211; Max Lauffer, "Memorandum: The Virus Research Program," May 22, 1950, University of Pittsburgh Archive.

    As a candidate for the position, Salk had submitted a wish list that included additional lab space and animal quarters, a secretary, a technician, a suggested annual salary of $7,500, and a joint appointment as "associate research professor." He did not, however, see these "requests" as "limiting factors" in considering him for the job. Indeed, Salk added, "I appreciate that you would be willing to do whatever [is] necessary within the capacity of your present budget." See Jonas Salk to Max Lauffer, June 27, 1947, Salk File, Edward Litchfield Papers, University of Pittsburgh Archive.

64. Jonas Salk to John Dingle, August 27, 1947, Folder 5, Box 4, Salk Papers; Carter, *Breakthrough*, 53.

65. Carter, *Breakthrough*, 54; Jonas Salk to Paul Stumpf, November 26, 1947, Box 4, Folder 8, Salk Papers.

66. Jonas Salk to Dr. W. S. McEllroy, December 9, 1947, Box 4, Folder 7, Salk Papers

67. Ibid.

68. Ibid.; Alberts, *Pitt*, 216.

Chapter 7

1. Benison, *Tom Rivers*, 405.

2. Harry Weaver, "A Formula to Determine the Cost of Research," *Journal of the American Medical Colleges*, July 1950.

3. Ibid.

4. Benison, *Tom Rivers*, 444–45; Harry Weaver, "A Formula to Determine the Total Cost of Conducting a Program of Research," in Medical Program, Series 8, Box 8, March of Dimes Archives, White Plains, N.Y. (hereafter cited as MDA).

5. H. W. Weaver to H. Van Riper, "Memorandum Re Payment of Direct Costs," February 1, 1951; Harry Weaver to R. W. Brown, October 17, 1952, both in Medical Program, Series 8 Box 8, "Indirect Costs, 1947–1959," MDA.

6. H. W. Weaver to H. Van Riper, "Memorandum Re Policies Governing Long-Term Grants," April 24, 1947, MDA.

7. Basil O'Connor to Thomas Rivers, July 21, 1947, Basil O'Connor File 6, Thomas Rivers Papers, American Philosophical Society, Philadelphia.

8. Quoted in Henry Lee, "No More Polio," *Pageant*, November 1953, 18.

9. Carter, *Breakthrough*, 61–62; also Harry Weaver to Jonas Salk, December 15, 1947, Box 4, Folder 8; August 13, 1948, Folder 5, Box 5, Jonas Salk Papers, Mandeville Special Collections, University of California, San Diego (hereafter cited as Salk Papers).

10. See, "Chronology of Events in Salk Research for Polio Vaccine," Jonas Salk File, Edward Litchfield Papers, University of Pittsburgh; Salk to Weaver, July 27, 1948, Salk Papers.

11. Salk to Weaver, August 24, 1948, Folder 5, Box 5, Salk Papers; Carter, *Breakthrough*, 107. Peter Salk, the oldest of the three sons, recalled: "My father made a point of walking through that ward. People would approach him in tears. 'Please, Dr. Salk, please save our child.' There was a pathos to this, a sadness that never left his mind." Author's interview with Peter Salk, November 22, 2002.

12. "Research Funds for Pitt Medical School," Box 296, Salk Papers.

13. "Neil Seidenberg, "Men and Scenes Behind Salk Vaccine," *Pittsburgh Post-Gazette*, April 12, 1955; Leonard Engel, "Climax of a Stirring Medical Drama," *New York Times Sunday Magazine*, January 10, 1954; "Vaccine's Name Irks Salk," *Pittsburgh Press*, April 12, 1955; "Age of Salk's Aides Averages Under 40," *New York Times*, April 12, 1945; "The Story Behind the Polio Vaccine," *Wisdom*, August 1956, 10–16; F. S. Cheever, "Leadership Qualities Draw Skilled, Devoted Workers," *Pittsburgh Sun-Telegraph*, August 4, 1959; "Salk Team's 'Mr. Inside' Honored for Work on Polio Vaccine," *Pittsburgh Post-Gazette*, August 9, 2001. Also Smith, *Patenting the Sun*, 115–17; Carter, *Breakthrough*, 69–71; Jonas Salk to Harry Weaver, August 24, 1948, Folder 5, Box 5, Salk Papers.

14. Harry Weaver to Jonas Salk, March 11 (two letters that day), 1949, Folder: 1949, W–Z, Box 6, Salk Papers.

15. Gordon Brown to Jonas Salk, June 17, 1949, Folder: 1949, A–C, Box 5, Ibid.

16. Ibid.

17. Thomas Francis to John Lavan, January 31, 1944, Box 51, Thomas Francis Papers, Bentley Library, University of Michigan; Cohn, *Four Billion Dimes*, 82.

18. See "Many Monkeys Needed in Vaccine," in M. Beddow Bayly, *The Story of the Salk Anti-Poliomyelitis Vaccine*, 1956, http://whale.to/vaccine/bayley.

19. Ibid.

20. Thomas Francis to J. N. Hamlet (Director, Okatie Farms), July 15, 1950; Hamlet to Francis, September 21, 1950, File: Monkeys, Box 5, Thomas Francis Papers; "The Unsung Heroes," *Newsweek*, April 25, 1955; Smith, *Patenting the Sun*, 121.

21. Carter, *Breakthrough*, 79.

22. Ibid., 81.

23. Jonas Salk to Albert Sabin, April 15, May 1, 1949, Folder: 1949, P–V, Box 6; Albert Sabin to Jonas Salk, June 20, 1951, Folder 3, Box 281; all in Salk Papers.

24. Paul, *A History of Poliomyelitis*, 234–35.
25. Albert Sabin to Jonas Salk, February 23, 1951; Salk to Sabin, March 1, 1951; both in Folder 3, Box 281, Salk Papers.
26. Friedman and Friedland, *Medicine's 10 Greatest Discoveries*, 133–52.
27. A. B. Sabin and P. K. Olitsky, "Cultivation of poliovirus *in vitro* in human embryonic tissue," *Proceedings of the Society of Experimental Biological Medicine*, vol. 34, 1936, 357–59.
28. Benison, *Tom Rivers*, 237.
29. Ibid., 446; Thomas Weller and Frederick Robbins, "John Franklin Enders," unpublished manuscript in author's possession; Simmons, *Doctors and Discoveries*, 266–69.
30. Paul, *A History of Poliomyelitis*, 378.
31. Weller and Robbins, "John Franklin Enders"; Frederick Robbins, "Reminiscences of a Virologist," in Daniel and Robbins, *Polio*, 121–25.

   Both Tom Weller and Fred Robbins came from prominent scientific families. Robbins's father, William, was a noted plant physiologist who supervised the New York Botanical Gardens. Weller's father, Carl, was a professor of pathology at the University of Michigan and a good friend of Salk's mentor, Thomas Francis.
32. Paul, *History of Poliomyelitis*, 374–75; Robbins, "Reminiscences," 126–28.
33. Robbins, "Reminiscences," 125–26; Simmons, *Doctors and Discoveries*, 268; Henig, *The People's Health*, 25–34.
34. Benison, *Tom Rivers*, 446–47.
35. Peter Olitsky to Albert Sabin, undated personal note, 1936, File 6, Peter Olitsky Papers, American Philosophical Society.
36. A. B. Sabin, P. K. Olitsky, and H. R. Cox, "Protective Action of Certain Chemicals Against Infection of Monkeys with Nasally Instilled Poliomyelitis Virus," *Journal of Experimental Medicine*, vol. 63, 193. Also Berg, *Polio and Its Problems*, 34–40, 41–42; Paul, *A History of Poliomyelitis*, pp. 247–248; Benison, *Tom Rivers*, 191–92; Berg, *Polio*, pp. 41–42. A thorough account of the Toronto incident can be found in Christopher Rutty, "The Middle-Class Plague: Epidemic Polio and the Canadian State, 1936–37," *Canadian Bulletin of Medical History*, 1996, 277–314.
37. Albert Sabin to Dr. Steiglitz, October 14, 1936, Box 3, Albert Sabin Papers, University of Cincinnati Medical School Archives.
38. Dorothy Horstmann Interview, April 26, 1990, p. 4, in "Daniel Wilson File," Dorothy Horstmann Papers, Yale University Archives. See also Corner, *A History of the Rockefeller Institute*, 385; A. B. Sabin and R. Ward, "Natural History of Human Poliomyelitis; Distribution in Nervous and Non-Nervous Tissue," *Journal of Experimental Medicine*, vol. 73, 1941. Also Berg, *Polio and Its Problems*, 71.
39. H. A. Howe and D. Bodian, "Poliomyelitis in the Chimpanzee," *Bulletin of the Johns Hopkins Hospital*, 1941, 149–81.
40. Dorothy Horstmann Interview, 17.
41. D. M. Horstmann, "Poliomyeletic in the Blood of Orally Infected Monkeys and Chimpanzees," *Proceedings of the Society of Experimental Biological Medicine*, vol. 79, 1952; J. F. Fulton to Dorothy Horstmann, February 19, 1953, Dorothy Horstmann Papers, Yale University Archives.
42. Paul, *Poliomyelitis*, 389.

Chapter 8

1. "Summer Season Brings Epidemics of this Uncontrollable Disease," *Life*, August 15, 1949, p. 47; Steven Spencer, "Where Are We Now on Polio," *Saturday Evening Post*, September 17, 1949, 26–27, 87–93.
2. "Polio Can Be Conquered," National Foundation for Infantile Paralysis, Public Affairs Pamphlet 150, 1949, 1.
3. Albert Sabin to Basil O'Connor, December 6, 1949, copy in Folder 1665, John Enders Papers, Manuscripts Division, Sterling Library, Yale University (hereafter cited as Enders Papers).
4. "Crusader by Accident: The Biography of Basil O'Connor," unpublished copy, March of Dimes Archives, White Plains, N.Y. (hereafter cited as MDA).
5. Jonas Salk to John Enders, September 17, 1949, Box 5, Folder 1949 (D–E), Jonas Salk Papers, Mandeville Special Collections, University of California, San Diego (hereafter cited as Salk Papers).
6. John Enders to Jonas Salk, September 26, 1949, ibid.
7. Frederick C. Robbins, "Reminiscences of a Virologist," in Daniel and Robbins, eds., *Polio*, 1997, 130; John Enders to Albert Sabin, December 8, 1949, Folder 1665, Enders Papers; Williams, *Virus Hunters*, 269. By early 1951, Enders was willingly sharing his material with Salk. See Enders to Salk, March 21 and April 12, 1951, Box 176, Enders File, Salk Papers. Enders's enthusiasm for "chemotherapeutic approaches" is described in a letter from David Bodian to John Paul, who was seeking information for a book he was writing about polio. See Bodian to Paul, May 8, 1967, David Bodian Papers, Chesney Medical Archives, Johns Hopkins School of Medicine (hereafter cited as Bodian Papers).
8. Paul, *A History of Poliomyelitis*, 233–39, 382–89. The best summaries of the work of Howe and Bodian can be found in: David Bodian to Dr. A. McGehee Harvey, March 5, 1975, unprocessed Isabel Mountain Morgan Papers; David Bodian, "Howard Atkinson Howe," 1976; Thomas B. Turner, "David Bodian," 1980; "Introductory Remarks: Bodian Symposium in Neuroscience," 1975; all in unprocessed Bodian Papers.
9. Paul, *History of Poliomyelitis*, 237; Howard Howe to David Bodian, October 15, 21, 1940, Howard Howe File, Bodian Papers; Carter, *Breakthrough*, 134.
10. Bodian to Harvey, March 5, 1975, Bodian Papers; Allen, *Thomas Hunt Morgan*, 100–101; "Research Award Nomination for Dr. Isabel Morgan," 1943, Isabel Morgan File 2, Peter Olitsky Papers, American Philosophical Society (hereafter cited as Olitsky Papers).
11. See Business Manager to Peter Olitsky, April 21, 1938, Box 4, Correspondence, 1935–64, Peter Olitsky File, Archive of Rockefeller Institute, Sleepy Hollow, N.Y.; Benison, *Tom Rivers*, 409.
12. Benison, *Tom Rivers*, 457.
13. Peter Olitsky to Dr. William Thalmeier, December 12, 16, 1953, Box 2, Folder: Assorted Correspondence, 1952–54, Olitsky Papers.
14. Author's interview with Eleanor Bodian, June 6, 2003.
15. Ibid.
16. Talk delivered by Walter Schlesinger at the Isabel Morgan Mountain and David Bodian Memorial Symposium at the Marine Biological Laboratory, Woods Hole, Mass., July 25, 1997, copy in author's possession.
17. Vaughan, *Listen to the Music*, 17–40.
18. Wilson, *Margin of Safety*, 142; Hooper, *The River*, 479–81.

19. H. Koprowski, T. W. Norton, and W. McDermott, "Isolation of Poliovirus from Human Serum by Direct Inoculation into a Laboratory Mouse," *Public Health Reports*, 1947, 1467–76.

20. Altman, *Who Goes First?* 126–58; Oshinsky, *"Worse Than Slavery,"* 190–93; Elizabeth Etheridge, *The Butterfly Caste: A Social History of Pellagra*, 1972, 3–39.

21. Vaughan, *Listen to the Music*, 1–2.

22. Charles Little, "Letchworth Village: The Newest State Institution for the Feeble-Minded and Epileptic," *The Survey*, March 2, 1912; New York State, Office of Mental Retardation, "Letchworth Village," 2003.

23. Vaughan, *Listen to the Music*, 6.

24. Hilary Koprowski, "Frontiers of Virology: Development of Vaccines Against Polio Virus," in appendix to Irena Koprowski, *A Woman Wanders Through Life and Science*, 1997, 297–303.

25. "Poliomyelitis: A New Approach, *The Lancet*, March 15, 1952, 552.

26. Benison, *Tom Rivers*, 461–69.

27. Carter, *Breakthrough*, 110; Vaughan, *Listen to the Music*, 15; Koprowski, "Frontiers of Virology: Development of Vaccines Against Polio Virus," 297–303.

28. Carol Saunders, "The Vulnerable Among Us: Protection of Children in Medical Research," *Research Nurse*, March/April 1996.

29. Paul Freund, "Introduction," in *Experimentation With Human Subjects*, xii–xviii; Altman, *Who Goes First?* 1–37.

30. David Bodian statement, May 6, 1960, in David Bodian File, Thomas Rivers Papers, American Philosophical Society.

31. Vaughan, *Listen to the Music*, 16.

32. Edmund Pellegrino, quoted in J. L. Melnick and F. Horaud, "Albert Sabin," *Biologicals*, December, 1993, 302.

33. Vaughan, *Listen to the Music*, 54–55.

34. Walter Schlesinger to Peter Olitsky, April 30, 1963, Box 3, Walter Schlesinger File, Olitsky Papers.

35. Interview with Albert Sabin, conducted by Arthur Zitrin, for the documentary "Albert B. Sabin: A Life in Science," copy on file in the archives of the New York University Medical School.

36. Ibid.

37. Ibid.

38. "William Hallock Park," *Medical Violet 1939*, 43, 163; "Remarks of Albert Sabin," *NYU Medical Quarterly*, 1987, 3; Benison, *Tom Rivers*, 359–62.

39. Interview with Albert Sabin.

40. *Bellevue Violet 1931*, 139.

41. National Foundation for Infantile Paralysis, *Facts and Figures about Infantile Paralysis* (Publication No. 59), 1947, 7–9; Paul, *A History of Poliomyelitis*, 445.

42. Albert Sabin and Arthur Wright, "Acute Ascending Myelitis Following a Monkey Bite, With the Isolation of a Virus Capable of Reproducing the Disease, *Journal of Experimental Medicine*, vol. 59, 1933, 115–17.

43. Benison, *Tom Rivers*, 234–35.

44. For the anecdote about Dr. Ledingham, see Peter Olitsky to Asa Chandler, September 16, 1954, Sabin File 2, Olitsky Papers.

45. Benison, *Tom Rivers*, 235; Albert Sabin to Simon Flexner, September 10, 1934; Rufus Cole to Simon Flexner, August 9, 1934; Business Manager to Peter Olitsky, October 1, 1934; all in Box 1, Folder 1, Albert Sabin Papers, Rockefeller Archive Center (hereafter cited as Sabin Papers, RA.)

46. Thomas Rivers interview with Richard Carter, quoted in Smith, *Patenting the Sun*, 147.

47. Igor Tamm, "Sabin at the Rockefeller," 1986, Box 1, Folder 4, Sabin Papers, RA; Walter Goebel, "Peter K. Olitsky," Peter Olitsky File, American Philosophical Society; Corner, *A History of the Rockefeller Institute*, 384–390.

48. Albert Sabin telegram to Peter Olitsky, September 12, 1935, Sabin File 7, Olitsky Papers.

49. See "Peter Olitsky Oral History," 58, Archive of Rockefeller Institute; Tamm, "Sabin at the Rockefeller," 5–6. "Report of Dr. Olitsky (assisted by Drs. Cox and Sabin)," *Scientific Reports of the Rockefeller Institute*, vol. 24, p. 86.

50. On Theiler, see Benison, *Tom Rivers*, 413–16, 464; Paul, *History of Poliomyelitis*, 263–69; Tamm, "Sabin at the Rockefeller," 6–7.

51. Following a modest pay raise, for example, he wrote the director this self-effacing note: "To be sure, when I look back at the things I have done, they seem so small and petty, so short of the mark envisaged that it becomes easy to lose heart." Sabin then promised to work even harder to realize "the ultimate purpose of it all"— the conquest of polio. Over time, however, Sabin came to question, and abandon, all of Flexner's main theories about the disease: that there was but one type of poliovirus, that it entered the body through the nose, and that it multiplied only in nervous tissue. See Albert Sabin to Simon Flexner, June 22, 1935, Box 1, Folder 1, Sabin Papers, RA.

52. Albert Sabin to Herbert Gasser, April 20, 1939, Box 1, Folder 1, Sabin Papers, RA.

53. A Graeme Mitchell to Peter Olitsky, January 23, 1940, Sabin File 8, Olitsky Papers.

54. *New York Herald-Tribune*, June 23, 1939; *New York Times*, March 10, 17, 1940.

55. Albert Sabin to Peter Olitsky, June 27, 1939, File 8, Olitsky Papers.

56. Albert Sabin to Peter Olitsky, June 6, 1939, Sabin File 7, Olitsky Papers; Albert Sabin to John Paul, May 14, 1941, Box 8 (1940–41), John Paul Papers, Yale University Archives.

57. Albert Sabin to Peter Olitsky, June 17, 1941, Sabin File 7, Olitsky Papers.

58. Peter Olitsky to Albert Sabin (no date), Sabin File 1, Olitsky Papers.

59. Sabin aimed to produce a vaccine for both diseases. He even brought back virus samples to the United States, hoping, he said, to run controlled experiments with "volunteers in some mental institution." As it turned out he used prisoners instead. Amidst great fanfare—"200 Convicts Risk Death in Fight on War Diseases" read one headline—Sabin "infected" his "volunteers." All survived, though some endured "considerable suffering." What the prisoners were promised in return—reduced sentences, additional privileges—was not mentioned. See *New York Daily News*, August 27, 1944; *Trenton Times*, August 28, 1944; Albert Sabin to Peter Olitsky, August 22, 1943, File 12, Olitsky Papers.

60. Sabin to Olitsky, August 22, 1943, Olitsky Papers; Albert Sabin, "Problems in the Epidemiology of Poliomyelitis At Home and Among Our Armed Forces," paper presented at the Rocky Mountain Conference on Infantile Paralysis, December 1946.

Chapter 9

1. Oshinsky, *A Conspiracy So Immense*, 95–96.

2. Alonso Hamby, *Man of the People*, 1995, 428–29; Eleanor Bontecou, *The Federal Loyalty-Security Program*, 1953, 35–72.

3. Jonas Salk's FBI Headquarters File Number is 121–22866. In 1942 an article in *Social Work Today* lauded Salk and others, claiming: "These men and women have made it possible for *Social Work Today* to strengthen and prepare itself for the supreme test of today." It called Salk a "leading cooperator."

4. Bontecou, *Federal Loyalty-Security Program*, 74–75.

5. See especially, Memo, August 8, 1950, Detroit FBI Office; Memo, August 16, 1950, New York City FBI Office; Memo, August 29, 1950, Los Angeles FBI Office, all in Salk FBI File.

6. Report of Special Agent, August 8, 10, 1950, Detroit; August 29, 1950, Washington; both in Salk FBI File.

7. "Jonas Edward Salk, Synopsis of Facts," August 30, 1951, Salk FBI File.

8. Report of Special Agent, September 8, 1951, San Francisco; September 17, 1951, Dallas; both in Salk FBI File.

9. Hiram Bingham, Chairman, Loyalty Review Board, U.S. Civil Service Commission, to J. Edgar Hoover, FBI Director, November 7, 1952, Salk FBI File.

10. Author's interview with Darrell Salk, February 18, 2003.

11. Memo, August 10, 1950, Pittsburgh FBI Office, in Salk FBI File.

12. Julius Youngner, Unpublished Memoir, 12; copy in author's possession.

13. On Donna Salk, see *Pittsburgh Sun-Telegram*, April 12, 1955, July 3, 1960; *Pittsburgh Post-Gazette*, July 24, 1959, December 30, 1960.

14. Jonas Salk to Harry Weaver, April 10, 1949, Box 5, Folder 5, Jonas Salk Papers, Mandeville Special Collections, University of California, San Diego (hereafter cited as Salk Papers).

15. Salk to Weaver, June 16, 1950, Box 91, Folder 8, Salk Papers.

16. Ibid.

17. Weaver to Salk, June 22, 1950, Salk papers.

18. See Jonas Salk for the Standards Committee, NFIP, "Immunologic Classification of Poliomyelitis Viruses," for Presentation at Second International Poliomyelitis Congress, September, 1951, Copenhagen, Denmark, copy in Polio Correspondence, 1952, General, Box 4, Albert Sabin Papers, University of Cincinnati.

19. Carter, *Breakthrough*, 114.

20. See "Polio Hits Basil O'Connor's Daughter," 87–93, in Cohn, *Four Billion Dimes*.

21. Carter, *Breakthrough*, 121.

22. Ibid., 141; Vivien Encel, *Australian Genius: 50 Great Ideas*, 1988, 55–57.

23. Youngner, Unpublished Memoir, 1–7; Neil Seidenberg, "Men and Scenes Behind Salk Vaccine," *Pittsburgh Post-Gazette*, April 12, 1955; "Age of Salk's Aides Averages Under 40," *New York Times*, April 12, 1945; author's interview with Julius Youngner, March 17, 2004.

24. Younger, Unpublished Memoir, 5–7.

25. Ibid. Also Troan, *Passport to Adventure*, 185–89.

26. Younger, Unpublished Memoir, 5–7. Also Benison, *Tom Rivers*, 542–43.

27. For an excellent description of Medium 199 and Connaught Laboratories' larger role in the polio story, see ch. 7 in Christopher Rutty, "Do Something! . . . Do Anything! Poliomyelitis in Canada, 1927–1962," Ph.D. dissertation, University of Toronto, 1995.

28. Wilson, *Margin of Safety*, 77.

29. Carter, *Breakthrough*, 106.

30. See Jonas Salk, "Studies in Human Subjects on Active Immunization Against Poliomyelitis," *Journal of the American Medical Association*, vol. 151, no. 13, 1088–93.

The Type III strain had come from Jimmy Sarkett, age thirteen. A clerk at the hospital had misspelled his name on the vial containing his sample—thus "Saukett."

31. Youngner, "Unpublished Memoir," 7–10; author's interview with Youngner; Carter, *Breakthrough*, 185, Troan, *Passport to Adventure*, 189.

32. Benison, *Tom Rivers*, 490–99; William McD. Hammon, "Standardization Problems Encountered in the Large Scale Manufacture of Poliomyelitis Vaccine in the United States," 1954, unpublished paper in author's possession.

33. Carter, *Breakthrough*, 131–36.
    Salk's technical presentation, at least, appeared to impress Sabin more than he let on. A few months later, Sabin wrote Salk to ask "whether or not you would be willing to have my associate, Dr. J. Wissner, come to your laboratory for a few days or longer, if necessary, to familiarize himself with the details of the tissue culture work as it being done by your group." Salk agreed. See Albert Sabin to Jonas Salk, March 18, 1952, Box 2, Albert Sabin Papers, University of Cincinnati.

34. There are conflicting accounts as to when Salk gave his vaccine to his own children—and to himself. Pittsburgh reporter John Troan, who knew Salk well, wrote: ". . . before heading off to Polk, the doctor administered the vaccine to himself, his wife, and their three sons." This would have been 1952. Salk biographer Richard Carter, who interviewed Salk at length in the 1960s, puts the date of the family inoculations in 1953, following the initial experiments at the Watson and Polk facilities. Donna Salk, while not recalling the exact date, claimed that her husband inoculated the whole family, including himself, in the family kitchen. Darrell Salk confirms this version. "I remember it well," he said. "Jonas came home one night, lined us up, and boom . . . that was it."
    Lawrence Altman, a correspondent for the *New York Times*, had trouble pinning down Salk about Salk's own vaccination. In 1970 one of Salk's aides told Altman that Salk had *not* taken his vaccine because he knew he had antibodies to polio. Several years later, at a scientific conference, Altman ran into Salk and posed the question directly. "I asked Salk why he hadn't taken his own vaccine when he had given it to his children. Even though he had antibodies, I said, he could have tested the safety of the polio vaccine by taking it himself. Salk then insisted that he had actually taken it. When I asked why he had told . . . a different version [earlier], Salk said it was because he didn't know why the question was being asked."
    To add to the confusion, members of Salk's laboratory claimed to have received the polio vaccine first, before any outside testing was done. Indeed, there is an undated photo in the March of Dimes Archives of Salk, right sleeve rolled up, getting a polio shot from a colleague. See Troan, *Passport to Adventure*, 196; Carter, *Breakthrough*, 170. For Donna Salk, see Seavey, Smith, and Wagner, *A Paralyzing Fear*, 202; author's interview with Darrell Salk, February 18, 2003; Altman, *Who Goes First?* 358–59.

35. See Commonwealth of Pennsylvania, "Mental Patients . . . Vaccine Research," August 10, 1944, Box 92, Folder 4, Salk Papers.

36. See Gale H. Walker to William C. Brown (Pennsylvania Secretary of Welfare), February 4, 1952, Box 92, Folder 4, Salk Papers.

37. Benison, *Tom Rivers*, 467.

38. Christine Kindl, "The Creation of a Cure: D. T. Watson Rehabilitation Hospital," *Pittsburgh Post-Gazette*, September 9, 1990; Smith, *Patenting the Sun*, 140–42.

39. "Volunteers Recount Their Participation in Historic Trials," June 24, 1995; "Polio Pioneers," July 2, 2002; both in *Pittsburgh Post-Gazette*.
40. Troan, *Passport to Adventure*, 193–95.
41. "Volunteers Recount Their Participation . . ." Using crutches to help him walk, he graduated from Franklin and Marshall College. "I could see that I just wasn't cut out for medicine," said Kirkpatrick, who went on to become an Episcopal priest.
42. Carter, *Breakthrough*, 139.
43. Salk, "Studies in Human Subjects," 1098; Carter, *Breakthrough*, 140.

Chapter 10

1. Cohen, *Shots in the Dark*, 31.
2. *Washington Post*, July 4, 1952; Memo from Roland Berg to Marguerite Clark, July 16, 1952, copy in Polio Epidemic File, *Newsweek* Morgue, Center for American History, University of Texas, Austin.
3. See Neal Nathanson and John Martin, "The Epidemiology of Poliomyelitis: Enigmas Surrounding the Appearance, Epidemicity, and Disappearance," *American Journal of Epidemiology*, vol. 110, 1979, 672–90.
4. Ibid., 675; Albert Sabin, "The Epidemiology of Poliomyelitis," *JAMA*, vol. 134, 1947, 750.
5. Sabin, "Epidemiology of Poliomyelitis, 755–756; also Monroe Lerner and Odin Anderson, *Health Progress in the United States*, 1963, 152–56.
6. Karl Schriftgiesser, "When 11 of 14 Children Were Hit with Polio," *Collier's*, November 29, 1952, 17–20.
7. Max J. Fox and John Chamberlain, "Four Fatal Cases of Bulbar Poliomyelitis in One Family," *JAMA*, March 28, 1953, 1099–1101.
8. T. Francis Jr. et al., "Poliomyelitis Following Tonsillectomy in 5 Members of a Family," *Epidemiologic Study*, August 22, 1942, 1392.
9. Alice Heaton, "A Friend—and Partner," *Good Housekeeping*, July 1953, 17, 209–10; "Basil O'Connor: One Man's War Against Disease," *Medical World News*, January 31, 1964; Dorothy Horstmann interview, 27, in Daniel Wilson File, Dorothy Horstmann Papers, Yale University Archives.
10. "Crusader By Accident: The Biography of Basil O'Connor," unpublished, copy, March of Dimes Archives; for various memoranda, see "Presidential Directives to Staff, 1942–1947," Box 3, Basil O'Connor Papers, MDA.
11. Beaton, "Friend—and Partner," 210; Troan, *Passport to Adventure*, 210.
12. Carter, *Breakthrough*, 144.
13. Benison, *Tom Rivers*, 499. Also "Joseph M. Smadel, M.D.," Lasker Foundation Award Winners, www.laskerfoundation.org/awards/library; Thomas Woodward, "History of the Commissions on Immunization and Rickettsial Diseases," http://history.amedd.army.mil/booksdocs/historiesofcomsn/section7.htm.
14. Benison, *Tom Rivers*, 496–98.
15. Troan, *Passport to Adventure*, 198.
16. Ibid.; *Pittsburgh Press*, January 27, 28, 1953.
17. "Vaccine for Polio," *Time*, February 9, 1953, 43.
18. Albert Sabin to Jonas Salk, February 9, 1953, Box 93, Folder 5, Jonas Salk Papers, Mandeville Special Collections, University of California, San Diego.
19. John Paul to Jonas Salk, January 28, 1953, quoted in Paul, *A History of Poliomyelitis*, 419.
20. Jonas Salk to John Paul, February 2, 1953, ibid.

21. Wilson, *Margin of Safety*, 85.
22. Benison, *Tom Rivers*, vii–xiii, 499.
23. Ibid., 499–501; Carter, *Breakthrough*, 150–51.
24. Carter, *Breakthrough*, 152.
25. Ibid., 156.
26. Ibid., 158.
27. A full copy of Salk's text can be found in the *Pittsburgh Sun-Telegraph*, March 27, 1953.
28. Ibid., *Pittsburgh Sun-Telegraph*, March 27, April 2, 1953.
29. Carter, *Breakthrough*, 176.
30. Benison, *Tom Rivers*, 502–3; "Basil O'Connor: One Man's War Against Disease," 12.

Chapter 11

1. Author's interview with Darrell Salk, February 19, 2003; author's interview with Peter Salk, November 22, 2002; Shirley Levine, "Dr. Jonas E. Salk—Scientist with a Mission," *Pittsburgh Jewish Outlook*, April 10, 1953.
2. Financial statement and employment list in, Jonas Salk to Dean W. S. McEllroy, January 10, 1953, June 10, 1953, Box 298, Folder 8, Jonas Salk Papers, Mandeville Special Collections, University of California, San Diego (hereafter cited as Salk Papers); Carter, *Breakthrough*, 212; interview with Don Wegemer, in Seavey, Smith, and Wagner, *A Paralyzing Fear*, 191–98.
3. Author's interview with Julius Youngner, March 19, 2004.
4. Younger, "Unpublished Memoir," 6–20.
5. "Joseph A. Bell: A Biographical Appreciation," *American Journal of Epidemiology*, vol. 90, 1969, 464–67; Paul, *A History of Poliomyelitis*, 422–23; Benison, *Tom Rivers*, 506–11.
6. Carter, *Breakthrough*, 177.
7. Joseph A. Bell, "Outline of Considerations and Tentative General Plans for an Epidemiologic Field Trial of a Poliomyelitis Vaccine," September 8, 1953, Folder 4, Box 123, Salk Papers.
8. Albert Sabin, "Present Status and Future Possibilities of a Vaccine for the Control of Poliomyelitis," unpublished, copy in author's possession.
9. Carter, *Breakthrough*, 179.
10. Benison, *Tom Rivers*, 509. Though Rivers admitted that the committee's excessive caution had made Salk's task much more difficult, he didn't mention that the committee had solicited—and then rejected—the "confidential" advice of Francis, the acknowledged expert in this field, who assured the members that the adjuvant in the polio vaccine was both safe and effective, with "none of the characteristics known to be associated with carcinogens." Francis went on to endorse the "human testing" of Salk's vaccine, saying that "the basis for my conclusions is related to the fact that I have had relatively close association with the work of Doctor Salk." See Thomas Francis to Harry Weaver, February 19, 1953, National Foundation File, Box 51, Thomas Francis Papers.
11. Carter, *Breakthrough*, 191–93.
12. Ibid., 177–78.
13. Harry Weaver to Basil O'Connor, August 29, September 1, 1953, Basil O'Connor Papers, March of Dimes Archive, White Plains, N.Y.

Some viewed Weaver's resignation as the result of a losing struggle with his direct superior, Hart Van Riper, the foundation's medical director, over the course of the coming trials. Weaver clearly expected to make the major decisions himself, after consulting with Bell and the Vaccine Advisory Committee. He saw no reason to confide in Van Riper, a pediatrician, whom he dismissed as a lightweight.

Van Riper was a power in his own right, however, close to Basil O'Connor and well connected in the medical community. His contacts with doctors, nurses, and public health officials were essential to the success of a national vaccine trial. On balance, O'Connor was relieved to see Weaver go. "He had piloted the ship, and brilliantly," O'Connor recalled. "Now that we were entering the port he gave the impression that he was the only person who belonged on the bridge." See Carter, *Breakthrough*, 181–85.

14. Benison, *Tom Rivers*, 511; Joseph A. Bell, "Outline of Considerations and Tentative General Plans," Salk Papers.
15. Carter, *Breakthrough*, 187; "Joseph A. Bell: A Biographical Appreciation," 466.
16. Thomas Rivers to Basil O'Connor, December 3, 1953, Basil O'Connor File 5, Thomas Rivers Papers, American Philosophical Society, Philadelphia.
17. Albert Sabin to Aims McGuiness, December 15, 22, 1953, Box 5, Albert Sabin Papers, University of Cincinnati (hereafter cited as Sabin Papers, UC).
18. Howard Howe to Albert Sabin, December 29, 1953, Sabin Papers, UC.
19. David Bodian to Albert Sabin, December 9, 1953, Sabin File, David Bodian Papers, Chesney Library, Johns Hopkins Medical School.
20. Thomas Francis to Albert Sabin, December 22, 1953, Box 5, Sabin Papers UC.
21. Carter, *Breakthrough*, 202–6.
22. Thomas Francis to Harry Weaver, December 29, 1953, Folder: NFIP, Box 51, Thomas Francis Papers, Bentley Library, University of Michigan (hereafter cited as Francis Papers).
23. Carter, *Breakthrough*, 205–6.
24. "Meeting of Advisory Group on Evaluation of Vaccine Field Trials—Hotel Commodore, New York," January 11, 1954, in Francis Papers.
25. Carter, *Breakthrough*, 203.
26. Ibid., 204.
27. Paul Meier, "Polio Trial: An Early Efficient Clinical Trial," *Statistics in Medicine*, vol. 9, 13–16.
28. Hart Van Riper to Carl Neupert, State Health Officer, Wisconsin, November 19, 1953, in File NFIP/Van Riper, Box 16, Francis Papers.
29. Hart Van Riper, "Brief Background Statement for the Polio Vaccine Trial," Francis Papers.
30. Thomas Francis Jr., "Evaluation of the 1954 Poliomyelitis Vaccine Field Trial," *JAMA*, August 6, 1955, 1266–70; Liza Dawson, "The Salk Polio Vaccine Trial of 1954: Risks, Randomization and Public Involvement in Research," *Clinical Trials*, 2004, 122–30.
31. Thomas Dublin to Hart Van Riper, "Preliminary Proposals for Enlisting State and Local Cooperation in the Field Trial," File: Dublin, Box 16, Francis Papers.
32. Ibid.

Chapter 12

1. Sarah M. Lambert and Howard Markel, "Making History: Thomas Francis, Jr., MD, and the Salk Poliomyelitis Vaccine Field Trial, *Archives of Pediatric and*

Adolescent Medicine, May 2000, 512–517; March of Dimes, "The Shot Heard Around the World: A Tribute to Jonas Salk Thirty Years Later"; Paul Meier, "The Biggest Public Health Experiment Ever: The 1954 Field Trial of the Salk Poliomyelitis Vaccine," in *Statistics: A Guide to the Unknown*, ed. Judith Tanner, 1989, 3–15; The quotes are from Arnold Monto, "Francis Field Trial of Inactivated Poliomyelitis Vaccine: Background and Lessons for Today," *Epidemiological Reviews*, 1999, 7–23; Marcia Meldrim, "'A Calculated Risk': The Salk Polio Vaccine Trials of 1954," *British Medical Journal*, 1998, 1233.

2. "Closing in on Polio, *Time*, March 29, 1954; Robert Coughlin, "Tracking the Killer," *Life*, February 22, 1954, Leonard Engel, *New York Times Sunday Magazine*, January 10, 1954; Carter, *Breakthrough*, 268–69.

3. Melvin Glasser, "M–Day for Polio," *Adult Leadership*, September 1954, 5.

4. Naomi Rogers, "Sister Kenny Goes to Washington: Polio, Populism, and Medical Politics in Postwar America," in Johnston, *The Politics of Healing*, 102, 335; Smith, *Patenting the Sun*, 249; Brandt and Gardner, "The Golden Age of Medicine?" in Cooter and Pickstone, eds., *Medicine in the Twentieth Century*, 21–37.

5. "Crisis and Cost," *Newsweek*, August 30, 1954; "Halts March of Dimes," *Business Week*, September 11, 1954, 56–57; Smith, *Patenting the Sun*, 300–301.

6. Glasser, "M–Day for Polio," 6.

7. "Discussion Guide for Manual of Suggested Procedures for the Conduct of Poliomyelitis Field Trials," in Dr. Dublin File, Box 16, Thomas Francis Papers, Bentley Library, University of Michigan (hereafter cited as Francis Papers).

8. Basil O'Connor, "A Message to Parents"; "Parental Request for Participation in Poliomyelitis Vaccination Field Trial," both in Francis Papers; Lambert and Markel, "Making History," 515; Smith, *Patenting the Sun*, 237.

9. "What You Should Know About the Polio Vaccine Tests of the National Foundation for Infantile Paralysis," Dr. Dublin File, Box 16, Francis Papers.

10. Parke-Davis & Company, "Parke-Davis at 100: 1866 to 1966," 1966; George Hook, "An Historical Evaluation of the American Drug Market Since 1900," unpublished Ph.D. dissertation, University of Pittsburgh, School of Pharmacy, 1955, 25–49.

11. Christopher Rutty, "Herculean Efforts: Connaught and the Canadian Polio Vaccine Story," http://www.healthheritaggeresearch.com/polio; Carter, *Breakthrough*, 184.

12. The problems with Parke-Davis came early. In September 1953, within days of Weaver's departure, Hart van Riper advised foundation officials to stop further shipments of live poliovirus from Connaught Laboratories to Parke-Davis until "this whole complicated problem can be discussed with Mr. O'Connor himself."

    The initial problems with Parke-Davis did mean, however, that the start of the polio vaccine field trials would have to be pushed back several months, to early spring of 1954. Salk, under intense pressure himself, was not averse to the delay. An interoffice memo from Parke-Davis, reports a phone conversation with Dr. Salk: "It was pointed out that we are running behind schedule now and that if we had to start testing all over again it will be impossible to have any vaccine ready before the first of next year. Dr. Salk said not to worry. It is much more important to find out how to handle this material in bulk and if they can't have the vaccine in time they will just have to postpone the study." The note from Hart Van Riper (September 17, 1953) and the interoffice memo (October 7, 1953) can both be found in Folder 1, Box 123, Jonas Salk Papers, Mandeville

Special Collections, University of California, San Diego (hereafter cited as Salk Papers).

13. Saul Benison, *Tom Rivers*, 514–15.

14. Ibid., also Carter, *Breakthrough*, 208.

15. Basil O'Connor to Jonas Salk, October 28, 1953, Folder 16, Box 251, Salk Papers.

16. Thomas Francis to Hart Van Riper, March 10, 1954, NFIP/Van Riper File, Box 16, and Francis Diary, April 1, 1954, both in Francis Papers.

17. Richard Nelson, MD, to Albert Sabin, April 16, 1954; Nelson to John Enders, April 16, 1954; Alfred Golden to John Enders, March 8, 1954, copies in Polio Vaccine File, Misc. Correspondence, 1953–1955, John Enders Papers, Yale University (hereafter cited as Enders Papers).

18. Sabin to Nelson, April 19, 1954, Sabin Papers, UC; Enders to Nelson, April 21, 1954; Mary Bradford to Enders, April 5, 1954; Enders to Bradford, May 22, 1954, Enders Papers.

19. Neil Gabler, *Winchell: Gossip, Power, and the Culture of Celebrity*, 1994, 470–72; Smith, *Patenting the Sun*, 256–58.

20. Carter, *Breakthrough*, 221; Public Health Service, "Technical Report on the Salk Poliomyelitis Vaccine," June 1955, 9.

21. Carter, *Breakthrough*, 221.

22. Ibid., 223–24; Benison, *Tom Rivers*, 533–34.

23. Michigan State Medical Society, "Statement for Immediate Release," April 5, 1954, copy in Box 15; Francis Diary, April 7, 1954; both in Francis Papers.

24. Troan, *Passport to Adventure*, 216–18.

25. Francis Memo, Meeting with Health Authorities, June 18, 1954, Box 21, Francis Papers.

26. "269,000 Needles," *Time*, May 10, 1954, 68.

27. Margaret Hickey, "Have We Won the Fight Against Polio?" *Ladies Home Journal*, December 1954, 25–26; "O Pioneers!" *The New Yorker*, May 8, 1954, 00; Smith, *Patenting the Sun*, 273.

28. Francis Diary, May 12, 17; June 2, 1954; Dr. Korns to Francis, May 26, 1954; R. B. Voight to Francis, June 3, 1954; Field Trial Irregularities Folder, Box 14, Francis Papers.

29. Francis to Van Riper, May 31, 1954, NFIP/Van Riper Folder, Box 16; Francis Diary, May 31; June 1, 1954, both in Francis Papers.

30. Francis Diary, May 31; June 1, 1954, ibid.

31. Francis Diary, June 1, 3, 14; July 1, 1954, ibid.

32. See Foundation Grants, CRBS, University of Michigan, 1954, March of Dimes Archives, White Plains, N.Y. (hereafter cited as MDA).

33. To complicate matters, Francis's wife, Dorothy, was involved in a serious car accident in July 1954. As polio writer Jane Smith described it, Francis arranged to send his son to Scotland and to have a friend drive his daughter to Wellesley College that fall, while thereafter interrupting "his work three times a day to visit Dorothy in the hospital." See Smith, *Patenting the Sun*, 287.

34. Carter, *Breakthrough*, 242–43.

35. Jonas Salk to Thomas Rivers, May 27, 1954, Box 1, Correspondence: Vaccines, MAD; Benison, *Tom Rivers*, 546–47.

36. Carter, *Breakthrough*, 210–11.

37. Ibid, 258.

38. Ibid.; author's interview with Julius Youngner, March 19, 2004.

39. Seavy, Smith, and Wagner, *A Paralyzing Fear*, 207.

40. *New York World Telegram*, March 30, 1955; *Pittsburgh Press*, April 3, 1955.

41. Williams, *Virus Hunters*, 1959, 314–15; Troan, *Passport to Adventure*, 222–23; Cathy Covert, "Reporters Sizzling Over Polio Chaos, *Editor and Publisher*, April 16, 1955; *New York Times*, April 13, 1955.

42. "A Quiet Young Man's Magnificent Victory," *Newsweek*, April 25, 1955, 64, 66–67; Frank Deford, *An American Summer*, 2003.

43. Basil O'Connor to Thomas Francis, April 12, 1955, Francis Papers.

44. Poliomyelitis Vaccine Evaluation Center, University of Michigan, "An Evaluation of the 1954 Poliomyelitis Vaccine Trials: Summary Report," *American Journal of Public Health*, Appendix, May 1955, 13, 49–50.

45. Williams, *Virus Hunters*, 314.

46. Introductory Remarks by Jonas E. Salk, April 12, 1955, in Folder 2, Box 123, Salk Papers.

47. Ibid.

48. Author's interview with Julius Youngner, March 19, 2004.

49. See "Salk's Regrets Are Few," *Pittsburgh Post-Gazette*, November 27, 1994; Richard Carter, *Breakthrough*, 279–80.

50. Carter, *Breakthrough*, 281.

51. Benison, *Tom Rivers*, 550; Carter, *Breakthrough*, 281.

52. Carter, *Breakthrough*, 281–82.

53. Paul, *A History of Poliomyelitis*, 433; Carter, *Breakthrough*, 273.

54. John Paul to John Enders, April 15, 1955, John Paul Correspondence File, Box 68, Enders Papers.

55. Paul Clark to Thomas Francis, April 28, 1955, Vaccination Examination File, Box 8, Francis Papers.

56. Carter, *Breakthrough*, 188.

57. Harry Weaver to Jonas Salk, May 1, 2, 1950; Salk to Weaver, June 27, 1950, Folder 1, Box 7, Salk Papers.

58. Author's interview with John Troan, March 18, 2004; author's interview with Julius Youngner, March 19, 2004.

59. Erik Barnouw, *Tube of Plenty: The Evolution of American Television*, 1975, 171–84; "See It Now: U.S. Documentary Series," and "Murrow, Edward R," in http://www.museum.tv/archives/etv.

60. See Alexander Kendrick: *Prime Time: The Life of Edward R. Murrow*, 1969, 35–36, 64, 344, 395; Smith, *Patenting the Sun*, 304–5; Joseph Persico, *Edward R. Murrow: An American Original*, 1997, 402.

61. Smith, *Patenting the Sun*, 304–5.

62. A transcript of this program can be found in Edward R. Murrow and Fred Friendly, eds., *See It Now*, 1955, 00.

63. Stephen Ryan to Marvel Whittemore, April 2, 1953; M. M. Sandoe to Ryan, August 5, 1953; Ryan telegram to Jonas Salk, September 17, 1953; Sandoe to Ryan, March 9, 1954; Sandoe to Ryan, September 18, 1956; in Patents, Salk Vaccine Folder, Box 4, Government Relations, Federal, MDA.

64. John Paul to Basil O'Connor, April 15, 1955, O'Connor Correspondence: Congratulatory Letters, 1955, Basil O'Connor Papers, MDA.
    O'Connor's younger daughter, Sheelagh, worked at a New Haven hospital where Dr. Paul had an office. Following the Ann Arbor announcement, she wrote her father: "Much chatter about whether or not Salk will get the Nobel Prize and much difference of opinion on this.... Saw John R. Paul at a distance

today and thought he was looking rather more pale than usual." See Sheelagh O'Connor to father, April 18, 1955, O'Connor Congratulatory Letters File, 1955, Basil O'Connor Papers, MDA.

65. Jonas Salk interview, in Academy of Achievement: A Museum of Living History, http://www.achievement.org.

66. Donna Salk interview, in Seavey, Smith, and Wagner, *A Paralyzing Fear*, 208.

67. Thomas Francis to Edward R. Murrow, April 22, 1955; Francis to Basil O' Connor, April 18, 1955; Francis to Thomas Dublin, April 22, 1955; all in Box 25, Francis Papers.

68. Thomas Francis to Paul Clark, May 11, 1955, Box 8; Francis to Dublin, April 22, 1955, both in Francis Papers.

69. Black, *In the Shadow of Polio*, 224.

Chapter 13

1. "A Hero's Great Discovery is Out to Work," *Life*, May 2, 1955, 27; "An International Hero Returns Home to Pittsburgh," *Greater Pittsburgh*, May 1955, 25–26; "A Quiet Young Man's Magnificent Victory," *Newsweek*, April 25, 1955, 64–65.

2. Marc Selvaggio, "The Making of Jonas Salk," *Pittsburgh Magazine*, June 1984, 43–51.

3. Office of the Clerk, U.S. House of Representatives, "Congressional Gold Medal Recipients"; *Pittsburgh Post-Gazette*, May 11, 1955.

4. Deborah Kurland to President Eisenhower, April 17, 1955; Harry Bellow to President Eisenhower, April 23, 1955; Frank Hodson to President Eisenhower, April 21, 1955; Mrs. Manuel Suarez to President Eisenhower; April 20, 1955; all in Central Files, General File, Box 1026, File GF 131-D-2, Jonas Salk Polio Vaccine, Dwight D. Eisenhower Presidential Papers, Eisenhower Library (hereafter cited as DDEPP).

5. Smith, *Patenting the Sun*, 356.

6. J. Edgar Hoover to Dillon Anderson, special assistant to the president ("personal and confidential by special messenger"), May 10, 1955, in Jonas Salk FBI File, 161-22356; S. H. Alex, Public Relations Counsel, National Foundation for Infantile Paralysis, to Office of Press Secretary James Hagerty, April 12, 1955, Official File 117-G, Box 601, DDEPP.

7. Carter, *Breakthrough*, 295. The reporter was Andrew Tully of the Scripps-Howard chain.

8. Supplements to the Citations Presented by the President to Dr. Jonas E. Salk, April 22, 1955, Official File, 117-G, Box 601, DDEPP; Wilson, *Margin of Safety*, 102.

9. Carter, *Breakthrough*, 294–296.

10. *Pittsburgh Press*, April 12, 1955.

11. Hobby, Oveta Culp, "The Handbook of Texas Online," http://www.lib .texas.edu.; Cary Reich, *The Life of Nelson Rockefeller: Worlds to Conquer, 1908–1958*, 1996, 513.

12. Dwight D. Eisenhower, *The White House Years: Mandate for Change, 1953–1956*, 1963, 92; Stephen Ambrose, *Eisenhower: The President*, 1984, 24. "Lady in Command," *Time*, May 4, 1953, 24–27; Reich, *Nelson Rockefeller*, 518.

13. Reich, *Nelson Rockefeller*, 517.

14. "The Problem Now Is Production," *Business Week*, April 16, 1955, 137.
15. Mayor Robert F. Wagner to President Eisenhower, April 13, 1955, Official File, Box 601, File 117-I-1, Salk Polio Vaccine, DDEPP; Robert Branyan and Lawrence Larsen, *The Eisenhower Administration, 1953–1961: A Documentary History*, vol. 1, 1971, 576.
16. John Rothenberg to President Eisenhower, May 24, 1955; Joseph Gould to President Eisenhower, May 19, 1955; Mrs. Thomas J. Flynn to President Eisenhower, May 18, 1955; Mr. and Mrs. Allan Miller to President Eisenhower, May 16, 1955; Elspeth Lee to President Eisenhower, May 13, 1955; all in Central Files, General File, Box 1026, File GF 131-D-2 (3), DDEPP.

    The gender issue cut both ways. A number of women wrote the president to complain that Mrs. Hobby was being victimized *because* of her sex. "I hope she won't resign and give those good for nothing men who are jealous of her any satisfaction," said one. "The women of this country do not want her to be replaced and we are very proud of her," said another. Mrs. Hobby also had the strong support of women's clubs throughout the country. See letters and telegrams in GF 131-D-2, Box 1026, DDEPP.

17. Percy Priest to Secretary Hobby, (n.d.), Official File, Box 601, File 117-I-1, DDEPP.
18. Karl Bambach (executive vice-president, American Drug Manufacturers Association) to Congressman John Bennett, May 27, 1955, DDEPP
19. See especially Robert Crichton, "How Canada Handled the Salk Vaccine," *The Reporter*, July 14, 1955, 28–32.
20. Spencer Klaw, "Salk Vaccine—The Business Gamble," *Fortune*, September 1955, 172.
21. Minutes of Cabinet Meeting, April 29, 1955, Cabinet Series, Box 5, DDEEP.
22. Homer Fritsch to President Eisenhower, May 9, 12, 1955, Official File 117-G, Box 601, File 117-1-1, DDEPP. On vaccine projections by the drug companies, see Report to the President by the Secretary of Health, Education and Welfare on Distribution of the Salk Vaccine, May 16, 1955, DDEPP.
23. *New York Herald Tribune*, May 2, 1955.
24. See handwritten notes to cabinet meeting of May 13, 1955, Office of the Staff Secretary, Records, 1952–61, Cabinet Series, Box 3, File C-23, DDEPP.
25. Douw Fonda to President Eisenhower, August 8, 1955, President's Personal File, 699, Box 27-B-3, Infantile Paralysis, DDEPP.
26. "Supplementary Notes," Legislative Leadership Meeting, May 4, 1955, Legislative Meeting Series, Box 2, File: Legislative Meetings, 1955, DDEPP.
27. Steven Spencer, "Where Are We Now on Polio?" *Saturday Evening Post*, September 10, 1955, 19–21.
28. Dr. Haas's comment is in Telephone Conference, National Institutes of Health, April 27, 1955, 3, copy in author's possession. The participants included Dr. Thomas Francis, University of Michigan; Dr. Joseph Smadel, Army Medical Center; Dr. William McD. Hammond, University of Pittsburgh; Dr. Howard Shaughnessy, Illinois Department of Health; Dr. David Price, Assistant Surgeon General, Public Health Service; Dr. Victor Haas, Director, National Microbiological Laboratory; and Dr. William Workman, Chief, Laboratory of Biological Control.
29. Ibid., 8–9.
30. Ibid.
31. Ibid., 11–12.

32. On Leonard Scheele, Office of the Surgeon General, "Leonard Andrew Scheele," http://www.surgeongeneral.gov/library/history/bioscheele.htm; David S. Atcher, "The History of the Public Health Service and the Surgeon General's Priorities," unpublished lecture in author's possession.

33. Frederick Goehringer, "The Effects of Government Control on the Manufacturers of Poliomyelitis Vaccine," Master's thesis, Wharton School of Business, University of Pennsylvania, 1957, 29–46.

34. University of California, Regional Oral History Office, Bancroft Library, "Cutter Laboratories, 1897–1972: A Dual Trust," 1975; author's interview with Dr. Paul Offit, Chief, Infectious Diseases, Children's Hospital of Philadelphia, October 3, 2003.

35. Klaw, "Salk Vaccine," 174; Carter, *Breakthrough*, 216–217.

36. *New York Times*, April 27, 28, 1955.

37. Neil Nathanson and Alexander Langmuir, "The Cutter Incident," *American Journal of Hygiene*, 1963, 39–44; "Epidemic Intelligence Service Claims Credit for Addressing Polio Vaccine Scare in the 1950s," http://www.whale.to/a/eis/html; Leonard Engel, "The Salk Vaccine: What Caused the Mess?" *Harper's*, August 4, 1955, 1–32.

38. U.S. Department of Health, Education, and Welfare, Public Health Service, "Technical Report on Salk Poliomyelitis Vaccine," June, 1955, 25.

39. Carter, *Breakthrough*, 326; Edward Shorter, *The Health Century*, 69.

40. *New York Times*, May 9, 1955.

41. Ibid.; Wilson, *Margin of Safety*, 109–10.

42. "Remarks by Senator Wayne Morse," *Congressional Record*, May 17, 1955, 6416–17; Carter, *Breakthrough*, 327–29.

43. "The Polio Story—It Boils Down to This," *U.S. News & World Report*, May 20, 1955, 30.

44. Greer Williams, "Polio Post-Mortem: What Really Happened," *Medical Economics*, August 1955, 144–52, 215–18.

45. John Paul to John Enders, June 28, 1955, Box 68, John R. Paul File, *John Enders Papers*, Yale University Archives (hereafter cited as Enders Papers).

46. John Enders to John Paul, July 11, 1955, Enders Papers.

47. Dorothy Sterling to Albert Sabin, May 3, 1955; Albert Sabin to Dorothy Sterling, May 14, 1955; in Box 2, Folder, Correspondence 1955; Albert Sabin Papers, University of Cincinnati (hereafter cited as Sabin Papers, UC).

48. Albert Sabin to William Workman, April 15, 1955, Box 2, Vaccine File 1955, Sabin Papers, UC .

49. Benison, *Tom Rivers*, 522–23; "Technical Report on Salk Poliomyelitis Vaccine," 34; author's interview with Dr. Paul Offit, October 3, 2003.

50. Williams, "Polio Post-Mortem," 147.

51. "Technical Report on Salk Poliomyelitis Vaccine," 9.

52. Shorter, *The Health Century*, 68–69; For Dr. Eddy, see ch. 3, footnote 28, p. 275.

53. This and preceding Youngner quotations are from his "Unpublished Memoir," 15–18, copy in author's possession.

54. "Technical Report on Salk Poliomyelitis Vaccine," 15–17, 49.

55. Wilson, *Margin of Safety*, 111–12; "Salk Vaccine: What's Behind the Story of Confusion?" *Business Week*, June 4, 1955, 90.

56. Williams, *Virus Hunters*, 1959, 336.

57. Hearings Before the Committee on Interstate and Foreign Commerce of the House of Representatives, "Poliomyelitis Vaccine," 84th Cong., 1st sess., June 22, 23, 1955, 171–73.

58. Ibid., 134–39, 168–70.

59. Ibid., 139–43, 173, 180.

60. Ibid., 177–228. The vote is summarized on 227.

61. John Enders to Albert Sabin, July 9, 1953, Box 79, Albert Sabin Folder, Enders Papers.

62. Carter, *Breakthrough*, 336–37.

63. Albert Sabin to Basil O'Connor, June 25, 1955, Box 3, Folder NFIP, Sabin Papers, UC.

64. Basil O'Connor to Albert Sabin, July 13, 1955, Sabin Papers, UC.

65. Albert Sabin to Basil O'Connor, August 1, 1955, Sabin Papers, UC.

66. Jane Krieger, "What Price Fame—to Dr. Salk," *New York Times Magazine*, July 17, 1955, 23.

67. John Enders to Jonas Salk, March 23, 1953, Jonas Salk File, Box 79, Enders Papers.

68. Carter, *Breakthrough*, 323; Krieger, "What Price Fame," 23.

Chapter 14

1. David Bodian et al., "Interim Report, Public Health Service Committee on Poliomyelitis Vaccine," *Journal of the American Medical Association*, December 10, 1955, 1445. The rate of polio for these six contaminated lots was 47 per 100,000 children, more than ten times the "normal occurrence."

2. World Health Organization Technical Report Series No. 101, "Poliomyelitis Vaccination: A Preliminary Review," 1956, 5; U.S. Department of Health, Education, and Welfare, Public Health Service, "Report on Poliomyelitis Vaccine Produced by the Cutter Laboratories," August 25, 1955, 1–6; Neil Nathanson and Alexander Langmuir, "The Cutter Incident," *American Journal of Hygiene*, 1963, 16–79.

3. Leonard Engel, "The Salk Vaccine: What Caused the Mess?" *Harper's*, August 1955, 33.

4. "Poliomyelitis Vaccination," 6; David Rutstein, "How Good Is Polio Vaccine?"*Atlantic Monthly*, February 1957, 48–51.

5. President Eisenhower to Secretary Oveta Culp Hobby, July 13, 1955, in Robert Branyan and Lawrence Larsen, *The Eisenhower Administration, 1953–1961: A Documentary History*, 1971, 583–84; Smith, *Patenting the Sun*, 368–369; Shorter, *The Health Century*, 70.

6. Starr, *The Social Transformation of American Medicine*, 338–347; Strickland, *Politics, Science, and Dread Disease*, 32–54; Smith, *Patenting the Sun*, 369.

7. See especially nationally syndicated articles by Marguerite Shepard in the *St. Louis Globe-Democrat*, February 14–21, 1956; also Eric Josephson, "Why The Dimes March On," *Nation*, November 10, 1956, 361–64.

8. "The Battle for Health . . . And Dollars," editorial, *St. Louis Globe-Democrat*, February 20, 1956.

9. See "An Open Letter From the Officers and Directors of the St. Louis Chapter of the NFIP," *St. Louis Globe-Democrat*, February 21, 1956.

10. Shepard, "Polio Fight Sold Like Hucksters Sell Soap," *St. Louis Globe-Democrat*, February 15, 1956.

11. For the battle between the AMA and the National Foundation, see Greer Williams, "Polio Post-Mortem: What Really Happened," *Medical Economics*, August 1955, 144–52, 215–18.

12. Ibid.

13. Ibid.

14. Gordon Leitch, M.D., "A Step Toward Socialized Medicine," *The Freeman*, December 1955, 776–78.

15. "The Cutter Polio Vaccine Incident: A Case Study of Manufacturers' Liability Without Fault in Tort and Warranty," *Yale Law Journal*, vol. 65, 1955, 26–73.

16. Melvin Belli to Jonas Salk, January 20, 1958, Box 108, Folder 7, Jonas Salk Papers, University of California, San Diego (hereafter cited as Salk papers); *Gottsdanker v. Cutter Laboratories*, 182 Cal.App.2d 602.

17. "Next: Live Vaccine?" *Time*, May 23, 1955, 50–52.

18. Peter Olitsky to Saul Benison, July 14, 20, 1963, Saul Benison File, Peter Olitsky Papers, American Philosophical Society, Philadelphia.

19. Wilson, *Margin of Safety*, 133.

20. Vaughan, *Listen to the Music*, 54.

21. Research Grant, Albert B. Sabin, Investigator, 1949–54, Box 12, Medical Program, March of Dimes Archives, White Plains, N.Y. Also Albert Sabin, "Oral Poliovirus Vaccine: History of Its Development and Use and Current Challenge to Eliminate Poliovirus from the World," *Journal of Infectious Diseases*, 1985, 423.

22. Robert Chanock, "Reminiscences of Albert Sabin," *Proceedings of the Association of American Physicians*, 1995, 117–18.

23. Wilson, *Margin of Safety*, 47.

24. See, for example, Stuart Blume and Ingrid Geesink, "A Brief History of Polio Vaccines," *Science*, June 2, 2000, 1593–94; "Polio Vaccine: Dead or Alive," *Medical World News*, May 20, 1960, 17–19; Paul, *A History of Poliomyelitis*, 441–456.

25. Albert Sabin, "Oral Poliovirus Vaccine," *Journal of the American Medical Association*, November 22, 1965, 874.

26. Albert Sabin to Robert Ward, March 15, 1954, Correspondence, 1940–1961 NFIP, Box 4, Sabin Papers, UC.

27. Albert Sabin to Gilbert Dalldorf, March 25, 1954, Correspondence, 1940–1961, NFIP, Box 4, Sabin Papers, UC.

28. Albert Sabin to Robert Ward, March 15, 1954, Sabin Papers, UC. Ward, a professor at NYU Medical School, was then running a rubella experiment at the Willowbrook State Hospital in New York City. Sabin wanted to run his polio experiment at Willowbrook as well.

29. Henry Kumm to Albert Sabin, March 22, April 20, 1954; memo from Basil O'Connor, April 22, 1954, Sabin Papers, UC.

30. Albert Sabin to Robert J. Huebner, September 30, 1954, Sabin Papers, UC.

31. Albert Sabin to Henry Kumm, December 14, 1954, Sabin Papers, UC; *Pittsburgh Press*, January 8, 1955.

32. Albert Sabin to H. M. Janney, November 19, 1954, Sabin Papers, UC; Albert B. Sabin, "Behavior of Chimpanzee—a Virulent Poliomyelitis in Experimentally Infected Human Volunteers," *American Journal of Medical Science*, July 1955, 1–8.

As noted earlier, it was standard practice for researchers to test their vaccines on themselves before using it on others. Drs. Park, Brodie, and Kolmer had done this in the 1930s. Koprowski and Cox had followed suit in the late 1940s. Salk had inoculated his wife and three sons as well as himself. Sabin also went first, although, contrary to press reports, he did not include his family right away. As a researcher, Sabin had attempted to experiment on institutionalized children in 1954. As a husband and a parent he would vaccinate his wife and daughters in 1957, when he felt more comfortable about the safety of his virus strains, and just before he began to test his vaccine on non-institutionalized children. As Sabin recalled, his wife and two daughters, five and seven years old, were all "triple-negative," meaning they had no previous exposure to polioviruses. "Because I could not ask other parents for permission to perform the necessary studies on the triple-negative children if I did not believe that the accumulated data were sufficient to warrant studies on my own family, the next phase . . . involved detailed studies with my own wife and children." See Sabin, "Oral Poliovirus Vaccine," *Journal of Infectious Diseases*, March 1985, 422.

33. Sabin, "Oral Poliovirus Vaccine," 423.
34. Albert Sabin to David Johnson, October 26, 1955, Albert Sabin to W. Ritchie Russell, August 2, 1955; in Polio Vaccine File, Box 4, Sabin Papers, UC.
35. Henry Kumm to Albert Sabin, January 25, 1955; Albert Sabin to Henry Kumm, January 28, 1955; Hilary Koprowski to John R. Paul, February 16, 1955; Minutes of the meeting of the Subcommittee on Live Virus Immunization of the NFIP, March 7–8, 1955; all in Oral Polio Vaccine: Correspondence, Lederle Laboratory, Sabin Papers, UC.
36. Vaughan, *Listen to the Music*, 50–51, 76.
37. Hilary Koprowski to John Enders, November 22, 1954, Koprowski File, Box 41, John Enders Papers, Yale University Archives.
38. Hooper, *The River*, 219.
39. Ibid., 223.
40. Ibid., 222; Gould, *A Summer Plague*, 171; Wilson, *Margin of Safety*, 164–66; Benison, *Tom Rivers*, 467–68; Vaughan, *Listen to the Music*, 73–74
41. Wilson, *Margin of Error*, 176–77; Vaughan, *Listen to the Music*, 85.
42. Albert Sabin to John Paul, January 23, 1957, Correspondence, Box 4, Sabin Papers, UC.
43. Albert Sabin to John Paul, August 7, 1956, Box 4; H. van Zile Hyde (chief, Division of International Health, Public Health Service) to Albert Sabin, January 19, 1956, "Russian Trip, 1956," Sabin Papers, UC.
44. Albert Sabin to H. van Zile Hyde, January 11, 1956, Sabin Papers, UC.
45. S. Byrne-Jones to Albert Sabin, February 20, 1956; Walter Rudolph to Sabin, March 8, 1956; Joel Warren to Sabin (n.d.), all in Correspondence, USSR Visits, 1955–56, Sabin Papers, UC.
46. See "Subject: Dr. Albert B. Sabin, Internal Security," June 18, 1956; "Subject: East-West Exchange Program," April 23, 1957; in Albert Sabin FBI File.
47. Dorothy Horstmann, "The Sabin Live Poliovirus Vaccination Trials in the USSR, 1959," *Yale Journal of Biology and Medicine*, 1991, 501–2.
48. David Langdon to Albert Sabin, September 11, 1957, in Correspondence USSR Visits, 1955–56, Sabin Papers, UC
49. Author's interview with Peter Salk, November 22, 2002.

50. See especially Paul Russell to Albert Sabin, February 11, 1957, General Correspondence, in Sabin Papers, UC; Saul Benison, "International Medical Cooperation: Dr. Albert Sabin, Live Poliovirus Vaccine and the Soviets," *Bulletin of the History* of Medicine, 1982, 473; Benison, *Tom Rivers*, 570–76.

51. Albert Sabin to H. van Zile Hyde, December 19, 1957, in Correspondence USSR Visits,Sabin Papers, UC; Dorothy Horstmann, "Report on a Visit to the USSR . . . to Review Work on Live Poliovirus Vaccine, August–October, 1959," copy in Box 1, Folder: USSR Trip, Dorothy Horstmann Papers, Yale University Archives.

52. Mikhail Chumakov to Albert Sabin, December 24, 1959, Chumakov File, Sabin Papers, UC.

53. Albert Sabin to Mikhail Chumakov, January 22, 1960, Sabin Papers, UC.

54. Years later, in describing his travails in developing his vaccine, Sabin put John Paul and Dorothy Horstmann at the top of his list of scientists who "advised me to continue and offered me their continued collaboration." See Albert Sabin, "Oral Poliovirus Vaccine," *Journal of Infectious Diseases*, March 1985, 420.

55. Horstmann, "Sabin Live Poliovirus Vaccination Trials," 499–500.

56. John Paul to Dorothy Horstmann, October 6, 1959, in "USSR Trip," Dorothy Horstmann Papers, Yale University Archives.

57. "Casual Notes: Report from Dr. Horstmann in Moscow," October 3, 1959, Dorothy Horstmann Papers, Yale University Archives.

58. Horstmann, "Sabin Live Poliovirus Vaccination Trials," 499

59. Benison, "International Medical Cooperation," 479.

Chapter 15

1. "Polio Isn't Licked Yet," Bulletin No. 10, National Foundation for Infantile Paralysis, March of Dimes Archives, White Plains, N.Y.

2. Thomas Rivers, "Research in the Expanded Program of the National Foundation," *Journal of the National Medical Association*, July 1960, 251.

3. "1959 Polio Vaccination Facts," NFIP Papers.

4. "Confidential Memorandum to Board of Trustees Containing a Proposal for an Expanded Program for the National Foundation for Infantile Paralysis," May 20, 1958, NFIP Papers (statements by O'Connor on the foundation's future direction that follow are from this document).

5. Basil O'Connor to Jonas Salk, April 22, 1960, copy in Jonas Salk File, Edward Litchfield Papers, University of Pittsburgh Archives (hereafter cited as Litchfield Papers).

6. Douglas Heuck, "Institute a Blueprint for a New Way of Thinking," *Pittsburgh Post-Gazette*, November 28, 1994.

7. Carter, *Breakthrough*, 404.

8. Edward Litchfield to Jonas Salk, October 28, 1957, in Jonas Salk File, Litchfield Papers.

9. Robert C. Alberts, *Pitt: The Story of the University of Pittsburgh*, 1986, 244–55.

10. "Dynamo at Pitt," *Time*, January 7, 1957, 64.

11. Quoted in Paull, *A Century of Medical Excellence*, 204.

12. Jonas Salk to Edward Litchfield, October 17, 1957, Jonas Salk File, Litchfield Papers.

13. Heuck, "Institute a Blueprint."
14. Jonas Salk to E. R. McCluskey, April 29, 1959, in Jonas Salk File, Litchfield Papers.
15. "Memo From Edward Litchfield: Subject: Jonas Salk," May 29, 1959, Litchfield Papers.
16. Ibid.
17. Stanton C. Crawford to Edward Litchfield, March 21, 1960, Litchfield Papers.
18. Edward Litchfield to Charles Zellers, March 11, 1960, Litchfield Papers.
19. *Pittsburgh Post-Gazette*, March 12, 1960; *Pittsburgh Press*, March 13, 1960.
20. Quoted in Paull, *A Century of Medical Excellence*, 220.
21. Hooper, *The River*, 29.
22. Wilson, *Margin of Safety*, 190.
23. Herald Cox to Peter Olitsky, January 5, 1960, Cox File, Box 3, Peter Olitsky Papers, Archives of the Rockefeller Institute, Sleepy Hollow, N.Y.
24. Herald Cox to Albert Sabin, April 10, 1959, Correspondence, Misc., 1959, Albert Sabin Papers, University of Cincinnati (hereafter cited as Sabin Papers, UC).
25. Health Commissioner, Hamilton County, Ohio, to Luther Terry, U.S. Surgeon-General, March 22, 1961, Folder 8, Box 127, Jonas Salk Papers, University of California, San Diego (hereafter cited as Salk Papers).
26. AMA, "The Present Status of Poliomyelitis Vaccination in the United States: Summary of the Council on Drugs," August 22, 1961; Ruth and Edward Brecher, "What's Delaying the New Polio Vaccine," *Redbook*, April, 1961, 133.
27. *Wall Street Journal*, August 25, 1960.
28. "Memorandum: Charlie Bennett to Dr. Rivers: Sabin Panel Appearance in Boston," Folder 8, Box 127, Salk Papers.
29. John Paul, "The Case for Live Poliovirus Vaccination," *Yale Journal of Biology and Medicine*, February 1960, 242–47; Alexander Langmuir to Albert Sabin, December ??, 1959, Correspondence 1959, Sabin Papers.
30. Thomas Rivers to Albert Sabin, November 16, 1959, Sabin Papers.
31. Thomas Rivers to David Bodian, February 14, 28, 1961, David Bodian File, Thomas Rivers Papers, American Philosophical Society.
32. David Bodian to Thomas Rivers, February 24, 1961, Thomas Rivers Papers, American Philosophical Society.
33. AMA, "Summary Statement of the Council on Drugs," April 22, 1961, copy in Oral Polio Vaccine, 1961, Sabin Papers.
34. Gould, *A Summer Plague*, 181–82; Carter, *Breakthrough*, 363; Brecher, "What's Delaying the New Polio Vaccine," 37, 127–34.
35. Geoffrey Edsal to Albert Sabin, February 7, March 24, 1961; Sabin to Edsal, March 28, 1961, Oral Polio Vaccine, Sabin Papers.
36. John Youmans to Jonas Salk, July 10, 1961, Folder 1, Box 128, Salk Papers; Carter, *Breakthrough*, 371.
37. Carter, *Breakthrough*, 375; *New York Times*, July 14, 1961.
38. Leonard Larson to Jonas Salk, August 28, 1961; Jonas Salk to John Youmans, September 26, 1961, Youmans to Salk, November 4, 1961, Folder 1, Box 128, Salk Papers.
39. There are numerous theories regarding the AMA's support for the Sabin vaccine. One is that its officers were still smarting from previous battles with Basil O'Connor and were out to punish him. Another is that the AMA was looking to demonstrate its civic-mindedness in a well-publicized, if relatively harmless, fashion—as the guardian of the nation's children. Some believed that the AMA

had been deeply compromised by the influence of the pharmaceutical lobby, which saw Sabin's vaccine as far more profitable than Salk's, given its ease of application and enormous global potential. And others viewed the AMA as bowing, understandably, to the wishes of the giants in the field of polio research, who strongly favored the Sabin vaccine at this time.

40. See Jonas Salk to Luther Terry (U.S. Surgeon General), August 3, 1961, Folder 8, Box 127, Salk Papers.
41. Mikhail Chumakov to Albert Sabin, May 6, 1963, Correspondence: Chumakov, 1960–69, Sabin Papers.
42. Albert Sabin to Peter Olitsky January 7, 1958, February 8, 1960, February 11, 1962, Sabin File, Peter Olitsky Papers, American Philosophical Society; Albert Sabin to John Paul, October 29, 1960, S File, 1960–65, John Paul Papers, Yale University Archives.
43. Hooper, *The River*, 480; Vaughan, *Listen to the Music*, 93.
44. Author's interview with Peter Salk, November 22, 2002.

Chapter 16

1. Douglas Heuck, "Institute a Blueprint for a New Way of Thinking," *Pittsburgh Post Gazette*, November 28, 1994.
2. Nicholas Wade, "Salk Institute: Elitist Pursuit of Biology with a Conscience," *Science*, November 24, 1972.
3. Carter, *Breakthrough*, 403; Julius Youngner, Unpublished Memoir, 25, copy in author's possession.
4. Youngner, Unpublished Memoir, 33.
5. Smith, *Patenting the Sun*, 374–78; Wade, "Salk Institute"; Joseph Burton, "Thomas Jefferson, Louis Sullivan, Frank Lloyd Wright, Louis Kahn and the Image of Democracy," Master's Thesis, University of Texas, 1975.
6. Wade, "Salk Institute"; George Johnson, "Once Again, A Man with a Mission," *New York Sunday Times Magazine*, November 25, 1990.
7. "Memorandum: H. E. White to Basil O'Connor, November 4, 1965, Salk Institute for Biological Studies, Box 1, File: Correspondence, Financing, 1961–1966, March of Dimes Archive, White Plains, N.Y. (hereafter cited as MDA).
8. Basil O'Connor to Board of Trustees, Salk Institute, March 9, 1966, MDA.
9. John McCloy (chairman, Board of Trustees, Salk Institute) to Melvin Glasser, May 25, 1972, Correspondence, 1964–1972, MDA.
10. See especially Elmer Bendiner, "Salk: Adulation, Animosity, and Achievement," *Hospital Practice*, June 1983, 194–218; "John Callaway Interviews Dr. Jonas Salk," Transcript Library, Fall 1981 (copy in author's possession). The quote from Salk is in "An Evolutionary Philosophy for Our Time" (copy in author's possession).
11. Author's interview with Darrell Salk, February 19, 2003; Bendiner, "Salk," 218; *New York Times*, June 18, 1970; Jonas Salk to Thomas Francis, March 26, 1955, Thomas Francis Papers.
12. Albert Sabin, "Oral Poliovirus," *Journal of Infectious Diseases*, March, 1985, 420.
13. "Out of Favor for 20 Years, the Salk Vaccine Makes a Comeback," *New York Sunday Times*, Week in Review, January 25, 1981; Sabin obituary, *New York Times*, March 4, 1993.
14. Stuart Blume and Ingrid Geesink, "A Brief History of Polio Vaccines," *Science*, June 2, 2000, 1593–94; Jonas Salk and Darrell Salk, "Control of Influenza and Poliomyelitis with Killed Virus Vaccines," *Science*, March 4, 1977, 834–47.

15. Author's interview with Darrell Salk, February 19, 2003; U.S. Census Bureau, "Statistical Abstract of the United States, 2003," No. HS–18, Specified Reportable Diseases—Cases per 100,000 Population, 1912–2001.

16. Darrell Salk's articles in this period include, "Eradication of Poliomyelitis in the United States, *Reviews of Infectious Diseases*, March–April, 1980, 228–42; "Herd Effect and Virus Eradication with Use of Killed Poliovirus Vaccine," International Symposium of Reassessment of Inactivated Poliomyelitis Vaccine, 1981, 247–55; "Polio Immunization Policy in the United States: A New Challenge for a New Generation," *American Journal of Public Health*, March 1988, 296–300.

17. See Web site of the National Academy of Sciences, membership lists of active and deceased members.

18. Sheryl Stolberg, "Hero With Something to Prove," *Los Angeles Times*, March 7, 1993.

19. Johnson, "Once Again, a Man With a Mission"; Mikail Chumakov to Albert Sabin," January 21, 1976, Sabin to Chumakov, February 14, 1976, Correspondence File, Individual, Chumakov, 1974–1992, Albert Sabin Papers, University of Cincinnati (hereafter cited as Sabin Papers, UC).

20. File: "Scientific Symposium in Honor of Albert B. Sabin's 80th Birthday," August 26, 1986, Box 18, Dorothy Horstmann Papers, Yale University Archives; *Biologicals*, December 1993; John Enders to Albert Sabin, January 28, 1985, Sabin File, John Enders Papers, Yale University.

21. On these honors for Salk, see, for example, *Pittsburgh Press*, February 3, 1979, April 15, 1983; Bendiner, "Salk" 194; "Proclamation 5335—Dr. Jonas E. Salk Day, 1985," Office of the Federal Register. Also, Cohen, *Shots in the Dark*, 88; Jonas Salk obituary in *Los Angeles Times*, June 24, 1995. Also, "The *Time* 100: Scientists and Thinkers," *Time*, March 29, 1999. The article on Salk was written by polio survivor Wilfrid Sheed.

22. Cohen, *Shots in the Dark*, 20.

23. Stolberg, "Hero With Something to Prove."

24. "AIDS Experiment Based on Salk's Theories," *New York Times*, February 12, 1988; Phillip Nobile, "A Shot in the Dark: Jonas Salk and the Quest for an AIDS Vaccine," *Bergen Record*, December 2, 1990; "Hopeful Talk from Jonas Salk," *Business Week*, June 21, 1993, 42. A detailed account of Salk's business can be found in Elinor Burkett, *The Gravest Show on Earth: America in the Age of AIDS*, 1995, 115–25.

25. Cohen, *Shots in the Dark*, 218–24; Salk obituary in *Bergen Record*, July 24, 1995.

26. Youngner, "Unpublished Memoir," 33–36; Douglas Heuck, "Salk's Regrets Are Few," *Pittsburgh Post-Gazette*, November 27, 1994.

27. "Albert Sabin, 86, Polio Researcher Dies," *New York Times*, March 4, 1993; Richard Lacayo, "The Good Doctor," *Time*, July 3, 1995.

28. *Pittsburgh Post-Gazette*, June 24, 1995.

29. See Web site of American Academy of Family Physicians, "Poliovirus Vaccine Options," January 1, 1999.

30. Author's interview with Darrell Salk, February 19, 2003.

31. Tom Curtis, "The Origin of AIDS," *Rolling Stone*, March 19, 1992, 54–59.

32. Editor Clarification, *Rolling Stone*, December 9, 1993, 39.

33. Hooper, *The River*, 244–83; Lawrence Altman, "An Improbable Theory on AIDS Is Put to the Test," *New York Times*, March 21, 2000; Michael Worobey et al., "Contaminated Polio Vaccine Theory Refuted," *Nature*, April 22, 2004, 820; "Editorial: Chimpanzees and Journalists," *Vaccine* 22 (2004), 1829–30.

34. Stephen Lehrer, *Explorers of the Body*, 1979, 404–5; Debbie Bookchin and Jim Schumacher, *The Virus and the Vaccine*, 2004, 60–62. On Dr. Eddy's earlier role in the Cutter incident, 230–31.

35. Thomas Rivers to Albert Sabin, June 16, 1960, Box 2, Sabin Papers, UC.

36. Bookchin and Schumacher, "Introduction," *Vaccine and Virus*, xiv.

37. Testimony of Dr. James Goedert, September 10, 2003, Web site of U.S. Department of Health and Human Services.

38. Dr. William Schaffner, chairman, Department of Preventive Medicine, Vanderbilt University, in http://www.consumerreports.org.

39. Sass, *Polio's Legacy*, 133, xiv.

40. Ibid., 72, 80, 101–2, 108–10, 116–17, 132. The quotation is on 123. For polio survivors and Type A personality, see Bruno, *The Polio Paradox*, 98–106.

41. Lauro Halstead, "Post-Polio Syndrome," *Scientific American*, April 1998, 00. The quotation is in Bruno, *The Polio Paradox*, 101.

42. "A New Scare for Polio Victims," *Newsweek*, April 23, 1983, 83; Donald Mulder, "Clinical Observations on Acute Poliomyelitis," 1–10, and M. C. Dalakas, "Post-Polio Syndrome 12 Years Later: How it Started," 11–18, both in *The Post Polio Syndrome: Advances in the Pathogenesis and Treatment*, ed. M. C. Dalakas, Harry Bartfield, and Leonard Kurland, *Annals of the New York Academy of Sciences*, vol. 753, 1995.

43. Halstead, "Post-Polio Syndrome," 43.

44. See Post-Polio Health International, "The Late Effects of Polio: An Overview," http://www.post–polio.org/ipn/lep/html; B. Jubelt and J. C. Agre, "Characteristics and Management of Post-polio Syndrome," *Journal of the American Medical Association*, July 26, 2000, 412–14. The quote is in Bruno, *The Polio Paradox*, 29.

45. Halstead, "Post-Polio Syndrome," 46.

46. Ibid. Also, "Reliving Polio," *Time*, March 28, 1994, 54–5; Mee, *A Nearly Normal Life*, 24; Richard Owen, "Foreword," in Sass, *Polio's Legacy*, vii–viii.

47. See National Park Service, Franklin Delano Roosevelt Memorial, "FDR's Struggle With Disability," http://www.nps.gov/fdrm/home/htm; Rosemarie Garland-Thomson, "The FDR Memorial: Who Speaks From the Wheelchair?" *Chronicle of Higher Education*, January 26, 2001, B11–12.

Epilogue

1. World Health Organization, "Global Polio Eradication Initiative: Strategic Plan, 2004–2008," WHO/Policy/00–05.

2. Rotary International, "History of PolioPlus," http://www.rotary.org.foundation; Huntley Collins, "Rotary Clubs Pump Millions into Effort to Wipe Out Polio," *Philadelphia Inquirer*, February 22, 1999; WHO, "Polio Eradication: The Final Challenge," http://www.who.int/why/2003; interview with Robert Keegan, February 16, 2004.

3. WHO, "Global Polio Eradication Initiative"; *New York Times*, May 27, 2004; "UN: Africa Condemned to Major Polio Epidemic," *Reuters Health*, October 8, 2004.

4. WHO, "Global Polio Eradication Initiative"; WHO, "Polio Eradication: Now More Than Ever, Stop Polio Forever," http:/www.who.int/features/2004/polio/en; *International Herald Tribune*, October 28, 2004.

Selected Bibliography

Manuscript Collections

David Bodian Papers, Chesney Medical Archives, Johns Hopkins Medical School, Baltimore

Dwight D. Eisenhower Presidential Papers, Abilene, Kansas

John Enders Papers, Yale University Archives, New Haven

Simon Flexner Papers, American Philosophical Society, Philadelphia

FBI File, Jonas Salk

FBI File, Albert Sabin

Franklin Delano Roosevelt Papers, FDR Presidential Library, Hyde Park, N.Y.

Thomas Francis Papers, Bentley Library, University of Michigan, Ann Arbor

Dorothy Horstmann Papers, Yale University Archives, New Haven

Edward Litchfield Papers, University of Pittsburgh Archive

National Foundation for Infantile Paralysis Papers, March of Dimes Archives, White Plains, N.Y.

Newsweek Research Archive, Center for American History, University of Texas, Austin

Basil O'Connor Papers, March of Dimes Archives, White Plains, N.Y.

Peter Olitsky Papers, American Philosophical Society, Philadelphia

Peter Olitsky Papers, Rockefeller Archive Center, Sleepy Hollow, N.Y.

John Paul Papers, Yale University Archives, Hew Haven

Thomas Rivers Papers, American Philosophical Society, Philadelphia

Albert Sabin Papers, Rockefeller Archive Center, Sleepy Hollow, N.Y.

Albert Sabin Papers, University of Cincinnati Medical Heritage Center, Cincinnati

Jonas Salk File, Archives and Special Collections, City College of New York

Jonas Salk Papers, Mandeville Special Collections, University of California, San Diego

Personal Interviews

Dean Allard

Eleanor Bodian

Robert Keegan

Paul Offit
Darrell Salk
Peter Salk
John Troan
Julius Youngner

Books

Allen, Garland. *Thomas Hunt Morgan: The Man and His Science*, 1978
Altman, Lawrence K. *Who Goes First: The Story of Self-Experimentation in Medicine*, 1987.
Altman, Nathaniel. "Hot Springs and Mineral Spas in North America," in *Healing Springs: The Ultimate Guide to Taking the Waters*, ed. N. Altman, 2000.
Benison, Saul. "The Enigma of Poliomyelitis: 1910," in *Freedom and Reform: Essays in Honor of Henry Steele Commager*, ed. Harold Hyman, 1967.
———. "The History of Polio Research in the United States: Appraisal and Lessons," in *The Twentieth Century Sciences: Studies in the Biography of Ideas*, ed. Gerald Holton, 1972.
———. *Tom Rivers: Reflections on a Life in Medicine and Science*, 1967.
Berg, Roland H. *Polio and Its Problems*, 1947
Black, Conrad. *Franklin Delano Roosevelt: Champion of Freedom*, 2003.
Black, Kathryn. *In the Shadow of Polio*, 1996.
Bonner, Thomas. *Iconoclast: Abraham Flexner and a Life of Learning*, 2002.
Brandt, Allan. *No Magic Bullet: A Social History of Venereal Disease in the United States Since 1880*, 1987.
Brandt, Allan M., and Martha Gardner. "The Golden Age of Medicine?" in *Medicine in the Twentieth Century*, ed. Roger Cooter and John Pickstone, 2000.
Brown, E. Richard. *Rockefeller Medicine Men: Medicine and Capitalism in America*, 1979.
Bruno, Richard L. *The Polio Paradox: What You Need To Know*, 2002.
Burnow, James G. *Organized Medicine in the Progressive Era*, 1977.
Carter, Richard. *Breakthrough: The Saga of Jonas Salk*, 1966
———. *The Gentle Legions*, 1961.
Chernow, Ron. *Titan: The Life of John D. Rockefeller, Sr.*, 1998.
Cohen, Jon. *Shots in the Dark*, 2001.
Cohn, Victor. *Four Billion Dimes*, 1955.
———. *Sister Kenny: The Woman Who Challenged the Doctors*, 1975.
Condran, Gretchen. "Changing Patterns of Epidemic Disease in New York City," in David Rosner, *Hives of Sickness: Public Health and Epidemics in New York City*, 1995.
Cook, Blanche Wiesen. *Eleanor Roosevelt, 1884–1933*.
Cooter, John, and John Pickstone, eds. *Medicine in the Twentieth Century*, 2000.
Corner, George W. *A History of the Rockefeller Institute, 1901–1953*, 1964.
Crawford, Dorothy. *The Invisible Enemy: A Natural History of Viruses*, 2000.
Crosby, Alfred. *America's Forgotten Pandemic*, 1989.
Cutlip, Scott. *Fund Raising in the United States: Its Role in America's Philanthropy*, 1965.
———. *The Unseen Power: Public Relations, A History*, 1994.
Dalakas, M. C., Harry Bartfield, and Leonard Kurland, eds. *The Post Polio Syndrome: Advances in the Pathogenesis and Treatment*, Annals of the New York Academy of Sciences, vol. 753, 1995.
Daniel, Thomas, and Frederick C. Robbins, eds. *Polio*, 1997.
Davis, Fred. *Passage Through Crisis: Polio Victims and Their Families*, 1963.

Davis, Kenneth S. *FDR: The Beckoning of Destiny, 1882–1928*, 1971.

———. *Invincible Summer: An Intimate Portrait of the Roosevelts Based on the Recollections of Marion Dickerman*, 1974.

De Kruif, Paul. *The Sweeping Wind: A Memoir*, 1962.

Dowling, Harry F. *Fighting Infection: Conquests of the Twentieth Century*, 1977.

Flexner, James Thomas. *An American Saga: The Story of Helen Thomas and Simon Flexner*, 1984.

———. *Maverick's Progress: An Autobiography*, 1996.

Freidel, Frank. *Franklin D. Roosevelt: The Ordeal*, 1954.

Freund, Paul. "Introduction," in *Experimentation with Human Subjects*, ed. Paul Freund, 1969.

Friedman, Meyer, and Gerald Friedland. *Medicine's 10 Greatest Discoveries*, 1998.

Gallagher, Hugh Gregory. *FDR's Splendid Deception*, 1985.

Goldberg, Richard Thayer. *The Making of Franklin D. Roosevelt: Triumph Over Disability*, 1981.

Goldman, Herbert. *Banjo Eyes: Eddie Cantor and the Birth of Modern Stardom*, 1997.

Gould, Lewis. *Grand Old Party: A History of the Republicans*, 2003.

Gould, Tony. *A Summer Plague: Polio and Its Survivors*, 1995.

Grob, Gerald. *The Deadly Truth: A History of Disease in America*, 2002.

Hawkins, Leonard. *The Man in the Iron Lung: The Frederick B. Snite, Jr., Story*, 1956.

Hellman, Hal. *Great Feuds in Medicine*, 2001.

Henig, Robin Marantz. *The People's Health: A Memoir of Public Health and Its Evolution at Harvard*, 1996.

Hooper, Edward. *The River: A Journey to the Source of HIV and AIDS*, 1999.

Howe, Irving. *A Margin of Hope*, 1982.

Hoy, Suellen. *Chasing Dirt: The American Pursuit of Cleanliness*, 1995.

Johnston, Robert. *The Politics of Healing*, 2004.

Karlen, Arno. *Man and Microbes*, 1995.

Kennedy, David M. *Freedom from Fear: The American People in Depression and War, 1929–1945*, 1999.

Kenny, Elizabeth. *And They Shall Walk*, 1943.

King, Lester. "Medical Education: The Decade of Massive Change," in American Medical Association, *American Medicine Comes of Age, 1840–1920*, 1984.

Klein, Aaron Klein. *Trial by Fury: The Polio Vaccine Controversy*, 1971.

Kolata, Gina. *Flu: The Story of the Great Influenza Pandemic of 1918 and the Search for the Virus That Caused It*, 1999.

Kraut, Alan. "Plagues and Prejudice: Nativism's Construction of Disease in Nineteenth and Twentieth Century New York City," in *Hives of Sickness: Public Health and Epidemics in New York City*, ed. David Rosner, 1995.

———. *Silent Travelers: Germs, Genes, and the "Immigrant Menace,"* 1994.

Lederer, Susan. *Subjected to Science: Human Experimentation in America Before the Second World War*, 1995.

Leff, Mark H. "Franklin Roosevelt," in *The Reader's Companion to the American Presidency*, ed. Alan Brinkley and David Dyer, 2000.

Lippman, Theo, Jr. *The Squire of Warm Springs: FDR in Georgia, 1924–1945*, 1977.

Lovett, R. W. *The Treatment of Infantile Paralysis*, 1916.

Ludmerer, Kenneth. *Time to Heal: American Medical Education From the Turn of the Century to the Era of Managed Care*, 1999.

Markel, Howard. *Quarantine: East European Jewish Immigrants and the New York City Epidemic of 1892*, 1997.

Martin, Emily. *Flexible Bodies: The Role of Immunity in American Culture From the Days of Polio to the Age of AIDS*, 1995.

McElvaine, Robert S. *The Great Depression*, 1984.

McMurry, Linda. *George Washington Carver: Scientist and Symbol*, 1981.

Mee, Charles. *A Nearly Normal Life*, 1999.

Melnick, Joseph R. "Enteroviruses," in *Virology* (2nd ed.), ed. B. N. Fields, 1990.

Meyerowitz, Joanne. "Beyond the Feminine Mystique: A Reassesment of Postwar Mass Culture, 1946–1958," in Joanne Meyerowitz, *Not June Cleaver: Women and Gender in Postwar America, 1945–1960*, 1994.

Oldstone, Michael. *Viruses, Plagues, and History*, 1998.

Oshinsky, David M. *A Conspiracy So Immense: The World of Joe McCarthy*, 1983.

———. *"Worse Than Slavery": Parchman Farm and the Ordeal of Jim Crow Justice*, 1996.

Paul, John R. *A History of Poliomyelitis*, 1971.

Paull, Barbara. *A Century of Medical Excellence: The History of the Pittsburgh School of Medicine*, 1986.

Plotkin, Susan, and Stanley Plotkin. "A Short History of Vaccination," in Stanley Plotkin and Edward Mortimer Jr., *Vaccines*, 1988.

Robbins, Frederick, and Thomas Daniel. "A History of Poliomyelitis," in *Polio*, ed. Thomas Daniel, 1997.

Rogers, Naomi. *Dirt and Disease: Polio Before FDR*, 1992.

———. "Dirt, Flies and Immigrants: Explaining the Epidemiology of Poliomyelitis, 1900–1916," in *Sickness and Health in America*, ed. Judith Walter and Ronald Numbers, 1997.

———. "Sister Kenny Goes to Washington: Polio, Populism, and Medical Politics in Postwar America," in Robert Johnston, *The Politics of Healing*, 2004.

Roosevelt, Eleanor. *This I Remember*, 1949.

———. *This Is My Story*, 1937.

Rose, David. *Images of America: March of Dimes*, 2003.

Rose, Mark. *Cities of Heat and Light: Domesticating Gas and Electricity in Urban America*, 1995.

Rosner, David, ed. *Hives of Sickness: Public Health and Epidemics in New York City*, 1995.

Rothman, David J. "The Iron Lung and Democratic Medicine," in *Beginnings Count: The Technological Imperative in American Health Care*, ed. David J. Rothman, 1997.

Salk, Lee. *My Father, My Son: Intimate Relationships*, 1982.

Sass, Edmund. *Polio's Legacy: An Oral History*, 1996.

Seavey, Nina, Jane Smith, and Paul Wagner. *A Paralyzing Fear: The Triumph Over Polio in America*, 1998.

Shorter, Edward. *The Health Century*, 1987.

Sills, David. *The Volunteers: Means and Ends in a National Organization*, 1957.

Simmons, John Galbraith. *Doctors and Discoveries: Lives That Created Today's Medicine*, 2002.

Sink, Alice. *The Grit Behind the Miracle: A True Story of the Determination and Hard Work behind an Emergency Infantile Paralysis Hospital, 1944–1945, Hickory, North Carolina*, 1998.

Smith, Jane. *Patenting the Sun: Polio and the Salk Vaccine*, 1990.

Spock, Benjamin. *The Common Sense Book of Baby and Child Care*, 1946.

Starr, Paul. *The Social Transformation of American Medicine*, 1982.

Sterling, Bryan, and Frances Sterling. *Forgotten Eagle: Wiley Post, America's Heroic Aviation Pioneer*, 2002.

Strickland, Stephen. *Politics, Science, and Dread Disease: A Short History of United States Medical Research Policy*, 1972.

Tomes, Nancy. *The Gospel of Germs Men, Women, and the Microbes in American Life*, 1998.

Traub, James. *City on a Hill*, 1994.

Troan, John. *Passport to Adventure*, 2000.

Vaughan, Roger. *Listen to the Music: The Life of Hilary Koprowski*, 2000.

Vinikas, Vincent. *Soft Soap, Hard Sell: American Hygiene in An Age of Advertisement*, 1992.

Walker, Turnley. *Roosevelt and the Warm Springs Story*, 1953.

Wall, Joseph. *Andrew Carnegie*, 1970.

Walzer, Judith. *Typhoid Mary: Captive to the Public's Health*, 1996.

Ward, Geoffrey. *A First-Class Temperament: The Emergence of Franklin Roosevelt*, 1989.

Williams, Greer. *Virus Hunters*, 1959.

Wilson, John R. *Margin of Safety: The Story of the Poliomyelitis Vaccine*, 1960.

Ziporyn, Terra. *Disease in the Popular American Press: The Case of Diphtheria, Typhoid Fever, and Syphilis, 1870–1920*, 1988.

Acknowledgments

I BEGAN MY RESEARCH for this book five years ago. Many people helped along the way. Professor Dan Wilson of Muhlenberg College, a kind, wise, and courageous man, spurred my interest in polio. Professor Shirley Eoff and her students at Angelo State University provided background material for the 1949 epidemic in San Angelo, Texas. Sydney Soderburg scoured the Eisenhower Presidential Library for documents relating to polio. I would like to thank the archivists and librarians at the American Philosophical Society, the Bentley Library at the University of Michigan, the Center for American History at the University of Texas, the Chesney Medical Archives at Johns Hopkins, the FDR Presidential Library, the Rockefeller Archive Center, the University of Pittsburgh, and the Yale University Library. I am deeply indebted to Maggie Yax, who skillfully led me through the boxes of the partly processed papers of Albert Sabin at the University of Cincinnati Medical Heritage Center, and to Lynda Claassen, who helped me navigate the Jonas Salk Papers housed in the Mandeville Special Collections Library at the University of California, San Diego. My largest research debt is owed to David Rose, archivist at the March of Dimes, for his skill, his interest in the project, his boundless energy, and his friendship.

I would also like to thank those who provided valuable input in other forms. Dr. Margaret McDonald, Associate Vice-Chancellor for Academic Affairs at the University of Pittsburgh, set up a number of key interviews, gave me a tour of the university's world-class health and medical facilities, and made my stay there a delight. Dr. Joan Heller

Brown, Chair of the Pharmacology Department at UCSD Medical School, offered similar kindnesses in San Diego. Dr. Darrell Salk spent many hours explaining the science of polio to me and reminiscing about his father. His insights and his generosity helped make this project a joy to pursue. Dr. Peter Salk added valuable pieces to the story. Dr. Paul Offitt, Chief of Infectious Diseases at the Children's Hospital of Philadelphia, shared information with me about the Cutter incident and critiqued large parts of the manuscript. Dr. Julius Youngner, Distinguished Service Professor at the University of Pittsburgh School of Medicine, provided vital first-hand information about the dynamics of polio research, critiqued the full manuscript, and had a knack for giving sound advice at the perfect time. Dean Allard and Eleanor Bodian offered insight into the career of Dr. Isabel Morgan and the workings of the Johns Hopkins Polio Group. John Troan, former editor of the *Pittsburgh Press*, recalled his days as a confidant of Jonas Salk. Robert Keegan of the Centers for Disease Control described for me the most recent global effort to eradicate polio.

At Oxford University Press I had the great fortune to work with a superb editorial and production staff. My gratitude to Peter Ginna for his keen editorial eye, his enthusiasm for the project, and his personal generosity can hardly be overstated. I owe him a debt that he alone understands. Furaha Norton managed various parts of the book process with a combination of warmth and efficiency that all authors should be lucky enough to experience. Joellyn Ausanka, a consummate professional, brought the book to conclusion with an extraordinary eye for style, nuance, and detail. My agent and good friend, Gerry McCauley, represented me with his legendary (and genuine) grace and skill.

Thank you to all.

Index

Note: Page numbers followed by "n" refer to notes; page numbers in **bold** refer to chapters.